The Crown and the Caged God

Book One:

A Time for Wrath

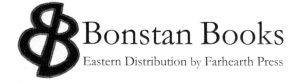

Bonstan Books
Eastern Distribution by Farhearth Press

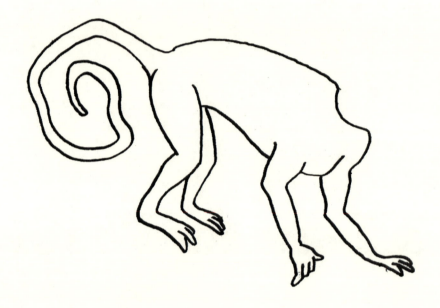

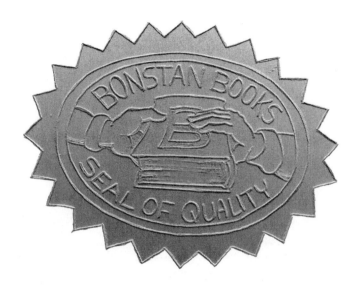

Copyright © 2024
Bonstan Books, LLC
United States Copyright on:
5/5 in the Year of Our Lord, 2024

All Rights Reserved

ISBN-13: 978-0-9913145-1-5

Thevro Chronicle

Laberyn Silent

By Irkov

Second Lufoa, Day Ten

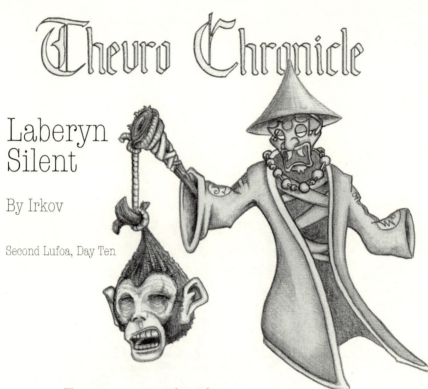

There was a time of mirth
  and an age of grief
In turn, we'll greet a time for wrath
As sparks rise, stars fall, and embers fade
  beyond the cage of the empty god

To sprout new seed from rain and rot
  the sweetest fruit must first lie down
Lifeless, it writhes; deathless, it dies
While lord, mortal, mother, and child
  all await the new crown's rise

Book of Druin, 33

At the first brush strokes of dawn on the second day of Second Lufoa, the Thorn Star arrived. It hung low over Laberyn, painting the sky with its menacing glow and staining the rising sun. Countless stories begin with similar portents, but it's been a long span since it last began.

Theuro Chronicle

Details of the present story remain sparse, as we have yet to receive the Rider's Report. However, the Pigeon's Perspective containing the First Five Facts has landed in the News Nest. Here is what we know:

1. The attack on Laberyn occurred at sunset on the second day of Second Lufoa, and the battle lasted well into the night.

2. The Nameless Hunt arrived at the city's border shortly before the loathsome lurker from Thorn was seen approaching.

3. The Hunt was aided by a roving band of Rodorites and Laberyn's bravest locals. Although the three armies displayed no collaboration, they managed to succeed, driving the sinister stalker back to Thorn.

4. The exact number of casualties is unknown, but it exceeds 1,000. All victims were either Laberi or members of the Nameless Hunt.

5. This is the fourth major clash between the macabre marauder and the Nameless Hunt since the *Chronicle* began chronicling the conflict.

In recent years, Gaea has spun her days and nights in peace. No bands of brigands descended upon our cities. No war was waged between our nations. Even the malignant nightmare from Thorn refused to invade. Night after night, as Gaea continued her eternal procession around the sun, all our fears went unfulfilled. And so, day after day, they slowly decayed.

The longer safety lingers, the more our hearts and minds are released from the captivity of our dread. Eventually, even the oldest terrors are worn as lightly as the shade: the insidious starspawn's sporadic bursts of slaughter are relegated to campfire stories. Our belief resides somewhere between grisly folklore and ghastly past.

But it doesn't remain there forever. In the end, that perennial malice always reblooms, and like the aloxa locusts' rise, it always consumes. This time, it was Laberyn, Gaea's musical capital, that was sentenced by the glow of the widow's lantern.

For the first time, that festive city of endless song was hushed to a fatal silence.

Thevro Chronicle

Countless fathers and mothers lost sons and daughters. And countless sons and daughters lost fathers and mothers. Husbands and wives, brothers and sisters, all torn apart in a night.

Across our Connected Continents, there may be seven distinct faiths that divide us. But there is also one that unites us: it is the fate of *every* Gaean to be ruled by the heart, that tender spirit seated on the throne of our souls, jailed within our ribs, forever beating its message of love. And today, thousands of hearts are broken.

The details of a Rider's Report need not be described to understand the depth of tragedy felt by the many. The mourning bell will be tolling for weeks to come. But in these dark and despairing times, we can still take solace in the words of Druin. Scrawled in the ancient, immutable language of the heart, the meaning is just as clear today: the longest night is always followed by dawn's bright sun, and so too does all grief ultimately give way to mirth. Thus, together, may we have the patience to let Time, the eternal alchemist, complete its transmutation.

> Upon the close of the deepest night
>   the monarch's rise still burns away all gloom
> The first dream may bloom the blackest sky
> But even in dark hearts
>   the mortal river renews its life
>
>   Book of Druin, 66

Part One:

A New Journey

One

Nyros, Second Lufoa, Day Ten. Afternoon.

The sun was still dreaming when I awoke this morning. I sat at the edge of my bed for at least half an hour listening to it snore out of my open window. Its metered breath rattled the dry leaves and plied the night frogs like old, creaky bellows. And I just stared into the empty air, its blackness fighting the brightness of a tremendously full moon.

The moon was winning the fight, its silver beams bleaching the shadows wherever they crept. But also parching the color from everything touched by the light, as though draining Gaea of her blood. Radiance may win the war, but it leaves behind a pale wreath. I guess that's the cost of battle, that silent struggle in the night's sky as eternal as gravity.

Those were my thoughts at the time. While I sat there. I hadn't yet escaped the gravity of my own sleep, that other dark world gentling pulling at my will, dimming my mind, drawing me in. I wasn't going to succumb; I was just loitering in that groggy orbit, waiting for my back to accept the upright posture I had forced it into. The posture that would permit me to get on with my day.

Most mornings, I wake up a few minutes later and emerge from bed a few minutes earlier. Today, it took longer for my body to cooperate with my will. Once it finally did, I went to the kitchen, lit a fire, warmed some water, and began preparing the grey nettles for my first cup of tea.

I did all of this slower and quieter than usual. As though my normal behavior – sighing, shuffling my feet, chipping my mug with a clumsy pour from the kettle – might awaken the sun before it intended to rise. And put it in a bad mood. My constitution is sour enough; I don't need nature adding additional acidity. If I'm going to enter that sacred place in my mind, where the tea feels free to communicate, the immediate world that's enveloping me – all the air and ambiance – needs to possess the right temperament. If not fully serene, at least in the same family tree.

I'm not explaining myself clearly. Let me start over:

I got out of bed before sunrise, went downstairs, made tea, and drank it. And I didn't make much noise.

As always, I triturated the nettle with my mother's medical pestle. In her medical mortar. It's at least a foot and a half across, and there's residue from ten thousand treatments in it. And every one of them was meant to be taken by tea. Nothing as crude as a poultice was produced with that pestle. So, what steeps in my mug is slightly different each morning.

I've had the mortar for a year and its potency hasn't diminished: every dawn comes with a unique cocktail. I sip the subtlest hints of nature's wonders… provided I pay close enough attention. Which I almost always do.

It's my first wholly alert activity of the day. And one of my favorite activities of any day. It's calm. Contemplative. The world holds a sort of peace in place for me. For a moment. But even for a moment, peace of mind goes a long way to remedy dispeace of body.

Especially this morning's mug: it had a trace of Mulgothan cilantro in it (very different from the variety that grows in my yard). It took me a few swallows to notice. After each one, my breath began to move more freely, as though the accretion of inner peace was reducing the usual friction lining my airway. Needless to write, I am currently indulging a marginal enhancement of self-acceptance. And that feeling is exactly what I needed to confront the events that followed.

As soon as I had identified the effect of the tea, and the herb responsible, the sun finally opened its eyes. And the first color-restoring rays landed on my porch. Which muted the last of the nightsnores. That's when I stepped out to fetch the *Thevro Chronicle*. Today's issue. With the Laberyn article.

I saw the title and immediately put it down. On my kitchen table. For five seconds. Then I picked it back up and read it. And then put it down again. For ten seconds this time. Then I picked it up again and reread it. And then I put it down for the last time. Then I took the kettle from the fire, replaced it with a pan, and went back outside to collect some eggs. From the hill. Which is a ten-minute walk to the west. Ten-minute hike, actually; the slope gets pretty steep. And isn't that what a hike is? A there-and-back walk across hilly terrain? This particular there-and-back took about twenty-five minutes. Descending the hill takes longer. (No one ever injures themselves going *up* Slippery Leaf Lane.)

The decision to eat eggs, the preparation of those eggs, and the eggs themselves were all carefully chosen. The kind of care that comes from childhood convictions.

There used to be a publication called *The Harker*. But nobody called it that. "Did you read this morning's *Poorman*?", hillians and flatties alike would ask. Originally dubbed "the poor man's Chronicle", it was eventually shortened to *The Poorman*. And it kept that disparaging appellation until it was defunct. And then nobody called it anything anymore. But before it lost its name, a new issue was published every Seros morning. And during one of those mornings, I remember reading an article – together, as a family – about Busik. It must have been almost thirty years ago. But I still remember.

Those antique blocks of *Poorman's* prose taught me about the heart-swaddling magic of a well-made omelet. That culinary interstice (not quite dairy, not quite meat) probably connects with my constitution more than most. But done right, no one can fend off the serenity that accompanies ingestion. There may be nothing in the chewable universe capable of comforting the chewer as deeply, I learned that day. And perhaps believed. And perhaps still believe, as I made one such omelet today. Or at least I did my best to replicate Busik's masterpiece. Unfortunately, there was no recipe printed within the article. It was mostly the seasonings that lacked replicable detail. There were five, obviously – the number of the East – but which five exactly? I can only guess. My choices (water basil, chives, snow garlic, parsley, and rosemary) may differ here and there. What I know for sure, however, is that my eggs were the same. Or at least they were from the same lineage. Descendants of descendants. That was the whole reason for the hike.

I returned home carrying the three best eggs the hill could offer me. Actually, they were the *only* three I found. But they were flawless. As though laid by feathered angels.

I pulled the pan from the heat and began to make my omelet.

As soon as it was perfectly-ish prepared, I set the table. I would prefer to put the pan directly on the table and eat out of that. But, crassness aside, I would feel too guilty ruining the woodwork that my great grandfather himself carved into the house. It's the one piece of furniture that can never be removed. The surrounding walls were built around it. Technically, the table can't be moved at all. Its pedestal base is a white elderwillow stump, around which the kitchen was built. The top of the table is unblemished and as smooth as the evening breeze. But if you look beneath it, in the roughly hewn underside of the wood is an engraving of my great ancestor's sigil. As though he were marking not just his property but his territory. For that reason, the table has never felt like it was mine. I'm more of a steward. And forever respectful in my stewardship, I set the table properly. A plate. A fork. A napkin. A glass. I was filling that glass with water when the first knock came at the door.

It was soft, but commanding. No hand other than Cyn's could have produced its tone. She was ready for today's instruction.

This is our sixth year together. Our last. When the year is up, she will ratify my legacy, and permit me a restful retirement, which I will spend riding Abbie, plucking my lute, and napping away perfectly serviceable afternoons. The kind of afternoon that gilds every leaf with beams poured onto them from the very pitcher of the golden sun. That's the kind of afternoon I will squander. Starting in the new year. Until then – for today, tomorrow, and a little over three and a half more months of two more seasons of one last year – I have a Cyn to teach and train.

I just checked my calendar: a hundred and ten days from now, Farhearth's infinitieth annual Science Faire ends. And so too ends my mentorship. And so too begins her career.

But we're not there yet. As of today, I'm still her mentor. And she still comes to my house every morning to continue her studies. And *this* morning, she ate breakfast with me. Or rather, she ate mine. My omelet. Not owing to a lack of manners. It would have been ill mannered had she refused, as I pretended to have made it *for* her.

"Have you eaten yet?", I asked, hoping she had. She usually has.

"Not this morning; I didn't have a chance."

"Then I'm glad your breakfast won't go to waste", I said, accompanied by a gesture meant to simultaneously direct her gaze and express insistence.

She sat down and ate.

Alas, I only brought three eggs back from the hill. So, I couldn't make a second omelet for me.

I will later. At some point, the effect of my tea will wear off. And I'll likely require some additional comforting. How much comforting? I'm not sure. Because I don't know how accurate the article is. Because it opens with that bungled Druin passage. I don't work in journalism and even I know it's a mistranslation, circulated as frequently and erroneously as "training to dance" or "don't wake the winnower". (It has five lines per stanza; Druin wrote six.) So I'm not sure how much faith I have in the facts that follow. But the *premise* – Laberyn was trampled by the creature from Thorn – is surely true. Which warrants anxiety. Which warrants an omelet. Which I don't have.

Instead of eggs, I sat beside Cyn with a bowl of butter berries. Which are neither dairy nor berry. They're nuts. People typically remove the red skin and mash them into a white, spreadable butter. Hence the name. But I didn't do that. I just ate them whole. Skin and all. Then I refilled my bowl, and anxiously ate that helping, too. I was about to refill it a third time when Cyn finished her omelet. So we left the kitchen and started the day's lessons.

As we studied, my thoughts kept wandering to the Laberyn article. And Cyn could tell I was distracted. She didn't say so, but I could tell she could tell. Which made for an awkward session. We were both ready for lunch half an hour early.

Lunch is when I planned to explain to Cyn why I seemed so preoccupied this morning. But before I had finished serving us, another knock struck the door, this one much bolder than Cyn's. Uniquely bold. I hadn't seen Rorrik in over a year, but no other hand could have produced that noise. The first crash of iron bones on redthorn wood said, "Hurry up, I've been knocking all day, and I'm too important to be kept waiting." The second impact almost read aloud, "In case you didn't already know, it's Rorrik, and I'm growing impatient." There was no third. His knuckles had already knocked everything they needed to say. To strike my door a third time would have communicated the rest of what he had traveled so far to tell me, spoiling its surprise. This was the sound of Rorrik holding back.

I think he expected to arrive before the article did. He assumed he could outgallop any riding messenger. And he assumed the deadeye doves would be unreliable (perhaps plucked from flight by a cloakwing stork). Rorrik's first assumption was correct – there's no way a rider of postal prowess has even reached the Sap Stone Bridge yet – but his second assumption didn't take. And that made me unsurprisable.

I didn't know the *details* of the story – too much paper to affix to a messenger bird's leg – and the rider who bears those minutiae won't make it to Thevro for a couple of days yet. But knowing the "Pigeon's Perspective" meant my sensibilities were already on guard. And that meant details wouldn't be startling enough to shock me. So, if Rorrik had delivered his third knock, he wouldn't have spoiled much.

Cyn opened the door.

Rorrik and Cyn already knew each other. Fondly enough, but only in passing. True to the nature of that relationship, Rorrik marched past her without greeting. As though the door had opened itself.

"Laberyn was attacked." Those were his first words.

He was sweaty. He smelled like the soils of three continents. And his gait looked like that of a man learning to use legs for the first time. But he spoke with the clarity and gravity of his fullest singing voice.

I'd forgotten how powerful Rorrik's voice can be. It surprises me every time he lets loose its thunder. Even outside of song, he fashions sentences like a Cinderheim smithy, each syllable crashing hard and ringing true.

I withheld my own first words and, instead, handed him the article. It had some mug rings and splatters of breakfast on it, but not much.

Rorrik acknowledged the title, read no further, and told me it had taken him eight days to ride from Laberyn to Estevro.

I know the distance between our cities. The most probable route is about 750 miles of hoof strikes. On varying, not-always-ideal terrain. The shortest possible distance, across some spans of worse terrain, is still over 600 miles. And Rorrik arrived before lunch on the eighth day. That's fast enough to win three consecutive Salt and Stone Circles. So he might as well have said, "Horses died to get me here." With that kind of pace, I assume he either left immediately and killed two, or waited until the next morning and killed three. (I hope he wasn't riding from stable to stable on martyr's mares.)

If he bore a tiny bit less pity – if just one more animal lay dead – and if he didn't conceal his final knock like a secret in his pocket, his fist may have struck with the purity of shock. But it didn't. I only felt relief. To see him alive and healthy... and filled with wrath.

Wrath is the entire reason he was standing in my kitchen on wobbly legs, breathing heavily, with at least thirty hands of dead horse stationed as periodic mile markers of his trip. That's not the pace of grief. He's not here to mourn; this is his effort to conscript my aid.

Still, I understand how important this is to Rorrik. It's his whole life, in a way. And has been *for* his whole life. As long as I've known him, killing the haunter of Thorn has been Rorrik's singular charge. And the Laberyn incident seems to have spurred it into a stampede. That's not the kind of resolution one stands in the way of. So I didn't. I just listened to his speech. Which ended with his insistence that I accompany him to the mouth of the black trees. "To confront that beast face to face", he finished. And then he paused as though he had asked a question.

"Does it even have a face?" Those were my first words. About five minutes into the conversation. Our first in over a year.

Rorrik didn't answer. He just smiled. At me. It was tender. Like a hug. But only his mouth was doing the hugging. His eyes continued to insist.

"You will be confronting that wraith, with or without a face, right beside me." He didn't actually say that. But he may as well have.

Before releasing his smile, he softened his eyes, turned his head, and aimed an expression of profound affection and understanding toward Cyn.

She received it accordingly.

It was a smile he gives to strangers, though. A perfect counterfeit of genuine attention. Rorrik has never set foot in the South. Not even to visit Lum. Nor has he learned anything about the continent Cyn and Lum came from. Because he doesn't see it as relevant to his ambitions.

But I know Rorrik is fond of Cyn. No matter what expression he gives her.

When that smile ended, we ate lunch. And I reflected on how strange life is. There's so much loss. So much unexpected turmoil. And unwelcome change. But along the way, some bridges never fall, some bonds never break, some birds always return. And somewhere in my heart, I believe Rorrik will always be the same.

After lunch, I excused myself, and I went upstairs to write. This.

But that's all the time I have. The sun is approaching its evening position, marking the post-day, pre-night hours. Which is when Cyn and I do our second session.

I'm sure I'll have a lot more to say next time I write.

And I'm sure I'll be up late.

Two

Nyros, Second Lufoa, Day Ten. Night.

It's nighttime now. Shortly before noon, Rorrik arrived with the conviction of a conqueror. Since then, he's had nearly ten hours to settle his thoughts… and he hasn't changed his mind. Or relented any of its urgency, brief recesses aside.

Before I talk about that, let me pick up where my last entry ended. Lunch. Where Rorrik's conviction was made clear, and our stomachs were made full.

To start this entry light-hearted (and heavy-stomached), I'll describe the food:

All I was planning on serving was a little bit of dried horrux and an excess of sunfruit, that brightly colored, blandly flavored staple of the East… and expensive delicacy everywhere else. It's too delicate to bother transporting, and the locals (me included) are hardly fond of it, but like so many other flatties, my garden insists on growing enough to nourish a village. So, owing to abundance alone, it cordially attends every meal. (Perhaps also owing to its patriotic color: Gaea grows nothing greener than a sunfruit; where else but the East would such tasteless greenness be the undisputable staple?)

After Rorrik and I finished our initial "conversation", I put a third setting on the table. Then I doubled the heap of horrux, tripled the girth of the green mound, and sat down.

That's when Rorrik, forever residing on the cusp of showmanship, pulled a duskfruit from his travel bag. *His* staple. From the central West. With a slow, reposeful motion and a half-restrained smile, he placed it on my plate.

To Cyn, Rorrik's change in temperament may have seemed abrupt. Like a gentle sun suddenly displacing a tempest. But that's Rorrik. He's always been that way, oscillating between extremes. Just listen to his music. Every song is a furious pendulum, swinging between quiet verse and inclement chorus. And each of them is true to his nature.

Before the look of surprise had finished assembling itself on my face, Rorrik pulled out *another* duskfruit. And then another. He placed one of them on Cyn's plate and the last one on his own. Then he sat down, grabbed a sunfruit from the pile, and took a bite.

"How?", I asked, while staring at the perfect purple bulb moping on my plate.

Rorrik finished chewing, swallowed his bite, and then said: "I expected to lose at *least* one, so I brought three." He took another bite, chewed some more, swallowed it, then finished his sentence: "And all three made the trip."

This was a treat for me, the duskfruit was. But it was a true novelty for Cyn, who had never even seen one before. I was almost envious of her experience. It's the most delicious gift from any tree… as long as you don't look at it. Because it is definitely the drabbest sight on any plate.

Those bruise-purple, tear-shaped bulbs give the impression that they're too depressed to reflect any light. To my knowledge, duskfruit scarcely makes it fifty miles past the thickets. Its flesh is resilient to the battering of transit, but a few days in an incompatible climate is sufficient to prompt its decay… when planted. When plucked, it rots faster than uncured meat.

Bringing edible duskfruit all the way to Estevro is considerably harder than transporting sunfruit (not in the form of tasteless jam) all the way to the West. What Rorrik did is the botanical equivalent of delivering ice to Cinderheim. I would be unsurprised if this were the farthest east an unspoiled bulb has ever traveled. And unless a couple of Salt and Stone winners have organized a complicated picnic in southern Thorn, this was the only time both fruits have coinhabited the same plate.

I almost expected to witness a chemical reaction upon their contact. They didn't react, but the flavors did pair matrimonially well. Every restaurant on Gaea would serve that pairing were it not impossible to do so. Or *nearly* impossible, I guess. That's the whole reason Rorrik brought the fruit. It was his pseudo-subtle way of conveying the haste of his trip. At the time, all it really conveyed was the taste of it.

Say what you want about the West and its ways, but one must admit: those farmers know what they're doing. If there's an agricultural entity that can change your life, it grows west of the thickets.

I say this as an Estevroan. I live in the baking co-capital of the world, and I remain reverent to the flavors of the West. (I'm conceding Thevro's status as Estevro's sibling capital even though all they eat is ripe cheese.)

As Cyn and I ate, Rorrik resumed his adventure mongering. The bequeathing of duskfruit was just an intermission. For the rest of lunch, he continued to insist, and I continued to resist.

And then we finished eating. And Rorrik settled down for a nap.

Not at the table. He made it to the bench on the porch. He would have gone upstairs, where the bedrooms are, but his legs could barely hold him upright. He'll need a full week to recover. He doesn't think so; he plans on leaving tomorrow. And said as much. But if he follows through on that plan, his body will surely betray its fealty to his will. To say nothing of his horse's body and will.

I asked him to stay for longer. "At least a couple of weeks", I said. "So we have the chance to talk on less urgent terms."

He didn't reply. And within a minute of not replying, he was sleeping. Deeply. This is a uniquely Western skill. When I go to bed, my waking mind chaperones my sleeping mind. Like a parent monitoring a child playing in the yard. "Don't go too far! Stay where I can see you!" Rorrik has no such supervision. His mind wanders without restriction, sails without anchor. And it went sailing on the bench on the porch for about four hours.

During this time, Cyn and I got in a short lesson, and then prepared a feast worthy of Rorrik's journey. Worthy of our reunion. Exclusively from the garden. That may sound modest, but excepting only The Aldsyn, the most diverse constellations of flora across the entire breadth of Gaea bloom in my backyard. It's almost entirely native-to-the-East plants, but their culinary offerings number in the hundreds. At least according to the *density* of diversity, I don't think my yard has an equal. I don't know many of the proper names of the plants – my mother and her father were the florists of the family, not me – but I know the flavors. And we ate a lot of them. Every color and flavor in season made it to the table.

Unlike lunch, dinner didn't begin with unabashed beseeching, rallying my aid for battle. In a way, dinner was more about the duskfruit than lunch was, despite eating none of it.

It was the *topic* of the duskfruit that served as Rorrik's invitation to reminisce. About the years we spent together at Farhearth. As students. When we were in each other's company every day. In particular, when we used to "borrow" wagons (some people might call this stealing, but we always returned them), and we would travel together during the breaks. Without a flip penny to our names. Sleeping under the open sky, eating whatever we could catch or find. Without any plan or expectation. Just journeying in whatever direction that felt right in the moment.

I hadn't thought about those jaunts in a long time. And I don't know that I could identify an age in which I felt more alive. Which is, I'm sure, the reason Rorrik brought it up, oscillating once again between impassioned wrath and tender remembrance.

His voice was soft. Sentimental. And every bit as poetic as his lyrics. Recounting our trips, his descriptions of the Western air filled my lungs as though I were inhaling something stronger than words.

That's what makes the West so special. It's not the terrain, all those sands and sloughs. It's the air. In our old adventuring days, I accompanied Rorrik half a dozen times through Lir, Laberyn, and Midrodor. And if I had been traveling blind, it wouldn't have subtracted much from the pleasure.

People who have not experienced Midrodor for themselves assume it's called The Oyster for its defensive shell, but as a fortress, it is not half the shell of Pendelhall. Others assume it is named for its fishing, but it could never compete with Ryndor. The Oyster is named for its air. It seems to filter all the waters of the world, distill their salts and tides, and dissolve their essence into its breeze. Stand on those cliffs, take the open skies into your lungs, and you will befriend the full expanse of the seas. Eyes add little to the experience.

The same is true of the rest of the continent.

We never went inside of Adonere, but along the low hills that flank it, there is a wind so pure, it must descend from some celestial paradise; to breathe is to share your breath with the stars.

In Lir, the purity of that wind is replaced by pollens, and every breeze is received as an offering, bearing the scents of the wildest flowers tamed.

And in Laberyn, the air was forever filled with songs: endless, twinkling melodies telling tales of great heroes and greater romances. And sometimes tales of Thorn. Those darker songs have long filled the air Rorrik beathed.

But it's not just notes filling its air. The *air* fills the air, too. And it's different. There's a scent that seems to come from the crying cloud. Like it soaks up the highest sky – absorbs the whole ethereal realm – and rains it down on Gaea below. It crashes on the roofs and roads and releases that empyrean expanse into the surrounding space, awakening the imagination that was slumbering in our lungs. When you breathe in Laberyn's sky-fallen air, you can't help but breathe out a lyric. That's the eyes-closed experience of that serenading city. Or it *was*, I guess.

As I dizzied myself with wistful emotions, Rorrik continued to nudge my sensibilities in the direction of adventure. One last trip together. It was a gentle nudging. I wouldn't have noticed but for the fact that I know Rorrik. He isn't sentimental in the way that I am. Or in the amount that I am.

I went to great effort to buy back my childhood home. From the people my parents sold it to when I was a teenager. Rorrik inherited his ancestral home, and he's never been there. Not since he was a toddler.

So Rorrik was not reminiscing for reminiscence's sake. He had an angle. One that was not natural to the geometry of nostalgia. And at the summit of my sentimentality, he deployed that angle, and spoke it slowly, plaintively, almost lyrically:

"All of this – the people, the cities, the air itself – will be gone. The only way you'll be able to revisit a familiar world then will be resuscitation of old, dead memories. And snatched back from the pale, nothing is ever the same."

It felt like a chorus in Rorrik's summoning song. After reciting it, he paused. Not briefly or passively. It was a fierce silence that gave no indication it would resolve on its own. It just kept lingering, uncomfortably, until I finally responded:

"Aren't there actual *militia* – at Midrodor, Eldergard, Pendelhall – that are better equipped to take this on? What is it you think *we* could do?"

Rorrik did not take a moment to collect his thoughts and formulate his argument. There were zero moments between the end of my question and the beginning of Rorrik's response:

"We've been in the Hundred-Years Armistice for well over a hundred years", he began. "Today's militaries are symbolic. At best, they defend. The only thing they *declare* is peace. And that's not going to kill the beast of Thorn. For that, I need *your* help."

Rorrik said this calmly, but there was fire in his voice. That kind of searing ambition that exclusively burns in youth... and, somehow, in Rorrik, who is a couple of seasons older than I am.

I did my best to contain and smother his flame while still enjoying its warmth.

My response ended with something like, "Maybe someday I'll join you, but now isn't the right time. For either of us. Haste feels like a path to remorse."

Rorrik responded.

I responded.

And so on. Until I said, "You don't have to leave. You can stay here longer."

Rorrik didn't respond to that. Not *verbally*, anyway. But the look he gave me accused my offer of having a patronizing tone. So, I clarified:

"I don't mean you're *welcome* to stay. Being welcomed implies you're visiting. And visitors never feel settled. Guests never really belong. And you have all the belonging of family. So what I meant was you should *settle* here. For as long as you want."

Rorrik nodded, which could be interpreted as "maybe" or "I think about it."

He gave the impression he was genuinely indecisive. Although I'm sure he was just wondering whether he'll need a few extra days to fan my flame.

Whereas I'm hoping a prolonged stay would do more to snuff his own.

One of us is going to be disappointed in how this ends.

But now it's late. Well past my bedtime.

I'll write more tomorrow.

Three

Eldos, Second Lufoa, Day Eleven. Morning.

Cyn isn't here yet. And Rorrik is still asleep. We were up late. So I may be unaccompanied until lunch. My lunch. Their breakfast.

Despite the late night, I still woke up before the sun. As I always do. Feeling groggy and listless. As I usually feel. But I also felt more anxious than I did yesterday. I'm not sure why.

I know the *source* of my anxiety: part of a major city was partly demolished. But I don't know why this morning kindled more concern than yesterday. Maybe I'm coming to terms with it. There's a kind of shock protection that accompanies surprise: the first strike of bad news is a superficial wound. But surprise doesn't armor me for long. One night's sleep generally disrobes me of its protection. And then, if the news continues to strike, it cuts deeper.

Maybe that's why I felt more anxious when I got out of bed. Although it does seem irrational: I'm two continents away, and I'm acquainted with no Labero other than Rorrik… and he survived. He's currently in the next room, asleep on the sofa. Silent but for his breath. Motionless but for his chest. A depth of sleep that is completely inaccessible to the fretful. And out of the two of us, he's the one with legitimate reason to fret. So why is it *me* feeling so anxious?

Recognizing all of this should have put the world at ease. But I still felt in need of some mood enhancement. So I made my tea carefully.

My mother didn't triturate without aim; the entire surface of her mortar was medicinally segregated. It was a map. Every bit as precise as my father's cartography. I'm not so particular. Most mornings, wherever the nettle falls is where I grind it.

This results in a different brew every time. This morning, though, I tried to grind the nettle in the exact same spot. To replicate yesterday's leaves.

This never works. The tea never heeds my will, but I did get a *similar* effect. Sort of. Not what I would call "mood mead" – it wasn't an immediate enhancer – but it did come from the same plant. Mulgothan cilantro. Except instead of the leaf, which I had yesterday, it was the seeds.

The seeds have a very different effect in the body. An effective compound, but only if it's taken habitually. Have it every morning for a month and you'll accumulate enough to feel the weight of the world lighten its load. And since the body doesn't metabolize the seeds very quickly, once that emotional uplift can be felt, it'll continue to be felt for a month following cessation.

Alas, I did not drink a whole month's tea this morning. So my mood remains unchanged. I wouldn't have been able to identify what I was drinking were it not for the sour taste: exactly like Sizarhorn lime seeds... which have no known medical property... which means lime had no business being in the mortar... which means cilantro is what I was tasting. "Mulgothan coriander seeds" to be exact. That's how it's recorded in apothecary inventories.

The sun finished cresting the horizon an hour ago. I finished my tea as it did. Then I spent the post-tea, pre-now hour walking in my back yard. Laps along the path that encircles my garden. Inside the fence of green wood that keeps the deer out. I had no fruit or flower to pluck. Nothing to do. Just walking, breathing in the air the garden was breathing out, and very slightly squinting against the still-rising sun.

It's my favorite time of day. And after my tea, it's my *second* favorite activity: orbiting my garden during the phase of morning when nature is at its most vibrant, but it can only be seen in the bottom hemisphere of my visual field. It's too bright to look up. At the roof of my sight, my lashes are hard at work, shielding the most blinding of the sun's beams. All I can see is the scattered dust from that collision, twinkling like a star-fretted heaven, hanging low in the sky. And I just keep walking. In circles. Being reminded that peace still lives in the world. And I can see it if I pay attention.

As I walked my laps, I had a thought. Or, rather, I thought about something Mizjak once said about knowing the mind of one's opponent. And I assigned it a different context. This:

You can come to know someone deeply if you understand their attention. Where is it aimed in any moment? What divides it? What diminishes it? What enlivens it?

For me, it's early morning nature that I attend to so keenly. And vengeance doesn't grow there. If someday the star-fretted roof of my sight is threatened with enveloping darkness, then sure, I'll reappraise the object of my keenest attention. But as this morning was perfectly gilded, I just can't be swayed by Rorrik's insistence. It's as though he has a congenital defect in contentment.

The two of us don't seem to be descended from the same stalk. Perhaps if you go back far enough, every branch is affixed to the same maternal tree. Some womb gave birth to all the critters that followed. But Rorrik's and my branches must have split long ago. Familial in our friendship, but unalike in our attention.

In a way, I'm the opposite of a yrtog. Their vision is based on movement while mine is based on stillness. That's what my mind is most attracted to. By comparison, Rorrik's vision seems to be based on vengeance. And it's not a casual glance; it's a baleful stare with unblinking eyes.

I do admire this quality in him, though. So charmed by his vitality, I used to join him all the time. Constant outings, musical performances, adventures of every kind. Back when Lum, Rorrik, and I were younger, the three of us were inseparable. And we were always doing *something*. I was usually exhausted or uncomfortable or feeling unsociable for the bulk of those experiences, but I still went. I was sure the one time I stayed behind I would miss something. Some spectacular, life-changing thing would occur while I was at home. Then I would have to hear "You should have been there!" for rest of my life. "I can't believe you missed it!" And so on.

Eventually, I came to appreciate what's actually important in life. Such as tea. And peace. And quiet.

As much as I would prefer a life of peace *and* quiet, if I can only have one, I'll take the quiet. I've been taking it all morning. Basking in its comfort. But it's coming up on noon. And I should have lunch ready by then. Lunch for me, at least. It'll be breakfast for Cyn and Rorrik. Cyn's probably on her way, and I'm sure Rorrik will reunify spirit and flesh soon (those Westerners really know what it means to slumber).

Enough tarrying for one morning. It's time to leave my desk and get on with my day. I'm sure I'll have a lot more to write later.

Four

Eldos, Second Lufoa, Day Eleven. Afternoon.

Cyn finally arrived. And Rorrik finally emigrated from slumberland. And we did finally eat.

I decided to serve my *personal* staple (different from that of my continental companions): the trendel cumber. Or at least that *would* be my staple if the vines weren't so stingy.

If my garden solicited my input before growing its bounty, it wouldn't be the sunfruit that multiplied fast enough to satisfy a hymog's appetite. It would be the trendel cumber; it's just as green, just as nutritious, and far more delicious. Like the sunfruit, it only grows in the East. *Unlike* the sunfruit, which grows abundantly here but is relatively unknown beyond, the trendel cumber barely grows *in* the East. And it's *completely* unknown beyond. So let me describe it:

It's a knobby cucumber that looks like a trendel snake. Or perhaps the other way around: the snake imitates the fashion of the cumber. Regardless of primacy and plagiarism, the miserly tithes offered by those creeping vines are nature's version of a doughnut. In shape only. Not flavor. Or crunchiness.

Most of the time, I eat them as I would a doughnut. A wet, crunchy one. But today, I put one cumber on each plate and stuffed their centers with diminutively diced rainbows of other fruits and vegetables. Slices of red and white radishes. Cubes of blue and yellow squashes. Something between slices and cubes of whiteish, yellowish bell pear. The purplest pomegranate seeds. Persimmon, apples, lychee, cherries, starfruit, and… I think that's it. Then I gathered some moon grapes and firepods, mashed them into a red molasses, and poured it over top. And finally, I topped that topping with three emerald primrose petals. Not for flavor, although they taste fine; rather, the placing of the petals was my attempt to imbue each dish with the spirit of Estevro… being the flower on the city's flag.

I'm realizing this sounds like a random combination of incompatible flavors. But it made for a good lunch. I don't know if it made for a good breakfast. Because I wasn't there. Cyn and Rorrik ate theirs a full hour after I ate mine. Which was a full hour after I set the table. I would have kept waiting, but my patience was being battered by boredom. And boredom always sharpens the pangs of my hunger. So I ate alone.

Then I spent the postprandial hour wandering around my garden, pretending to groom it, but really just grazing for dessert.

When I was a child, I thought my mother's gardening was pointless. Doesn't everyone grow vegetables?, I wondered. Can't we just walk to the market to get whatever we need whenever we need it?, I kept wondering. What's the point of having our house engirdled by a dense, waist-high wilderness?, my wondering was given a voice, and that voice had a cheeky tone.

That was my thinking back then. I would have been just as happy with no yard at all. Because without a yard, there wouldn't have been any yard-related toil demanded of me.

"Make sure you pull the weeds up by the roots!", my mother would remind me from the other side of the garden. She couldn't see my technique, but she knew what I was doing: hurriedly yanking the tops off so I could be excused from my garden duty as quickly as possible.

"Remember to get the roots!", she would shout three minutes later. Not unnecessarily.

I would grumble a bit, then begin pulling up an occasional non-weed by its roots. Not out of incompetence, but a desire to *appear* incompetent.

"Don't remove *those* ones!", my mother would scold me as soon as she saw. "Those are tomato plants", she would explain, after seeing my face embossed with a perfect brow of confusion. "But… there aren't any tomatoes on it", I would justify as sincerely as possible.

"It's too early in the season", she would explain – again – and then release a little exasperation: "Didn't we have this same conversation last week?"

"I'm sorry", I would say, followed by my attempt at a cunning excuse: "I can't tell the difference. No matter how many times you point it out to me."

After a few more performances, I was eventually pardoned from any future obligations in the garden. Until I was about thirty, when I began *volunteering* my toil. And I never unvolunteered it.

Today, I have come to appreciate the value of nurturing one's own nature. Especially if you don't have to nurture it very hard. Which I don't. Not nearly as hard as I remember. Evict a few trespassing weeds each week, and the rest of the garden maintains itself.

And there's a lot of garden performing its own upkeep. Practically every nut, fruit, vegetable, and seasoning native to the East has a home here. But it's not a farm. Farms are places where nature is enslaved for economic gain. That's not my garden. Nor is it a collection of crops so foreign to the region that I'm forced to fake a remote climate with imported soil or the brokering of sunlight or complicated watering schedules. None of that.

My garden thrives with neglect. Because its leafy residents lived on this continent long before people did.

Most of them, anyway. I do have a few peculiar plants. There are five or six that I've never encountered anywhere else. But the rest of my grounds are covered by the greens (and reds, yellows, purples, and in-betweens) that planted *themselves* here. Without coercion from me.

I write this because I think it says a lot about my *own* nature. I think *everyone's* relationship with Gaea reveals their character and values. Maybe I'm wrong. I'm just thinking of this now. I haven't done any laps on the thought yet. But indulge me as I work my philosophy out on the page:

In the West, the residents spend half their day gardening. In the East, those half-days are spent yarding. Remarkably different behavior.

Western gardening is a *collaboration* with nature. Even in Lir, the residents serve an almost enzymatic role. They're facilitators, assisting only the seeds which would have sprouted on their own… without any help… eventually. The gardeners – ever dutiful in their catalysis – simply speed along Gaea's will.

In the East, it's different. The residents intervene. Long ago, they penned Gaea in a reservation, segregating the natural and unnatural worlds. Today, nothing outside of Nemus is held sacred. So, there's no blasphemy in its manipulation. Easterners insist on nature working *for* them, rather than the other way around. In doing so, they construct completely unnatural yards. So people can point and say, "Look how pretty *that* yard is."

This is one of the many stark distinctions between Easterners and Westerners. And I don't align with either distinction; I'm split between servant and master.

I've long wondered if I inherited this interstitial constitution from my mother. A hereditary feature no less biological than hair color. My mother was both gardener *and* yarder as well. So was her father. And his. To my knowledge, he's the one who first nurtured this dense, waist-high wilderness. And he's the one who first settled in its location, along the border of the hills and flats.

And he's the one whose life decisions neatly divided those two worlds. And now, all these years later, it's me who lingers in that space, balancing between competing gravities. Waiting for that perfect, peaceful divide where I truly belong to open and greet me. And welcome me inside. Until then, the foot of the foothills is where I'll stay.

And that brings me back to the immediate matter:

Why would I go adventuring alongside Rorrik when I know there's no destination that would bring me as much contentment as home?

To me, windows are suitable lenses through which adventures can be viewed. Figuratively. In the sense that I experience more pleasure listening to Rorrik recount his tales than I do in experiencing them myself. It's a burden to be on the other side of that lens. Always marching somewhere, carrying around some cumbrous duty day and night. It's hard on the knees. Again: figuratively.

But literally, too. Some days, I prefer to receive actual sunlight through glass. It softens the beams, likens them to bathwater. And bathing in them feels like the perfect balance of indoors and outdoors. Not quite committing to either. Experiencing the elements without braving them.

Standing outside, unshielded, under the midday sky, is not as meditative as sitting next to the window, eyes closed, feeling the sun's soothing warmth. And breathing it in, and out, and back in. And listening to those breaths.

Only there, can I hold my most subtle, intimate thoughts up to the light for inspection. Turn them over silently in my mind. Handle them so delicately. Scrutinize them so completely. Many of my favorite thoughts have been shaped through the windows. Especially the window in front of me now. The one above the desk in my bedroom, with the row of stones lining its sill. Souvenirs of my old journeys. Adventures beyond the glass.

It's been a long time since I last "adventured" beyond the East.

That's what I was thinking about when I returned from my walk. I was eager to head upstairs and write it all down, but Rorrik had already woken up and Cyn had already arrived. They ate their trendel cumber breakfasts together, and were standing at the sink cleaning the dishes when I walked in.

After some perfunctory "good morning"'s, Rorrik launched into a ten-minute recruitment speech. Which was followed by some back-and-forthing where I resisted his summons.

Rorrik was clearly well rested. It was an inspiring performance. Never has a military general rallied his troops with more spirit or skill. But I had just finished wandering around my garden. Reflecting. Deeply. About gardens. And windows. And the kind of contentment that only home can provide.

I had been nurturing those thoughts for a full hour when "good morning" happened, so Rorrik's bidding didn't stand a chance.

Or at least that's what I thought when it began. But I'll tell that story later. Tonight. When I sit down to write my next journal.

At the same desk.

In front of the same window.

Which, at that hour, will be blackened by its effort to barricade my room from the night's chill, instilling a feeling of coziness.

And why would I leave that behind?

Five

Eldos, Second Lufoa, Day Eleven. Night.

I'm back in my bedroom, which doubles as my writing chamber, sitting beside my black window. And looking at the row of memory stones on the sill.

All those agates and jagged nuggets of striped feldspar and the heart-shaped chunks of chert I've taken from my younger adventures. Sitting alongside a linear constellation of rocks, minerals, and crystals I *can't* identify. All of them kept as relics to remember those journeys by. I like how the sun and moon illuminate them differently, dressing my recollections in different attire.

But tonight, I'm not writing about any of those experiences. I have too much to say about the present evening. Any day I spend with Rorrik, even if we do nothing but nap and eat, seems to clutter my mind and consume my paper. By bedtime, my hand is too cramped to continue writing and my journal has fallen behind. So I'll pick up where my last entry left off: Rorrik's recruitment speech.

One is simultaneously inspired and exhausted by the vigor of Rorrik's ambition. Maybe that's what a night of Western-deep sleep will do. If I slept like Rorrik, maybe I, too, would pursue my dreams. But pursuit is so… active. It's so tiring. At least for the no-longer-young, it is.

I've watched a lot of people depart their youth, that fleeting paradise we're all destined to squander. Some depart eagerly, others reluctantly, but we're all evicted eventually. Then we spend our remaining years in reminiscence, smoldering a former flame. The fire has gone cold, but it continues to emit a constant cloud of stories. "Remember the time" or "Remember when we" precedes every exciting sentence. I've found this to be true for most people.

Rorrik is not one of those people. He's the only exception I know. Still today, his life is all fire, no smoke. And every passing year, it seems to grow hotter. At this point, I wonder if death is hearty enough to extinguish it. And today, the full flame of his ambition is blazing in the direction of Thorn.

I could feel its heat during his kitchen sink recruitment speech.

He insisted that we breach its boundary together. And confront its denizen together. And greet certain death… together.

It's hard for me to respond to bidding of this kind. Because I like being perceived as the type of person who is capable of that sort of adventure. Capable of accompanying Rorrik on *any* of his countless campaigns. I like the lionheart he sees when he looks at me. Vibrant, tireless, courageous. Pretending to be that person feels invigorating. But the feeling doesn't last… because I quickly come to terms with the fact that I'm *not* that person. Not anymore. Rorrik is just conflating his memory of me with the version who's standing on the opposite side of the kitchen table. Which, for me, is the ideal proximity; I can savor the warmth of his aura with no risk of harm. It's like standing near a hearth fire. Standing *in* the fire, though? Actually *accompanying* Rorrik on one of his quests? That sounds unpleasant. I take more pleasure in reflecting upon experiences than I take in experiencing them as they unfold. I've been close companions with Rorrik and Lum since we were teenagers. We've done a lot of unfolding together. I've journeyed enough miles and undertaken enough trials to spend another two lifetimes living off the dividends of my memory. Even my windowsill is running out of room for additional stones.

I said something like that to Rorrik, overdoing the fire theme. "These days, mine is all but snuffed", I finished. To which he replied, "Your flame is fine. All it needs is some kindling."

In my response, I kept talking about combustion. Sometimes I get stuck on a metaphor. I can tell there's a gem in there somewhere; it just needs more cutting. So I keep up the lapidary work, to the exasperation of my audience, until I finally carve out the shape of my thought. Then I polish it with a sheen of quotability… which I failed to do in this case. I never figured out what I was trying to say. Despite saying a lot. I concluded my rambling monologue with something like: "I'm content watching Cyn's spark grow. It won't be long before she burns brighter than either of us. Except her fire won't burn this city to ash. I'm not so sure about yours. But I know my time has passed."

That was my attempt to end the conversation. It didn't work. No matter what I said, Rorrik had a rejoinder queued up. All of them were clear, persuasive, and fraught with urgency. Clarity and persuasiveness are difficult to take on, so I addressed the last one: "This situation feels too tense for me. It doesn't seem like an ideal time to make important life decisions. We should wait until the immediate conflict blows over."

Queue Rorrik's rapid rejoinder: "Life is far too breezy to remain idle. It blows away every memory that lacks emotional weight. Without heavy experiences, you'll find your later years barren. And this is one you won't forget."

I didn't respond. I just stared at him. For about six blink's time.

Not because I had nothing to say. But because I had too much. Rorrik was just being dramatic, trying to persuade me with flair, but his argument struck me in a philosophical way.

Every day, as I sit by myself, I revisit sentimental destinations in my mind that the winds of time have yet to blow away. I practically have paperweights on my windowsill to keep them secure. Although many of those memories are of heavier experiences, and they'd be unforgettable *without* a souvenir.

That's not where my socially withdrawn pondering ended. I began to wonder about the places we go to experience nostalgia. And why we must visit alone. If we're accompanied by anyone who wasn't present when the memory was built, visitation desecrates its hallowed grounds. If sentimentality is not kept secret, it decays. So we keep our most precious memories hidden, folded in our hearts.

But eventually, there comes a time in which we stop folding new memories. We stop taking risks, stop being emotionally present.

Every memory we will ever hold dear has already been formed. At that point, each one we spoil permanently erodes our emotional realm. One by one, our kingdom gradually diminishes into nothing. And then we die.

That was the circuitous path my thinking took while I stared and blinked, silently, in Rorrik's direction.

I hadn't yet responded. But Rorrik could tell I was about to. And he could tell my response was going to be an argument. And that its theme would be something like, "I already have two lifetimes of sentimentality stowed away; further adventure is wasted on me." I intended to say something like that, and I was inhaling the breath that would say it when Rorrik interrupted my intention:

"Coziness is not a virtue."

That's all he said. But he said it decisively. There was no question implied; it was a declaration. And I received it as an invitation for *more* introspection.

I tilted my head a few degrees, squinted a little, and stared into a *new* abyss of my own making. And Rorrik continued to be unfazed by my adjournment from the conversation. He knows my tendency.

Whenever a new idea is subjected to my custody, I take it apart, separate every component, inspect them individually. Turn them over, feel their edges, hold them up to the light. Then I reassemble them in a novel way, hoping to glean some small profundity from the examination. So that I might understand human nature better. So that I might learn how to think and behave in more productive or compassionate ways. Perhaps even live a tiny bit better.

The present idea, which I began to dis- and re-mantle, was coziness.

Somehow, the cruelty embedded in the feeling had never occurred to me. It's not enough that you feel safe, warm, and free of strife and strain. Someone else must be experiencing those things.

Coziness requires comparison. It's an emotion of relativity; it depends upon worse conditions being endured by others. Sitting beside a hearth fire in the middle of Arzox, looking at the snowfall outside is only cozy because of how unpleasant and generally uninhabitable the climate is on the other side of the window. It wouldn't arouse the same sensation if the multitudes of life all around you were basking in even greater comfort rather than suffering the bitter frost.

With that in mind, it's worth wondering whether the horror from Thorn terrorizing a city two continents away does more to increase coziness than deplete it. "By divine grace, my home remains unharmed", or some such gratitude. "Permit me a moment to luxuriate in the solace", my gratitude indelicately lingers. It's worth wondering whether Rorrik knocking on my door impairs my comfort more. I'm not saying that's how I feel. I'm just considering the possibility. As honestly as I can. Critical introspection is the one menace against which I have no fear.

I never came to a decision. I might have, given enough time. But Rorrik lacked the patience to let my reflection arrive at a conclusion. After about fifteen seconds, he began to expound on his statement.

But I didn't let him get very far. My interruption went something like this:

"You ate half a pound of horrux yesterday and seemed to suffer no remorse. And that pleasure is no less grim if you consider its implications. But nor is it worth repudiation."

Rorrik and I volleyed the point for several minutes, neither of us letting the other's argument land. And in the end, neither of us succeeded in convincing the other of our position. But I do think my reasoning was better.

It went something like this:

Our emotions, just like our sinews, are the handiwork of evolution. Rorrik's beseeching makes me anxious because anxiety kept our ancestors alive. In an age before cities, trepidation kept people out of peril's grasp. At least long enough to pass those trepid tendencies to their progeny. Coziness seems to come from the same place. When peril can be found trampling in our midst, it is not only negative emotions – like anxiety – that reinforce our avoidance. Self-preservation is also fortified with positive emotions. Such as coziness, which is what you feel when you find safety in a dangerous space. Is it worth reflecting on the implications of our coziest indulgences? Sure. Just as it's worth acknowledging the mother of the horrux we ate. The slaughter of her offspring bears a tragedy which takes nothing from the taste of the meat. So, whether it's the crackle of a fire or the flavor of our food, satisfaction is not indivisible from depravity, and a tiny hint of happiness need not haunt us.

Or something like that.

Rorrik was unmoved by my reasoning. Just as I was unmoved by his. After ten unbudging minutes, we agreed to let our futile volley fall. At which point, I excused myself, went upstairs, and wrote my afternoon journal.

Since then, I've continued to reflect on our exchange. And I have some additional thoughts.

First, I think there are two different cozinesses. And I think the distinction matters. There's the type that stems from a favorable imbalance of fortune. The type I already described: the feeling of warmth amid frigidity, safety in a dangerous space. There's *that* version of coziness – the common version – which is thoughtlessly relished by every Easterner. And then there's the Western version. Not the *whole* West. Just Adonere. Although I've never been inside the city, I know the expression they've long held sacred. It's the last line of an ancient hymn they still whisper to themselves every night like a prayer before bed. Once, I heard it pronounced in Old Adonian. Only once. It was like hearing a sorceress incant a spell of restoration. The sound of its syllables transcended song; it would be profane to call it "poetry". None of that magic survives translation, unfortunately, but I'm told the meaning is preserved. More or less. In Orfric, it translates to "I am home, I am whole." And that union of homeness and wholeness comprises a coziness that doesn't even consider the outside world. It is not relative to the experience of others; it is a state of reflection aimed entirely inward. To me, that's a much purer kind of coziness. Although I don't think it's the version I feel. Still, I thought it was worth acknowledgement.

Secondly, and lastly, I appreciate the flame Rorrik spent the morning fanning, stoking the spirit of those perfect days of stifling poverty and loud enemies. Together, we were beset by struggles – impossible trial after impossible trial – constantly fighting with the full extent of our faculties. Then celebrating the seeming miracle of our victories. I cherish that age. How could I not?

Today's struggles are different. Lethargy, apathy, back pain. These are quiet enemies. They bear all of the strain but none of the noise. Shepherd's fever may be more lethal than an arena lion, but no ovation awaits our triumph. Similarly, no song has ever been sung about the hero who vanquished his idleness. Victory only inspires when it prevails over that which roars. And today's opponents don't even snarl. The only sound is a sigh released from the afflicted as we slouch and succumb to one more nap.

In the end, senescence may harbor more sadness than untimely death, but it lacks the suddenness that moves the minstrels and bards.

And so, day after day, we strive on, without pomp or praise, until we finally give in to those silent lions.

With that dispiriting thought, I'm going to stop writing. My hand is cramping, and my journal is still behind. I've only made it through the afternoon… effectively completing my *previous* entry.

I'll catch up in the morning. I'm too tired to go on.

At the moment, all I can do is sigh, succumb, and do my best to show grace in defeat.

Goodnight Gaea. May all your inhabitants be safe, comfortable, and full of coze (the Adonian kind).

Six

Seros, Second Lufoa, Day Twelve. Morning.

Yesterday, when I was done writing my afternoon journal, I came downstairs, walked into the front hall, and encountered a goose. It was sitting near the front door amid the scattered pairs of shoes. We made eye contact, the goose and me. And then I walked past it, into the parlor, where I made eye contact with Rorrik, who mentioned – unnecessarily – that his goose was in the hall.

This is my attempt to catch up to the present moment. No time to mention last night's sleep or this morning's tea. No recollections of old thoughts or mulling of new ones. I'm just trying to unpack yesterday's events so I can confront today's without the burden of luggage.

"Gyfur's in the hall", Rorrik said. And I wondered if he thought it possible that I didn't notice. There's no other way into the front parlor (the sitting room with the hearth) than past Rorrik's goose. And to get past it, I had to walk *around* it; it was exactly in my way, sitting as determinedly as a mother warming an egg.

"I assumed he was here somewhere", I politely lied.

The truth is I'm surprised that I was surprised to see Gyfur in the hall. It's a believed-to-be-extinct breed of waterfowl that's completely flightless, nearly walkless, and perfectly companionable with Rorrik. This particular one has been Rorrik's companion for as long as I've known him. Longer, actually. And Rorrik just left his home for good. Presented with similar circumstances, I would never leave Abbie behind, and our bond is a briefer one. Rorrik even has a custom-made saddle with a seat for Gyfur built into it. So, "I assumed he was here somewhere" was not merely polite; it was also practical.

Rorrik didn't respond to my polite and practical fib. Cyn did. "Does its name make sense to you?", she asked me, and I knew what she was asking.

"It does, but I've spent a lot of time in the West. You can scarcely travel a mile beyond the thickets without encountering a horse. A truly majestic one. And then another. And another. And then a whole galloping herd of equally impressive creatures. Eventually, you've seen so many that their majesty appears ordinary. And every single one of them is named Solyre. You get used to it."

I guess the difference is nobody ever sees a gyfur. Rorrik's aside. I've never seen another. I would have never heard of the breed were it not for his.

I don't know how close to extinct it is. A dozen of them? Fewer? I would call it "endangered", but I suspect no living gyfur exists in a state of present danger. It may be banished from the air and clumsy on land, but that downy hunk of brawn can swim with the vigor of a Rivervalan tugboat, and unless it's pierced with a pretty thick arrow, it'll live to a hundred.

"How do you distinguish one from the other?", Cyn asked.

"A gyfur is considerably smaller with feathers and webbed feet while a solyre has a thin coat of hair and long legs with hooves."

Rorrik hadn't misunderstood her question. He was just being Rorrik.

Cyn needlessly clarified: "What I intended to ask was how you tell one solyre apart from the others? Abbie isn't named Lybax. Each of us isn't named Person. If you own more than one horse, wouldn't individual names permit clearer communication?"

Instead of answering the question that was asked, Rorrik chose to explain that Westerners don't *own* horses. They *bond* with them. It's different. He neglected to mention that Westerners buy and sell horses all the time... which seems an awful lot like ownership.

The conversation continued for a few more minutes. To no resolution or satisfaction. Then Rorrik took Gyfur outside. To play in the yard with Abbie. My goat and his goose are just as friendly as Rorrik and I are. They seem to share all of our fondness with none of our disputes. Or at least I assume that to be true.

When Rorrik came back inside, Cyn and I were in the study. The other parlor. Which doubles as my library. That's where most of our lessons and academic conversations take place, sitting opposite one another at the inglenook.

When Rorrik joined us, Cyn and I were sitting in our usual spots discussing the essays and aphorisms of Aetheldorf. That's what she's reading now.

Cyn has gone through practically every book I own. The only works left are the probably-wrong, the almost-certainly-wrong, and those that lie beyond the boundaries of rational thought, where plenty of wisdom resides if you're adventurous and unoffendable enough to trudge through those wilds.

That seldom-trodden path is where Aetheldorf resides. That's where society has cast his works, anyway.

On an average day, Cyn reads at least a hundred pages. And it's not novels. These aren't pages that can be turned lightly. They're heavy-lettered tomes on the natural sciences. Mostly. Some histories, too. A tiny bit of linguistics. Plenty of philosophical theses, which is what we've been doing lately. And no shortage of statistics and foundational research methods. But mostly biology. I send her home with a new book every few days, and we spend most of our morning and afternoon sessions discussing the latest one.

"Why not Farhearth?", Rorrik asked. Then he followed his question with a justification: "For every book in *your* library, theirs must have a thousand."

If Rorrik had stuck around Farhearth long enough, he would have known the answer. But he didn't. So I explained. And it went something like this:

Cyn may have been able to attend for coppers on the crown. But even that expense would have been a waste. And much more than tuition, it would have been a waste of *time*. Most of the great professors have left. Few remain. The culture can no longer sustain them, so they expel themselves before the over-powered students can level the charge. Annual turnover must be 90%. And the latest faculty use the latest books, which are never as good.

Writers today try too hard to appear "new"; the effort ensures their work is dated at the moment of publication. In part, it's the examples and analogies they use. Practically every page contains a reference to a current event, desperately flagging the recency of publication. Like a crone in Lonvarakan stage makeup portraying a beautiful maiden, these books are playing a role. In this case, that role is: "I'm brand new and I understand you! Look: I can relate to *today's* day-to-day experience!" It only takes a few encounters for the archetype to become a stereotype.

While I find this obnoxious, it's the books' content that does the true harm. The proportions of attention. The latest discovery is assigned enormous importance... even though it's unlikely to be true and even less likely to be interesting. Which is why it's decorated with so much stage makeup.

We think of jewels as aging into their value. Heirlooms gain preciousness with each successive generation's inheritance. Aetheldorf's *Aphorisms* is one such heirloom. And it's been removed from all Farhearth libraries. Another heirloom: Gundric's *Life of Mizjak*. That one has been relegated to Stables from its old once-prominent shelves in The Library.

Gundric – Mizjak's squire for a single year – was a female with a male's name. Being a male with a female's name, I've long felt an arbitrary connection. Like people who own the same breed of horse, or two foreigners who both emigrated from the same town. There's no commonality deeper than the veneer. But we all cling to *something* to find connectedness. And I connected with Gundric's veneer long ago.

She was Mizjak's last squire, and she wrote every day of their year together. Journal entries chronicling her daily lessons. Then she published each month of those journals as its own volume. If you study all twelve, you've learned more than you would with an entire Farhearth education these days.

Rorrik studied all twelve. He knows them better than I do. So I emphasized their absence from any program's curriculum in my answer to "Why not Farhearth?"

"Did you have her read the first volume?", Rorrik asked.

I shook my head in the direction of "no" and then said, "She read it anyway. I bet she can beat you in the begats."

The first book was almost entirely ancestries. Family trees from root to leaf. That and a childlike giddiness. Gundric's uncontainable excitement to be squiring for Mizjak was apparent on most pages. What *didn't* appear in the first volume was Mizjak's lessons. Scarcely a quotation until the second book. That's when the series got good.

"Cyn knows all twelve well enough to work as a scrivener without a source", I finished. And Rorrik seemed satisfied. He reclined in his chair and began listening quietly to Cyn and me.

Then he began to quietly ignore Cyn and me, as he pulled out two books of his own. *The Three Sisters*, which I'm familiar with, and *Even in Dark Hearts*, which I'm not.

I've always wondered if the sisters are supposed to represent lufig, lufir, and larlic. The mushrooms. The story is about three adventurous sisters whose bizarre journeys end in ruin. It's a familiar tale: those who dine on dreamveil need not *go* experience the great, wide world; they can *stay* experience an even wider world. But every time we embark on such a journey within the mind, the drug steals a sliver from our soul. Just a sliver. The loss cannot be felt. It's as invisible as a week of aging. But after a couple of decades of sacrificing slivers, we wake up to find half of Nemus hewn from our world.

I was about to ask Rorrik his thoughts on the matter. But then he opened the *other* book, removed a bookmark, and squinted at the page it had marked.

"An inscription from the author?", I asked, referring to his bookmark. It was a folded-in-half sheet of paper that was sealed with green wax and bearing someone's huge signature.

"A description of a horse", he said, and I didn't pry further. I just said, "huh", which communicates both acknowledgement and closure in every language. And I meant it. Further discussion would have cut into my conversation with Cyn. And our time is short. The Pendelhall Tournament is right around the calendar's corner. The Opening Ceremony is in seven days. Another four until her audition.

It's getting close. Now is a terrible time to dawdle.

So Cyn and I returned to our studies. We pondered and plumbed *Aphorisms* until deciding we'd been productive enough. And we were ready for dinner.

Rorrik spent our study session in silence, but as soon as dinner was served, he resumed pushing for my partnership. But he took a different, subtler tack.

Rather than play court reporter to his oral argument, transcribing it in full, I'll just say this: it was almost musical. His argument was. It had movements. Rhythms. Tones. But all of them up-tempo and bright. No dissonant notes of anxiety. No minor key remorse. It wasn't a sad ballad; it was an anthem of hope. Of optimism. Of wonder.

I understand optimistic musicians. One pass through Laberyn and you'll meet a thousand. And they all have a sense of wonder. Every new song might be "the one". Tomorrow's could be the catchiest or most sentimental melody in the canon of music. So how could you ever put your instrument down? There's too much possibility to abandon the treasure hunt.

That's Rorrik's outlook in everything. I get it. But for me, the only durable optimism I hold is in Cyn's future. Not ours. And I said as much to Rorrik:

"I think we should put our adventure mongering aside. If anyone is going to reclaim that land, it's not going to happen with might and weapons, but mind and its wit. And I don't think it's our generation that will do it. It's Cyn's."

"She's welcome to join us", Rorrik said plainly. Non-musically.

I turned and looked at Cyn. Not to extend an invitation. But as a gesture to Rorrik. As if to say, "I have other priorities now." But when I looked at her, I saw her brow furrow, and then furrow some more, crocheting its curiosity onto her face. As though she were entertaining the possibility. "Maybe I *do* want to help; tell me more", her expression said.

I turned back to Rorrik and asked, "How would we even do it?" in an overtly pessimistic tone. A *deservedly* pessimistic tone.

Weapons can't fell Thorn's monster any more than axes can fell its woods. And at the foot of those trees, the black brambles are even less welcome to intrusion. They're like teenage heirs of great wealth: the tiniest disturbance is met with fierce vengeance. The bloodshed is not commensurate with the disruption of its peace. It's best not to cross either of them: rich teens *or* the black brambles.

In response to my "How would we even do it?" question, Rorrik recounted some Charwargian rumors about secret clues buried in old fables.

But it was getting late.

I lacked the mental energy required to critically appraise the latest folklore.

"This feels like a conversation for another time", I said. In a firm tone.

Rorrik honored that tone for the rest of the day. But this morning marks a new day. And Rorrik arose earlier than usual. And Cyn arrived just as early. They've been outside for the last three pages of this journal. I should get out there and join them before he teaches her anything too heroic.

Seven

Seros, Second Lufoa, Day Twelve. Afternoon.

After finishing my last journal, I went downstairs and made breakfast. While we ate, Rorrik told us what happened in Laberyn. In gruesome detail. I will summarize, leaving out those details:

Uncountable people died, and many of them were young. Which is somehow more tragic. If you die at twenty-three when life expectancy is twenty-four, that doesn't arouse as much grief as dying at twenty-three when life expectancy is two hundred.

Among those who fell in battle, many were soldiers – both Rodorites and Nameless – but most were Laberi. Mobs of musicians swinging lutes and flutes and lyres wherever shovels, sickles, and pitchforks weren't available. The image of a minstrel dueling with his woodwind seems simultaneously humorous and heartrending… which makes me wonder if this was Rorrik's embroidery of a more colorful tapestry. After all, he is – both above and before all else – a singer. Which means his kitchen table regalings always involve *some* emotional magnification as they pass through the lyricist's lens. But with Rorrik, you can count on one thing: the most unbelievable parts of his story are true. Always. He never bends those details. Because it is only the unbelievable that we subject to verification. It's the *unimportant* details – the parts no one would bother to verify – that are fashioned from figments of Rorrik's imagination. And used as pigments to paint a more poignant story.

That seems to be how all of the celebrated histories have achieved their rank. And how half of the famous fables have maintained their station on modern shelves. They possess a single and singularly outrageous fact propped up with innumerable fictions. Each tiny fib changes the interpretation of the foundational fact a little bit more. And more. And more. Until it finally means something else entirely. And nobody thinks to verify those tiny details because the outrageous part has already passed the scrutiny of a dozen critics. So why bother questioning the trivialities?

Here's the outrageous truth from Rorrik's report: there was a clash between Laberyn's locals, a roving brigade of Rodorites, a swarm of Nameless soldiers, and the shambling calamity from Thorn. Countless people died. Rorrik was not one of them. But he could have been. And this is becoming a frequent experience; Rorrik seems haunted, practically hunted, by that skulking malady.

Every time it vacates its mysterious glade, death follows. In the present case, the bulk of the dying befell the Nameless Hunt. But there was no shortage of Laberi who fell beside them. And Rorrik knew many of them personally. Which invigorated his need for vengeance. And drove him to implore my aid.

Instead of biting that bait, I asked, "How did you know they were Nameless? As opposed to Rodorites or some far-from-home band of Pendelians?"

"A Nameless runt is taller than any Rodorite in the Guard. You know that."

I actually don't know that. I've *heard* it before. But I've heard a lot of things. Such as: Nemusenex's roots burrow so deep into Gaea that they come out the other end! Or: The North used to be just like every other continent until the creature from Thorn blanketed it in snow! I don't trust everything I hear. Nor did I contest the present claim, though. Instead, I asked, "At a distance can you really tell how tall anyone is?"

"I wasn't at a distance. I was close enough to see the sigil."

By this, he meant the wandering flame. The mark of the Nameless. The fire that was broken in two. Half of it was claimed by the tyrant of Thorn; the other half burns on that isolated jungle-topped plateau. And then wherever the story goes from there. Some ageless rivalry between the Hunt and the beast that must have a hundred fictions propping up its central fact.

If it weren't for that sigil, I wonder if anyone could distinguish them from ordinary Gaeans. Ordinary *large* Gaeans. The seldom-home farmhand down the street, the burly patron in the market, the lone traveler on the Grass Road who could swap roles with his horse and pull his carriage even faster. If any of them were Nameless, how would you know? They'd be perfect imposters.

I was lost in this thought when Rorrik reiterated his call to action. And I attempted to avoid that call. Again. This time with a protracted exposition on back pain. The subject bores every listener so thoroughly I've come to use it as suit of rhetorical armor. Whenever I'm besieged by requests for my service, I can wear out even the most energetic solicitor.

I seem to be the only person in the world who is fascinated by the topic. Not anatomically or physiologically, but philosophically. How it renders its victims invisible in a way. Males and females both, although for entirely different reasons. Among men, some injuries augment their attractiveness. A sprained ankle. A broken arm. A gash across his chest. What society deems less handsome is a *missing* ankle, a *boneless* arm, a gash across one's *lung*.

The former collection of wounds seems to indicate toughness, bravery, and the promise of full recovery. A promise of *future* demonstrations of toughness and bravery.

The latter collection may transmit toughness and bravery, but not recovery. So we don't lionize the sufferers. Instead, we sympathize with them. And sympathy rarely intensifies sexual desirability.

A prominent scar across a chest or limb is worn as jewelry. A necklace of a kind. Just as gold chains signify the wearer's prosperity, the gash is a symbol of gallantry signed into our flesh. Both are exhibited with pride. But if that gash is carved into an organ, its signature is a stigma we attempt to hide. Because potential paramours seldom swoon over a man's internal ornaments, however valiant their acquisition. Even orthopedic injuries – ankles, knees, necks – risk being unattractive. Which returns us to the subject of back pain. *My* back pain. Although it was earned in martial training, it communicates no such ruggedness. Back pain is similar to baldness, I guess, as it signifies oldness far more than valor. By comparison, the coppersmith's apprentice down on Tinkers' Row, has ornate grids of longitudes and latitudes streaked across his arms. From burns. Not because smithing cookware is a perilous profession. He's just clumsy. *Pathologically* uncoordinated. But that fact extinguishes none of his allure. He has throngs of admirers. Which, to me, confirms that we're a flawed species.

I wonder if lions and bykuls and rykils and the rest of Gaea's great predators occasionally suffer the same fate. A hunter once so mighty and majestic, wholly consumed by thoughts of the hunt, now mopes dejectedly around with debilitating back pain. Or hip pain. Or a misbehaving knee. Are they still feared by their prey and venerated by their herd? Or are they merely pitied by both? Or, fearing cultural demotion, do they hide it? Withhold their wincing and pretend everything is fine?

I'm not an apex predator, so I just limp when it's a limping day. And grumble to anyone willing to endure my grumbling. These days, that's Cyn, the only one who can tolerate the topic. Rorrik couldn't. When I started describing what "not a good back day" feels like, his enthusiasm was numbed to a halt. Which ended his recruitment speech. Sorry, Rorrik. Even if it were a "good back day", you're trying to roll a rooted rock.

Eight

Seros, Second Lufoa, Day Twelve. Night.

It's night now. Later than I usually write. Because Rorrik and I spent the evening playing music. And it was a long evening. Filled with long songs. The kind of songs that could have been short, but I didn't want them to end. So I'd insist we drag them out. Stretch a solo for eight more measures, add a second bridge, a third, repeat a chorus just one more time. And when they finally did end, we'd immediately start another.

It had been years since we last played together. We used to play all the time. In our early days, we probably exchanged more notes than words. Music was practically our primary language. It seemed to account for the bulk of our communication. Lum, too. It was always the three of us. Like a major triad. The root, the third, and the fifth. Rorrik, dependable leader, serving as the root. Lum, flawless in his musicianship functioning as the perfect fifth. And me, lingering in the middle, the major third. Tonight's *dyad* – just Rorrik and me, no Lum to be heard – did feel very slightly bereft. But Rorrik has such a powerful presence, even his solo performances have the fullness of five throats and ten hands. His rhythms gallop like a wild solyre, that thundering cadence you feel in your chest. And his voice is huge. Most people need accompanying vocals to fill out a thin presence. Not Rorrik. He can eclipse a choir with a single breath.

I accompanied him, sitting in the front parlor by the hearth, but my part was minimal. It didn't *sound* that way; when you complement an already-beautiful melody, the listeners – or listener in this case, Cyn being the only one – seem to credit you a portion of the underlying chords in addition to your overlying notes. That credit is short-lived. My role is forgotten the moment the song ends. Rorrik's isn't. His credit exits beyond the room. In culture itself. More than a few of his songs are known in the taverns of two continents. And he's not completely unknown in the South, despite having never been there.

In the East, there are probably a dozen recognizable songs. In the West, there must be twice that. An Estevro dozen (a dozen for you, a dozen for me; twenty-four in all). Far more than any of his contemporaries.

What's funny is that Rorrik doesn't actually *influence* any culture. At least not in the way that his contemporaries do. To influence, one must be imitatable. And Rorrik is not.

Neither is Lum, but for a very different reason. Lum is the most technically talented of the three of us. The most mechanically masterful. Among the most proficient the whole Gaea over. He is more than a musician; he is a mathematician. It takes a Higher Licentiate from Farhearth to understand the intricate equations buttressing his compositions. That's why he's so hard to imitate.

By comparison, Rorrik isn't really a musician at all. He's more of a magician. According to the fundamental tenets of music theory, his songs should be terrible. On paper, the compositions are nonsense. Which is why he never writes them down. And no bard, troubadour, or minstrel has ever performed one in a pleasing way. Not for a lack of effort; the effort just lacks humanity.

With other musicians, it's the song itself people want to hear. Any performer in possession of the sheet music is as good as another. This isn't the case with Rorrik. His songs can't be sung by another. Even though they seem so simple. It's not as though he's writing them in the key of H. He conveys his magic through the normal channels. The notes and words are easily written, easily read, easily played. But some part of those songs escapes translation. When performed by another, every note is bland, every lyric devoid of life.

What makes the experience emotional is Rorrik himself. His performances are so peaceful. And so restless. At the same time. There's this rending tenderness in his aggression, and a fierce aggression in his tenderness. Even the slowest, quietest moment of his slowest, quietest song holds a furious intensity. And the fastest, loudest moment of his fastest, loudest song carries a calm introspection. Every measure contains such feeling, such meaning. It's as though imprisoned emotions, held captive for a lifetime, are finally escaping. Sometimes, they sneak quietly from those secret places held deep within. Other times, they trample violently out, breaking through the ribs jailing his heart. Often, both forms of expression occur in the same song as he transitions back and forth between verse and chorus. Back and forth between gentle, angelic harmony and wailing animal in a trap – that raspy, piercing screech you can hear from a mile away and feel from the next town.

At the peak of those performances, you can see Rorrik's knees buckling beneath the weight of his words. But he's determined to carry them clear to the end of the song. And he always does. He always delivers. And *that* is a magic that cannot be replicated.

It's not new to me, Rorrik's music. We've been playing together since we were teenagers. But this was Cyn's first time hearing him play. It was the perfect environment for it: a subdued parlor performance.

If his voice is so restrained it barely carries beyond a campfire, you miss out on some of the emotion. And when he's performing at full volume, and fuller intensity, trimming an eighth from every fourth measure to gallop a hoofbeat ahead of the expected pace, something strange happens to first-time listeners: they throw up. They have to leave the venue to collect themselves. Take a few breaths, restore their guts, reassemble their wits. It doesn't happen to everybody. But even if it's only one in ten people, that's one in ten more than explanation can account for. Name another musician whose first song in a set induces vomiting in twenty audience members. I doubt Rorrik has a peer in this rather bizarre capacity.

Tonight's playing had no such force, but no less adventure. That's really what Rorrik's music is: an adventure. The initial note, which breaks the idle air, is the first step out of the house.

Not all of life's adventures are enjoyable. Like surviving a hymog attack. That may enliven your pulse, but you derive no pleasure from the experience. Other adventures are enjoyable but aren't worth repeating. Like the first semester as a Farhearth student. And then there are those adventures that you want to repeat over and over again. That's what Rorrik's songs feel like.

With his right hand, he summons the solyre, a rhythm galloping fearlessly across the open landscape. And with his left hand, his notes go exploring. And they don't necessarily tread the traveled paths. Often, they go wandering off into anxious or gloomy spaces. And listening starts to become tense or downhearting. It starts to wear on you, test the stamina of your emotions. And right when your heart can't take any more, the song turns. It begins to find its way home. Gradually at first. With subtle hints of restoration. And then triumphantly. But briefly.

Those endings hit the listener hard. They feel like they've earned it.

They went adventuring alongside him. They faced struggle, felt its strain, and in the end, prevailed. At the peak of that sensation of emotional triumph, Rorrik plays his last note, and leaves the listener with silence.

Those are the adventures Rorrik's songs take you on. They're no less riveting the fifth time. Even more excitement is felt during the sixth. There's a spirit that invades you, makes you believe you're younger than you are. As we age, our senses of wonder and adventure grow less limber than our backs. Every year, our joints and curiosity *both* lose a little more elasticity.

Ordinarily, I neither feel young nor old. I'm somewhere in-between.

But when I hear Rorrik's music, I instantly become a teenager. In my mind.

Even the oldest listener is thrust back in time, overcome by all the excitement and eagerness that exist only in youth, that impermanent province Rorrik still presides over. He never surrendered his impractical ambitions, never traded his confidence for caution.

Every other thirty-six-year-old bard sings his notes like a sixty-six-year-old biting into a handful of nuts: ease into it for fear of a cracked tooth. "There might be a piece of shell in there, so I had better bite gingerly until I'm sure it's safe."

Rorrik has no such hesitation. He belts out his lyrics with no consideration of a broken tone. He bites down on that opening note like a child with a mouthful of chocolate.

And he is no more inhibited, no less ravenous, in his pursuit of his nemesis from Thorn.

That was the point of tonight's adventures. They were another call to action. Spoken in a much more sentimental language: that of our shared youth. But if he keeps up this pursuit, he's going to chip more than a tooth, crack more than his voice.

Ambition is a long and destructive road, lined with the wreckages of resolve. Our bodies are broken, our hope is creased and ruffled, our lives are wasted along the way. Maybe the pursuit gives people a sense of purpose, but it's a form of slavery. Of bondage. Forever wearing their ambition as shackles. What emancipation is there but death?

That's not a road I want to travel. And I worry Rorrik's body will soon litter the wayside. And I said as much. And it didn't matter. Because there's no changing Rorrik's mind.

Nine

Aldos, Second Lufoa, Day Thirteen. Morning.

It's early. Cyn has yet to arrive. Rorrik has yet to rouse.

I slept okay. About five hours. Average for me. Less than that and I have difficulty focusing. And even more difficulty writing.

I started keeping a journal when I left home for Farhearth. Half my life ago. There must be a thousand pages containing every observation I ever made and lesson I ever learned. As a student. As a faculty member. And beyond.

I would have studied Language and Literature when I was in school – most Estevroans do – but I considered writing too precious to undertake as a labor. I was afraid it would be contaminated if a wage were affixed, or expectations were assigned. By comparison, the natural sciences are cold and calculated. There is no spirit that can be contravened by external demand. Forcible toil takes nothing away from it. So that's what I chose to pursue as a profession. But every night, when my studies and labors were finished, I would take out a sheet of paper and begin to write. For nearly two decades, I never missed a day. Until two months ago. When I stopped writing altogether. I don't know why. I guess I felt like I had completed the journal. Everything I had ever learned was contained in a pile of paper that must have consumed an entire river larch. Instead of starting in on a new tree, I sorted what I had written, put it in a box, wrapped that box, then put the wrapped box in the closet. It's still there. I plan to give it to Cyn after the Pendelhall tournament.

I hadn't written since. Until a few days ago, when I saw the *Chronicle* article and felt compelled to work through my thoughts. And the only way I know how to do that is with a pen.

But I also feel like I'm entering the final act of my life (to put it in Lonvarakan terms). The first act was my youth, in which I was too young to understand the emotions that throttled me. And the hormones doing the throttling. The second act was my education and early career as a professor. Coming to understand the body and its functions: how it builds, breaks, repairs, decays, and ultimately fails. And teaching every hormone that was responsible for the prior act's throttling. But Cyn is my final student, and we're concluding our final year together. So this act of my life is passing. And I don't know what comes next. In a way, starting this new journal is my attempt to find myself.

My previous journals – the whole larch's worth – were mostly about science. The first five years were bad. And the next five weren't much better. There's still plenty to learn from those pages, though. Maybe it seems pompous to give Cyn *my* writing as a gift. As opposed to the collected works of Gundric or Maren or Rouska. But that isn't the point. The lesson is a biographical one. Consider music:

Hearing a minstrel's canonized song doesn't teach me as much as listening to the hundred obscure and often terrible songs written before the famous one. It's the only way I can learn how the artist reasoned with tones and timing. The only way I can understand how the famous song was eventually devised. No one sails straight into brilliance. That's a hard-to-reach harbor. It takes a thousand hours of slogging before it can even be *seen*. Learning the footwork in fencing, or the finger positions on the fretboard, or the opening positions in regnavus. The fundamentals. You can't play without them. But *inspiration* comes at other times. When the circuitry of the mind fires in ways we never predicted. Both of these roles – inspiration and pragmatism – are essential and must be nurtured. Without the former, you have a lute instructor at a Farhearth preparatory guild. Without the latter, you have a lunatic caroling in the town square. Neither writes a masterpiece. But everyone who *does* accomplish mastery writes a hundred other songs first, each one sailing a bit closer to the harbor. And you learn by studying the voyage, not the mooring.

That's why I'm giving my journals to Cyn. Not because there's a masterpiece at the end, but because she's embarking on a similar journey, and it may be of some use to know how I navigated mine.

I was a Pendelhall tournament winner, a Ranked Professor at Farhearth, and I had two auditions for the Pendelhall Medic role. And two failures, but I made it to the rings twice, and during the second year, I had the Elyem Ring for my opening post.

By showing Cyn precisely how I got there, I think she will better understand her own course. And it won't be long before she passes me. When she does, I want her to move beyond me in every way. Reading my journals would all but guarantee that. Everything of value that I ever learned is in there. The early writing is foolish at times, but it's interesting in its own way. Humor and charm grow more freely when they aren't vigilantly chaperoned by wisdom.

This journal feels different. I don't plan to give it to anyone. I don't suppose it'll ever be read. I'm just letting my thoughts meander onto the page, trying to figure out what to do with my final act. But now, it's time to get on with my day. I see color on the horizon. The sun is coming soon. And so is Cyn.

Ten

Aldos, Second Lufoa, Day Thirteen. Afternoon.

During our morning session, Cyn and I finished our discussion of *Aphorisms*.

You'd never know at the beginning, but by the end, it's about the might of humility and the consequences of confidence. A lesson that really should be retained in the Farhearth curriculum. Nearly every student is now beaming with, and arrested by, their pride. So sure they've already arrived at mastery, they'll never even begin the journey.

Cyn's and my final conversation about *Aphorisms* was the perfect conclusion to our peripheral studies. There's never been a more comprehensive analysis of that work. I doubt Aetheldorf himself considered the implications of his words as thoroughly while writing them. It was mostly Cyn doing the talking. I just listened, nodding in agreement with her points. We finished well before lunchtime. And rather than start a new topic, we decided to prepone lunch (or whatever the opposite of postpone is).

We went out to the garden to gather some food. Cyn plucked a few berries from my macramog vine, held them out, and said, "Aetheldorf's acorn."

I gave her a confused look. I knew what she was referring to: the closing lines of the book. But what did macramog berries have to do with it? Cyn explained:

"In the absence of light, the vine keeps climbing. Once it reaches the light, it blooms and never climbs again. But should it confuse darkness with light, it ceases its search, and in doing so, stunts its growth. The perils of self-assurance." Then she ate one of the berries.

I smiled. And she interpreted the gesture correctly: there's nothing else I can teach you that you can't learn for yourself.

In the spirit of that closure, we picked every ripe "peril berry" on the vine, then went to the kitchen to invent a dish that uses them.

Rorrik wasn't there. "Let me find Rorrik", I said to Cyn, and then wandered around downstairs, poking my head into every other room. No Rorrik.

I went upstairs, looked in his room, and confirmed what I had suspected: Rorrik was gone. He left this morning. Before I got up. Which must have been *really* early.

His bed was made, and the rest of the room appeared similarly undisturbed. As though no one had stayed in it. Except for the long note on his pillow. Rorrik had left detailed instructions on how I could follow him. But I had better make haste if I want to catch up. And should I sacrifice moral duty for coziness, choose cowardice over conquest, then would I mind keeping Gyfur safe for the time being? "He'll be fine in the yard eating grass, but for your sake, keep the green gate closed; if he gets into the berries, he'll just nap, but onions, leeks, shallots – any kind of allium – and he'll make a mess." Then, instead of signing his name, he drew a picture of a headless monkey. A bad line drawing, but I knew what it was.

I should have known he would be gone. Because of last night's music. That was his final effort to conscript me into questdom. By serenading me into a questy mood.

During those songs, I'm able to see the world through his perspective. I can't articulate it here – I can't explain his reasons with words – but I'm given a glimpse at the *feeling* of those reasons. The emotions that make up his mind. And I shared them for a moment.

Rorrik's music has always had that effect. It communicates its message clearer than conversation. If there's such a thing as magic, I think that's it. It's the phenomenon of one creature coming to understand something by means other than experience. Achieving deep clarity about the deepest matters by someone else simply expressing it. And expression takes many forms. Words are one medium. Melody is another. If I knew anything about choreography, I'm sure that would be another. Unfortunately, most people don't express themselves masterfully. So the world is short on magic.

On the subject, Rorrik believes dreaming is another mode of communication. "With whom?", I've asked him on numerous occasions. And regretted asking when his whimsical answer began to hint at correspondence with some netherworld. "Every night, we're given spectral glimpses of its prose", he declares with religious conviction, launching us into a well-practiced debate.

"I don't doubt the *usefulness* of dreams", my counterargument begins. "As a form of productive rumination. An act of grooming what we already know. Tidying our thoughts so we can make better sense of them."

Rorrik then argues that the contents of dreams are frequently focused on people we have yet to encounter, places we have yet to travel, events that have yet to occur. And in response, I posit that dreams can also serve as dress rehearsals. Our minds generate random, often bizarre situations so we can simulate courses of action without real-world consequences. That way, should you ever find yourself in similar circumstances in your waking life, you won't be a complete novice.

We've had this conversation innumerable times, and neither of us has budged our beliefs. Although I've just realized there is one additional quality of sleep that's worth acknowledging: as long as Rorrik is lurking in his netherworld, he seems to be at peace. No matter where his corporeal bulk lies. It's when he's awake that he's constantly anxious to leave. He spends his life imagining vines pressed into his back. And so, without warning or a wave goodbye, you just find him gone. Although I guess last night's music did serve as a warning and a wave. They were the sort of songs that mark endings. Full of mirth. Full of grief. Full of wrath. The full breadth of human emotion fit to pitch and rhythm.

To Cyn, Rorrik probably appeared merry and exuberant. And not much else. But I know him better. I understand the reason he pursues wrath over the rest of his natures. At dusk on the day he was born, that prowling pestilence left the Crown of Thorn. And visited Adonere. And never has there been a bloodier bridal shower. His village wasn't densely populated to begin with, and the death toll was not small. The bell rang for a week. And it tolled for his mother. Along with countless others orphaned by the battle, Rorrik was raised in the guilds of Laberyn, where he spent his formative years learning to lean into those moods for the sake of his music. So today, when Rorrik looks up and sees Thorn's star hanging overhead, it's a reminder of what that nightborn widower took from him. And the recent massacre at Laberyn was received as a promise that the beast is not done taking. But Rorrik is done being taken from. He may appear merry and exuberant, but inside, he roils.

I was never at risk of joining him. That's his quest, not mine. But I wonder if my ten-year-old self would be disappointed in whom he became twenty-six years later. Growing up, I wanted to be a tracker. Whenever an adult asked me the boringest of all questions, "What do *you* want to be when you grow up?", I was certain of my answer. It had nothing to do with bounties; all I cared about was traveling. I was so much more interested in exploration than memorization. But then I grew up and became a professor. And all of my aspirations of exploration were replaced with exhausting memorization. After a few more years, I traded that life for quiet conversations at home and strolls through my garden. But I don't regret the course my life has taken.

When I returned to the kitchen, the house felt suddenly quiet. And suddenly lonely. Cyn felt it, too. "Did Rorrik leave?", she asked.

"Leaving is what he does", I said. Then, as we ate, I explained how Rorrik became who he is:

When Adonere was attacked, he was left with nothing but his name and his home. And he has since abandoned both. Still today, as a musician, he uses a different name practically every time he takes the stage. Almost like he's hiding from his identity, making it harder for that devil in Thorn to stalk him. That's not the explanation Rorrik gives for his everchanging name. He claims it's so he can play in front of smaller audiences who are surprised rather than expectant. He does the same thing with fencing: every time he competes in a tournament, he registers himself under a traditional Rivervalan name: Olgof or Olseg or Olnuk or some such. That makes more sense: the fencer with a known opponent has an advantage. Real names are recorded in the annals, so plenty of people register with pseudonyms. But Rorrik uses pseudonyms in everything. And it's the thousand names he's used *outside* of the rings that make me wonder. And it's the fact that he discarded his home more completely than his name. He's never even been there. But, if the rumors are believed, and Adonere is untouched by time, I'm sure his cottage looks the same as it did the day it was vacated.

After lunch, Cyn and I sat at the table for another hour talking about Rorrik. And about the West. And its ways. I know vengeance isn't the *only* reason Rorrik makes the choices he does. There's an Old Adonian expression he often quotes: "Only the heart can protect memory from time." Although he incants it in Old Adonian. Something something *grif* something something something something *gael*. I don't remember how it goes, but I remember it being poetic. And I remember the meaning: advancing age steals memories of the mind, but emotions remain long after they're claimed. And Rorrik is always on some adventure, filling his chest with new emotions. The present one just happens to be deeply vengeful. Which isn't an emotion that can be subdued with reason.

"What if he's right?", Cyn asked. "About the creature from Thorn. If every Northerner is living in constant dread, is Rorrik's mission more important than our studying?"

It was a brief and direct question, but it raised so many points that were worth addressing. By my count: six. And it took the entire post-lunch hour to work through them. It went something like this:

First and least important point: by Northerner, she meant everyone north of the South. That's the Southern definition of the word. To my knowledge, there has never been an attack in the South. They have a different scourge, and nobody lives in "constant dread" of it.

Second: constant dread. Whenever that "northern" ogre goes marauding, the stories that follow are spectacular and terrible. And the losses of life are heartbreaking. But incidents like this rarely happen. On a ten-year average, shepherd's fever kills more people. So does dysentery. And attacks by other wildlife (collectively). The death count from this *particular* animal exceeds any other, but that probably ranks it somewhere between enteritis and snake bites in terms of gross mortality. And if mortality is what we fear, it seems prudent to prioritize the causes of it.

Third: making decisions based on our constant dread. Fear is a deeply rooted emotion. Everyone sees tragedy on the horizon. Rorrik may be unique in his urge to confront it, but not in his anticipation of it. Probe anyone on the matter and they'll admit fear of impending doom. But people have impended that doom for centuries. And how doomed have the last hundred years been? Every decade continues to be better than the one that preceded it. So why do we continue to make this prediction when year after year it fails to come true? One recent catastrophe – however catastrophic – does not promise endless disaster ahead.

Fourth: is Rorrik right? If he can destroy that aberration of nature lurking in Thorn, he can rid Gaea of all future *unnatural* disasters. That would save a lot of lives, and it would permit Rorrik to use his own name without feeling exposed. Both worthy aspirations. But I get the impression Rorrik is chasing his tail here. Round and round, growling and biting at what's stalking him from behind, neither quite catching the other. I find it funny when Abbie does this. The tail seems to be the only appendage she views as "other", and periodically torments. She never bursts into an unprovoked frenzy over a hind limb. It's always the tail, and it's never caught. Same with Rorrik. He periodically bursts into a frenzy, hunting the creature he perceives as hunting him, and neither ever catches the other.

Fifth: the likelihood of success. Cyn has regularly traveled the coast of Thorn. She's seen the black trees. "Trees" is a euphemism. The heart of Gaea, where the creature makes berth, is trellised with a matrix of unbreakable black ribs. There's no crossing. And no other way in. There's a single vein that exits: the Crooked River. To enter, one must sail against a silent, indecisive current. Its directions cannot be predicted, its force cannot be overcome, and the black branches rip holes in every vessel that wanders too near the banks.

Impressive ships steered by impressive captains have braved that winding, upbound course. The river returned all but one to the bay half sunken and fully wrecked. There's an ancient fable about one boat that made it inside. One boat that never returned. Even if the tale is true, I doubt it will be Rorrik who succeeds in sailing the second vessel. He doesn't even own a canoe. He'd have to draw the creature out. And how would he do that? Stand at the mouth of the river and yell? If anyone could bellow to the river's end, it's Rorrik, but the whole endeavor seems futile to me. Exactly as futile as it seemed every other time Rorrik endeavored it. He always returns. And when he does, *something* is different. *Something* has changed. But it's never been this. No matter how committed he is to its pursuit, the taunting tail is never caught.

Which brings us to the final point: studying. That baleful specter is not going to be killed by a soldier with a sword. Or by a Pendelian brigade armed with a thousand swords. Or any other technology or strategy known to us today. If Gaea is ever going to be liberated from its desecrator, it will be the result of great learning. And great learning follows meticulous studying. Studying is the means by which we accomplish everything of meaning. And the most meaningful achievements always come as a surprise. We can never predict the exact gifts learning will bring. So that's the course Cyn and I will continue to pursue while Rorrik continues a pursuit of his own.

And now it's time for Cyn and me to resume the day's lessons.

Eleven

Aldos, Second Lufoa, Day Thirteen. Night.

Cyn and I studied well into the afternoon, which more than made up for our truncated morning session. Aetheldorf was a nice respite from physiology, but it's time to focus on Cyn's research. Her dissertation, basically. As though she were completing a Magister's Degree. Her topic is cellular metabolism. Every cell breathes; the lungs just make a scene of it. This has been known for years. What is less known is the metabolism of cellular *healing*. Until this ignorance is remedied, every branch of recuperative medicine is unreliable, every treatment a practice of faith. Cyn's work will go a long way to inform clinicians and, just as importantly, it will expand our understanding of the natural world. Who knows what that will lead to?

We'll submit her abstract – a few hundred words outlining the scope of her project – to Farhearth after the Pendelhall tournament. A few weeks later, we'll find out whether it's accepted at the annual Science Faire. Assuming it is, we'll return the last week of Second Elyem so Cyn can present her work.

I'm not sure what branch she should submit it to. It doesn't fit snuggly into any of the Eastern divisions of practice: physician, apothecarist, or herbalist. Once upon a time, all three were considered equal in reputation. Today, the physician is typically perceived to be the most reputable. But in many ways, I hold them in the lowest regard. Although I *can* appreciate the criticism of their peers, the herbalists and apothecarists:

The herbalist thinks every patient has a therapy, every therapy is a plant, and every plant on Gaea is a solution for *something*. They put so much trust in vegetation, some of them get quacky about it. Reading tealcaves, for instance. Practitioners of this bizarre diagnostic test claim the shape of those clumps can foretell our medicinal destiny. But this kind of quackery isn't common; most herbalists have comprehensive backgrounds in botany. They simply believe that nature is the key to health optimization. Survival is one matter; *thrival* is another. To truly thrive, we must become "one" with nature.

Contrasting that view, the apothecarist believes nature is the *problem*, and it must be neutralized. Manipulation is medicine. This field of study does not promote a balanced view of biology. All of their training is in alchemical allopathy, and all of their treatments are aimed at destroying the natures inside of us. But most apothecarists adhere to a needle-narrow scope of practice.

The physician, by comparison, doesn't factor in nature at all. While this may earn them a second helping of the public's respect, it doesn't help the patient. Instead of systematically investigating the cause of an illness, the physician simply thinks of *himself* as the solution. Or herself, but the himselves tend to be more pathological in their hubris.

Herbalists and apothecarists may hold strong thoughts about the importance of nature, but at least they don't regard themselves as the answer. "I'm a walking, talking panacea", physicians all but proclaim out loud. "And I'll only heal those who bow in reverence!"

That's a longwinded way of saying: I don't know what division of medicine Cyn should submit her work to. All three are in need of some renovation. In time, I trust Cyn will do that renovating. But first, she must secure her position as the Pendelhall Medic. She auditions in ten days. For two days. And then she'll serve that role for two years. I'm almost certain. Who could possibly outcompete her?

After her tenure as the Pendelhall Medic, she plans to return to Cinderheim. I'll miss her when she goes. And I'll allow myself to believe she'll miss me. But it really is the right place for her. In her hometown. Among her family. That's where she'll figure out how to heal the world of its most threatening ailment. Whatever that is. And then move on to the second most threatening ailment. Then the third. And on down the ladder until she finally relieves humanity of enteritis, the monster from Thorn, and snake bites. Civilization will be transformed, and I'll get to bask in the satisfaction that I set that transformation in motion.

And, of great *personal* importance, I will have actualized my life's foremost purpose: to do for someone else what Abendroth did for me.

I had no idea how to navigate education – personally or professionally – until Abendroth showed me how. She took me to Farhearth for the first time. She got me admitted. While I was a student, she employed me in a position with tuition remission. Then she guided me through the mazes of Farhearth's curriculum. And she showed me every loophole and secret passage through its even-more-circuitous political configuration, enabling me to circumvent any obstacle I might encounter as a student or employee.

Along the way, she taught me how to teach, publish, and succeed. She taught me how to think. And when she died, I suddenly had to think for myself. Which was harder than I thought it would be. But I couldn't have asked for a better mentor.

During our final semester together, I was working on a dissertation I had little interest in. Just trying to slog my way to completion. Because I thought the topic would be well received by the scientific community. "It might be", Abendroth said. "But school is brief. Careers are much longer. And if you're apathetic about this topic as a *student*, it's unlikely to be a fulfilling career that's built on it."

"I've learned so much about chronogeography, though" (a pretentious word I had coined for the field of study I was attempting to invent), "It would be such a waste to give it up now."

Abendroth pointed out that I had lost my interest in the topic the moment I had finished learning about it. When all that was left was dissemination. Toil, in other words. "And changing the direction of your *labor* takes nothing from your *learning*. The work you've done on chronogeography is already worth it. Look how much you've learned. For the rest of your life, those lessons will pay valuable dividends. In ways you never expected. But for now, you have a dissertation to complete. And dissertations shouldn't be about community reception; they should be about personal passion. If you pick a topic you're more passionate about, you can start over completely and still finish sooner."

Her words sounded wise. But I remained committed to my first dissertation. Until she died. And I found myself thrust into independence. Independent thought, independent decisions, independent everything.

There comes a day in which every student must advance to that stage.

Mine came abruptly. And devastatingly.

At first, I felt lost, having been separated from my guide. And I felt hopeless. How could I ever navigate Farhearth's convoluted mazes on my own?

For a couple of weeks, I was paralyzed with grief and panic. But then I began to realize: I knew every loophole and secret passage in the curriculum and configuration of the university.

I knew exactly how to graduate.

I knew how to teach and publish.

I knew how to succeed.

Abendroth had prepared me for all of this. So I began my journey.

The first thing I did was abandon my dissertation. I started over completely. And I published that new project in half the time it would have taken me to complete the original. The following semester, I was hired as a professor. Unranked, second tier. But I found it easy to build upon the foundation I had established with my second dissertation. Passion seemed to perform all the tasks of toil. With little effort, and no apathetic slogging, I accumulated enough publications that, in under four years, I became a Ranked Professor. I had grown into the person Abendroth had prepared me to be. The tragedy is that she never had the chance to see what her mentorship had made.

And then I quit. And I started a new journey. Mentoring Cyn. And today, Cyn is nearly ready to move on. And I'm fully ready to experience the joy of watching her career blossom. I don't know if it makes sense to anyone else, but that's when I'll feel like I've fulfilled my personal oath to Abendroth.

Cyn's dissertation is on the energy expense of tissue regeneration. Of course, she's emphasizing evolution.

If you're a Harthy by way of Estevro, there are two colleges available to you: Language and Literature (studying the magic of Orfric) or Apothecarial and Natural Sciences (studying evolutionary biology). If Farhearth had a culinary school, there'd be a third option. But it doesn't. So our choices are limited.

An occasional student does study Geology and Horticulture, but scant few. And scanter fewer earn degrees in Theology and Ethics. Both of those tend to be Western disciplines.

Cyn's dissertation topic lies at the heart of Apothecarial and Natural Sciences. And it was chosen purely out of passion. Which makes her an honorary flatty.

This is the last academic step in the long, winding staircase to independence. The last step in which I get to play the role of her guide. As an official student, one submits their dissertation to *Farhearth Frontiers* at the end of the ninth year. If it's accepted at the annual Faire *and* published in the corresponding journal, the student has met the final criterion for graduation. And is formally granted the highest degree. Nine years. Cyn and I did it in six. And during those six, we covered twice as much material. Every worthwhile book ever published.

But we're not *quite* done. We still have this one final step before she emigrates to the land of professional independence. So, what's left? What masterpiece of scientific literature have I chosen for our last series of lessons together?

My dissertations.

Not out of self-importance, but because the best way to learn how to publish a dissertation is by reading *other* dissertations, both published *and* unpublished, so the comparison can be made. And, as it happens, I have both.

First dissertation first: "Natural Order of the Rykub, Garlok, and Pitikos: A Study of Chronogeography." Terrible title.

At the time, all wildlife was classified as either nocturnal or diurnal. But that seemed to be a rather crude stratification. The day is long. Investigating diurnal species in the Rivervale region, I divided the day into three categories: sunrise, midday, and decline. And I found animals that were neatly segregated into each. Unfortunately, I got carried away with their names. Misnomers, all. Being from Estevro, I decided that was meaningful, and I tried to combine linguistics and biology into a single manuscript. Which meant I had twice as much to learn. Initially, I was hungry. So I learned and learned and learned. Until I was full. Then I began force-feeding myself information. Until I was stuffed. And I found myself sick of the subject before writing my first word. If I'm asked to describe food when I'm starving, I can craft words that will make an audience salivate. If I've just finished eating to the point of self-loathing, my descriptions of food lack all flavor. And that was my problem with this dissertation. When I finally started writing, the facts were sound, but the prose was bland. And I was never going to season it. So I put it away. For years. Until today. When Cyn and I began going through it. And she was so engaged in the discussion, it nearly renewed my interest in the work.

We only spent a minute on the misnomers, for fear of losing that engagement:

Rykub comes from rynkub, meaning "water cat", but the five-letter naming convention of the East amputated its n. That's not the misnomer. Kub is. It means cat. And you'd have to trace this creature's lineage a *long* way back before it crossed an intersection with anything feline. The same can be said about the "nest bear" (lok means bear, which this creature is not) and the "burrowing bird" (kos means bird, which this creature is not).

The biology is more interesting. And Cyn and I spent much more than a minute discussing it:

All three species *are* diurnal, but they have starkly different circadian rhythms likely consequent of predatorial adaptations. The "bear" hunts the "cat"; the "cat" hunts the "bird"; and the "bird" blinds the "bear" (plucks out its eyes). It's the biological equivalent of Natural Order, that old schoolyard game: wood dams water, water extinguishes fire, fire burns wood.

All three animals are interesting, but the rykub is the one really fascinates *me*. Because of its unique skeletal muscle system.

It can produce normal, voluntary muscle actions, but its *reactions* are largely involuntary and produced by external sensory stimuli. To put it plainly, its movement is based on vision.

Humans have *some* unconscious motion control. For example, we have brain regions that assist in coordinating muscle activity with sensory processing. This wasn't my discovery. That knowledge came from cruel experimentation. From an earlier age. All my experiments were done on the already deceased. And what my work revealed was that approximately half of the rykub's brain consists of ancillary regions that coordinate muscle actions with visual stimuli.

My second discovery involved their spines. In the human spine, there exist "central pattern generators", which regulate rhythmic muscle contractions. This enables us to walk without much higher brain control. What I found in the rykub's spine, however, was something else entirely: an intricately woven network so comprehensive, most locomotion likely originates there.

And my final discovery involved communication between the muscle fibers and those spines. In humans, there are deeply embedded "spindles" within individual skeletal muscles. These produce reflexive contractions in response to elongation forces. This has been understood for decades. And ignored for just as long. Because it's not that interesting. Because we're not rykubs. In a rykub's limb, there is more involuntarily innervated muscle tissue than there is consciously controlled mass.

Rykubs are not encumbered by the sluggish pace of voluntary recruitment. And this grants them the fastest reaction time of any known species.

Why would this trait develop?

Evolution. It was an arms' race between the rykub and its prey, the pitikos. If the pitikos were quicker, not only would the rykub lose its meal, but it may also lose its eyes.

That's as far as Cyn and I got into that dissertation today. She'll read the rest tonight. I sent it home with her. But she did express interest in publishing. Not just the rykub part, but the whole thing. After her current dissertation is in print in *Farhearth Frontiers*, of course. I don't want to scatter her thoughts in so many directions, she can't escort any of them across the finish line.

Cleaning it up would be an enormous amount of work. It's a jumbled tome of pointless trivia. I spent half a chapter on the topic of Natural Order. How fascinating its history is (it isn't; I was just trying to be a completist) and how it gives us an interesting way of viewing the three animals (it doesn't; I was just trying to be original). Again, it would be an enormous amount of work to prepare it for publication.

But I think it would be worth the effort. Because Cyn and I would be going through it together. And that would provide the perfect closure for the first two phases of my life.

Then she'll be on her own. And so will I.

But before we go our separate ways, we still have a Pendelhall tournament and a Farhearth Science Faire to attend.

Two more days at home, and then we leave.

I'm beginning to feel anxious. Mostly for Cyn. But also, about the trip itself. Ever since the *Thevro Chronicle* article came out, rumors of additional attacks, like small aftershocks, have been radiating through town. Including multiple reports of attacks on the road between here and Pendelhall.

I don't trust any of those stories, but that doesn't make them easy to ignore. Because the outrageous truth at the center, what those stories are hinged on, is true. This, I know because of Rorrik. The *Chronicle*, too, but I don't always trust that paper's facts. What I trust is that they'll report them eloquently. And if that means some truths have to be reconfigured, well, that's okay. Because their priority is not accuracy; it's reputation. And curating a noble reputation is only *partly* accomplished by casting hillians in the brightest light in every story. The rest of dignity management lies in the sentences that tell those stories. Not only are Thevro and its people necessarily portrayed in graceful ways; the language doing the portraying must uphold that grace.

Eloquence of this kind functions as a window into the souls of those writers. Inside, you can see insecurity hard at work. Like a frantic seamstress, weaving and weaving and weaving. Story after story after story.

What would people find if they looked into my soul? They'd probably see the inner mechanics of my anxiety. And realize I'm mostly just anxious about Cyn's audition.

After almost six years, it's almost here.

Twelve

Lyros, Second Lufoa, Day Fourteen. Morning.

I slept for about three hours. The rest of the night I spent lying still, listening to the branches rattle and frogs grumble beyond my window, just waiting for morning to come. And it finally came. Or at least it *started* to arrive. Night hasn't finished departing, but that in-between space – neither night nor day – felt like the right time to begin writing.

Having gone to bed thinking about the rykub, garlok, and pitikos, and having been awake for most of the night entertaining a wandering mind, I've been reflecting on my own chronobiology. I feel like I live in the times between night and day. I'm neither diurnal nor nocturnal.

If I stand outside under the full sun, I feel oppressed by nature, as though it's trying to shoo me indoors where I belong. "Scram!", it shouts with brightness and heat. And after the sun sets, when it's time to enter that great, slumbering kingdom, I'm not welcome there either. I stand on the porch and knock. And wait to be let in. But nothing happens, so I knock some more and keep waiting. All I want is refuge from the waking world. But that wish is seldom granted. *Sometimes*, it is. Once in a while, I'm permitted access to slumberland. As though the eternal doorman has a lapse in his vigilance, and I manage to sneak past him. But most nights, I just lie there, awake.

Last night was one of those nights. Which means I'm really tired today.

But I smell butter.

I smell butter being fried in a pan.

I thought I heard noises earlier. Downstairs. But I wasn't sure. Now I am. And I'm sure it's the noises of Cyn cooking breakfast.

I wasn't hungry until the scent reached my room. Now I'm ravenous.

I wonder if she arrived so early because she knows my mood will be experiencing a post-Rorrik lull. And she intends to remedy that with some breakfast cheer. She's right, if that's the reason she's here.

Now that Rorrik is gone, I do feel emptied of community.

We never feel lonely before revelry. Only after. In the way that I don't really feel hungry until I'm presented with the sights or smells of food. Then I find myself famished. But I wouldn't have noticed the feeling if it weren't shown to me. Once those pangs are felt, however, any food will do.

I think community is similar. When one friend leaves, another can stand in and barricade the gravity of that yawning void. So we don't get sucked into its mopey vortex. I think that's what Cyn is doing. But as I write this, I can hear the silence of Rorrik's absence. And I'm breathing butter in every breath. So I'm currently feeling famished of both food *and* friends.

And for some reason, my mind is wandering toward thoughts of Lum, whose antics could plug up any void. I wish he could have been here for the reunion. Although he couldn't have contributed much to our fruit spread. (My mind isn't wandering far from thoughts of food.)

There's no good fruit in the South. Or at least no good fruit that's *unique* to the South. Along the Sizarhorn Strait, the citrus and figs are identical to what grows in Thorn, except they're drier than cured horrux meat. In Moonkruug, there are carrot berries. Which don't taste terrible. But they're poisonous if eaten to satiety. Near the lavalands, it's just drought grapes and molten fruit. Which are both unique – you won't find them in any habitable climate – but no one has ever pretended to enjoy their consumption. Unless the alternative is starvation, there's no reason to put them in your mouth. Drought grapes taste like tanned animal hides rolled into tiny, shriveled spheres. And molten fruit is even worse. It can barely be considered comestible. But it's definitely com*bustible*. When cut open, it smells more like meat than fruit… because it cooks itself as it ripens. The growth rate is faster than any kid in puberty, and the process is essentially the same: rapid catabolism fuels rapid anabolism. And metabolism is a hot process. If you touch the outer shell of a molten fruit at the peak of its maturation, you can burn yourself. Stand in an orchard and the air feels like an oven. Hence the colloquial name, "furnace fruit".

I'm not a botanist, but I suspect they're related to the trees in the lichlands, which get even hotter. Or so I've heard. I've never been there. But I *have* seen, smelled, touched, and tasted the molten fruit. The seeds won't sprout without some internal combustion, and that usually renders its meat inedible. Unless you enjoy charred fruit cinders.

"It's a *delicacy*" (a word that conflates scarcity with flavor) is the closest thing to a compliment they're eligible to receive.

Unless the rumor can be trusted.

This rumor: if a molten fruit grows to maturity *without* cooking, it will be the most delicious thing you've ever eaten ever. Ever. It's that good.

Just ask any hillian at any Cookery Banquet. They'll regale you with fanciful tales of ripe molten pulp served raw.

Apparently, a Thevro chef once achieved this on the day of the competition.

When did this culinary miracle occur?

The hillians can't agree on a year. But it definitely happened!

I have my doubts.

If this hill-held rumor had truly rumed in real life, how did they manage it? Did they charter a fleet of ships to haul Northern snow to the lavalands, and then pack the trees as their fruit ripens? Even if that were possible, it doesn't sound profitable.

Yet, "The accomplishment alone is sufficient for victory!", they'll bellow if you fail to produce a deferential response. "And you think some local *omelet* can compete with *that*?", they'll add if they find out you're a flatty.

If ripe-and-raw molten fruit *was* served, there's no record of what it lost to, but the omelet is the *other* pouzo that unjustly unseated their pyloe. Which is why egg dishes are generally regarded as unpatriotic in Thevro.

I've been writing about food for half an hour. And there are now additional scents wafting up to my room. Onions and cookies.

I'm too distracted to keep writing.

More later.

Thirteen

Lyros, Second Lufoa, Day Fourteen. Afternoon.

After writing my morning journal, I came downstairs and found breakfast already made. Scrambled eggs from the market with some diced vegetables from the yard. And lots of butter. From my pantry.

But Cyn was also baking caravan cookies. Travel food. She ground up nuts to use as the base, and added buckwheat, flax, honey, and some other flours and seasonings I didn't have in my yard or pantry. She bought everything yesterday and brought it this morning. Getting ready for our trip.

No one could ever accuse Cyn of underpreparing. Or failing to be the first one fully prepared. For everything. In this case, we're going to be traveling together for a couple of days in a couple of days. What would have happened if she left me in charge of food? Waterskins aside, it would be nothing but bags of nuts and dried horrux meat. So she's doing the packing. And she's doing it two days in advance. That's Cyn.

Even when she's sick. A few weeks ago, she caught something that had her nearly bedridden. If it were anyone else, they would still be ridden in bed. But not Cyn. What did she do during her ailing days? Quadruple her reading.

The day I met her, a smith told me, "If the reaper don't lock up her coffin, she'll climb out for another day's work." It didn't take me long to believe it. Most people have a healthy fear of mortality, but I get the impression the "reaper" is more afraid of Cyn.

After breakfast, while the travel cookies cooled, we finished our discussion about my first dissertation. As expected, Cyn made every salient observation. And she explained them well. But she also had questions. Especially about the pitikos.

Yesterday, while she was at the miller's shop buying flours for the cookies, she mentioned our upcoming trip to the shopkeeper.

"Beware the blindin' birds, lass", he cautioned her with that old expression. Then he elaborated: "It's not just Wargees spreadin' the rumors. These days, it seems everyone buyin' bread's tellin' a story about the terror lurkin' nearby. Death's emissary, they're callin' it. And they say it ain't much of a negotiator."

The shopkeeper was clearly referring to the dweller of Thorn – that ghoulish recluse that's supposedly out there on the loose. But it was the expression that caught Cyn's attention: beware the blinding birds.

"Was that about the pitikos?", Cyn asked me.

"It was. Although I doubt he knew that. It's a well-known expression from a little-known creature. All people mean by it is to mind your surroundings, don't let your guard down, keep your eyes and ears open. That sort of thing. Although ears are more important than eyes in this case."

Then Cyn and I discussed the pitikos. And the noise it makes.

It's not stridulation, like the trill of a cricket. It's the high-pressure passage of air through a chamber in its thoracic cavity. The flapping of its wings plies a secondary diaphragm, which behaves like a set of bellows. But the air enters one channel and exits through another. In between, in the central chamber, there's a cartilaginous ball that rattles around, creating vibrations, which we hear as the signature screech of a pitikos in flight. That's *how* the noise is made. The more interesting question is *why*. What selective advantage is there in warning its prey?

Cyn had some clever ideas – concepts I hadn't considered – and she expressed interest in publishing them together. I suggested we defer that interest until her dissertation in print. Then perhaps we can reconsider publication.

She and I spent the rest of our morning session discussing her current project, and I had the increasingly rare experience of feeling useful. Someday soon, I will have nothing more to teach her. The last conversation in which I impart anything of value will be behind me. And I have no way of knowing when that time will come. So I cherish each of these moments as though they were my last. Including today's… which very well could be my last.

I invented a patient for us to diagnose: a Rivervalan fisherman named Oldug. He comes to Cyn during late Lufoa, and reports waking up one morning with upper extremity pain. Only on his dominant side. "I slept on it wrong", he said. "But it's been a week, and it doesn't seem to be improving. And I need that arm for work."

The Delta fishermen's high season is winding down in late Lufoa, indicating the patient's rotator cuff will have just endured several months of excessive rowing and casting. I didn't mention that part to Cyn. I wanted to see if she bit the red herring I cast as bait. About sleeping on it wrong.

She didn't. "Isn't that just Cliwen's tendinopathy?", Cyn said in a tone that dismissed further consideration.

"What do you mean by that?", I asked.

"Accumulated microtrauma that causes degeneration without inflammation."

"What do you mean by *that*?"

She kept explaining, and I kept asking her to explain further. Until we finally arrived at gaps in her understanding. Gaps in Cliwen's understanding, too. And everybody else's. "All we know about anything is the surface", I said. "There is no topic that has been fully excavated. No matter where you dig, if you do so sincerely, your shovel will always strike mystery."

Cyn was receptive. As she always is. And I was eager to make the most of what may be my last opportunity to play mentor. So I continued:

"We think we understand Thorn and its treillage of black trees because we've described its qualities in books. And we think we understand the North and its snows because cartographers have assigned names to everything visible on the surface. In doing so, they've emancipated the mysteries beneath from the custody of our curiosity. The same rule holds true in the natural sciences. When people know the name of a condition, such as Cliwen's tendinopathy, they stop digging. As though they've learned all there is to know about it. But it's a mistake to confuse names with knowledge. In this case, knowledge of the mechanisms responsible for the imbalance between degeneration and regeneration in Oldug's shoulder. We're getting into the crux of your work: when, where, why, and how do catabolic signals predominate? The physician who festoons his correspondence with flashy syllables does more to flaunt than inform. And knowing the name of the person who first characterized a phenomenon never reveals understanding of the phenomenon itself."

Cyn was smiling the entire time, apparently enjoying the conversation even more than I was. As soon as I paused long enough to permit interruption, she said, "The apothecarist with an answer to everything and nothing." Then it was me doing the smiling.

She was referring to *Second Botany* by Ezryn, Second Gardener of Lir. It's not a book we formally studied. Or even informally. I allude to it on occasion, but we've never discussed it. The copy I own – my mother's antique edition, which has enough marginalia to constitute a second book – isn't even in my library. I store it in the solar, the only room dustier than my cellar.

Still, I shouldn't have been surprised that Cyn tracked down a rare copy in her spare time and studied it scrupulously. What else would I expect after I briefly, casually, and vaguely mentioned it once or twice?

The line Cyn quoted comes from a late chapter: *The Futility of Vanity in Botany*. It begins: "The wiseman who memorizes the name of every flower that has ever grown lacks the wisdom to grow any of them." It then goes on to allege the same about apothecarists who have an answer to everything and nothing.

"I'll be right back", I said to Cyn. And I went to the solar to find the book. It took some searching, but I found it. The first thing I did was fan its pages while inhaling the aroma of an earlier age. Then I returned to the inglenook, flipped open to the penultimate chapter, *The Study of the Second Poetry*, and read a passage aloud:

"The artist reviles the anatomist. For he sees any examination of the flower's form as a deformation of its beauty. In scouring its anatomy, one strips it of all poetry. But to the Gardener, there are two poetries. There is that of color, shape, and perfume. And then there is a deeper calligraphy, which chronicles how the Flower is born, how it drinks from the rains, how it copes with the Night, and how it reasons with the Sun."

"Absent any rhyme or rhythm, that remains a wonder far more wonderful", Cyn said. It was the next line in the book. Which she evidently memorized. Now I was *really* smiling.

This is one of the earliest publications to describe science as a noble pursuit. As opposed to an enemy of faith and beauty, reducing all miracles and magic to chemicals and mechanics. I would have included it in Cyn's curriculum if the rest of the book wasn't so explicitly botanical. With no wider application or philosophical interpretation. (The final chapter is *Understanding Ragwort*.)

I guess, in a way, it *was* included. Inadvertently, but not insignificantly. Cyn and I spent an hour this morning discussing it. Mostly the wider applications. And philosophical interpretations. Ezryn wrote it centuries before the advent of modern medicine, but sometimes it feels like today's physicians are exactly whom he was describing. The white coats who memorize a thousand names of afflictions and therapies but learn nothing of value. In the clinic, all they are is poets attempting to disguise their ignorance with decorative syllables. It's no wonder malpractice is so common; what ailment has ever been cured by showmanship?

That's the summary of Cyn's and my conversation.

Afterward, we went outside and fenced. Vigorously. We do this at least once a week. She's preparing to be a combat medic. *The* combat medic. That's a difficult job if you don't know combat. And how can you learn if you don't participate? Consider the lute. You can read about it, watch performances, and discuss it all day. But unless you're actually practicing the instrument, you'll never learn to play.

That's why Cyn is decorated with the calluses of combat. Also, the exercise is good for memory. So we incorporate it as often as I have the energy.

Although this was the first time since Rorrik arrived. If he hadn't just finished the equivalent of three Salt and Stones, I would have insisted he and Cyn train together. He's the most talented fencer I know. But now he's gone. And Cyn and I are back to our normal structure. Which includes fencing. Which wore me out. So I'm going to lie down for a few minutes before our afternoon study session.

Fourteen

Lyros, Second Lufoa, Day Fourteen. Night.

Evening has barely started to arrive. And I'm already in my bedchamber. Our afternoon study session was shorter than usual. We mostly chatted about my second dissertation. The published one. And how I came to do it. After abandoning my first project, I couldn't afford another false start; I needed a topic I would see through to completion. So I returned to my roots. Literally and figuratively. I read my mother's work on the selective pressures of plants. She was a medical botanist both before and after her time as the Pendelhall Medic. (Back when there used to be a distinction between medical botany and herbalism.) There were several unpublished works and one paper that was printed in *Farhearth Frontiers*: "The Specificity of Floral Adaptation". Looking for inspiration, I read them all. And I found what I was looking for.

The premise of my mother's work was environmental fitness. Gravity may be consistent everywhere on Gaea; that is the burden born unto all botany. But the wind, sun, and rain differ greatly depending on longitudes, latitudes, and altitudes. And the vegetation that thrives in any region is that which is most compatible with the stressors found there. Excepting yards and farms, everywhere you look, you see plants exhibiting remarkable appropriateness to the conditions of their wilderness. An almost miraculous suitability to that territory's pressures and hazards. In a word: fitness. That's what you find growing in the wilder landscapes of Gaea.

My mother chose a coastal sand plant, a green lea shrub, and an inner-forest tree species to study as models of floral fitness. And she focused mainly on mechanical properties that influence structural integrity. Such as root depth and width, stalk thickness, the weight of seed-bearing structures at the ends of the branches, geometric patterns of those branches, and so on.

Rigidity of stem, stalk, and trunk, for example, depends on wind direction and speed, as well as the density and stature of its shadow-casting neighbors. How high must a plant reach before receiving its light? The dandelion that climbs too greedily upward is sure to topple, and bend into a sulking posture, no longer aiming its face to the sun. But a stubbornly stiff stem is likely to break with Gaea's gustier breaths. Pliability may be unnecessary in the stillness of the inner forest, but coastal plants must be limber enough to perform gymnastics with the erratic winds. Thus, plant development differs in different settings.

My mother selected three distinct settings for her research. But she didn't immediately study the plants that grow there. Instead, she documented the unique environmental pressures in those regions. Then she devised the ideal characteristics of plants that would thrive in each. And *then* she surveyed the plants themselves. And she found exactly what she had predicted to find.

What is true in plant mechanics, I reasoned, is surely true in skeletal muscle physiology. My first dissertation scratched at this concept but didn't quite cut through its crust. In my second attempt, I broadened my geography and narrowed my focus. I picked three distinctive species – one from the East, one from the West, and one from the South – with muscular systems that were perfectly calibrated to their environments: a mollusk, frog, and a bird. But not just any mollusk, frog, and bird.

From the East, I described the Delta Reef scallop, colloquially referred to as otters' bane. Like all bivalve mollusks, it has adductor muscles that close the valves of its shell. Like all other scallops, this species has striated adductors for swimming and nonstriated adductors for clamping. But unlike all other shellfish, the Delta Reef scallop is utterly unshuckable. So long as it's living, no amount of prying will part its valves. The hungry otter could sooner part a stone. And the grandiose chef, hoping to extract live flesh, could sooner serve the meat of a molten fruit ripe and raw. When an otter or a human contracts a muscle, there's a rapid onset of force decay because our survival doesn't depend on static endurance. But that *is* a major selective pressure for the bivalve mollusk. So while water weasels and pearl collectors may put up a commendable fight, the Delta Reef scallop always outlasts their best effort.

From the West, I described the nokfrosc. It's a dark purple frog that resides in the northwestern sloughs. Look closely at any rotten log floating through the murky shallows and you'll find one. Sitting as still as a statue. But for its black tongue plucking lamp flies out of the air. Also lurking in those marshes are the frogs' predators, however. Notably, the bogbear, a colossal nocturnal hunter that can submerge its immense bulk beneath the surface of the swamp. Only its nose and eyes are visible as it slowly drifts toward its prey. So listless it appears lifeless. "Nothing to worry about here; I'm just a clump of detritus floating past", it seems to convey. Until it floats into striking distance, and it bursts from the stillness like a thousand pounds of wet, carnivorous lightning. It seldom succeeds in catching its snack, however. Because nokfroscs are far more explosive. They can soar from the floor of the swamp to the branches that weave its roof in a single leap. There is no known creature with greater muscular power. Or worse endurance. In my heat capturing experiments, I found the nokfrosc to consume as much energy in a single contraction as the Delta Reef scallop does in a week of unremitting isometric exertion.

Lastly, from the South, I described the angel wren. For its unrivaled capacity in dynamic muscular endurance. Unrivaled among extant creatures, anyway. The last of the chameleon lorikeets died around the time I was born. While the lorikeets flew among the living, no animal had a more arduous itinerary. Or at least a *verified* itinerary ("the lunar albatross isn't called the wanderer for nothin'; it soars all the way to the antipode isles!" is almost certainly a myth). The daily journey of the lorikeets may have been legendary, but those legends were substantiated by Farhearth ornithologists. The birds would depart from the woods near Eggtog Cemetery, pass through the realm of the nokfroscs, and land in the heart of Mulgotha. Without stopping. At thirty miles an hour, that's twelve hours in the air. Upon arrival, they would feed, sleep, awaken at first light, and then begin their return trip. Back to the Eggtog woodlands. Where they would feed, sleep, and wait for the next morning's light. At which point, they would depart for Mulgotha again. Back and forth, back and forth, half their lives spent aloft. Until they went extinct. And the angel wren was promoted to the rank of Gaea's Stamina Champion. Their daily boomerang migration is no trifling feat. From their nesting ridge to their feeding reef, it's a little over a hundred miles (depending how far into the reef they go). And they make this trip – from ridge to reef and back – every day of the year. At about twenty miles an hour, they spend perhaps eleven hours a day aloft. And the metabolism supporting this lofty activity differs markedly from the aforementioned oyster and frog. The wren expends so much energy in flight, one would expect a lean and sinewy physique. But dissection reveals curiously greasy musculature. Curious until one considers: fat yields far more energy than carbohydrate per unit of weight, making it the preferred substrate for aerial endurance. The *individual* wren may grow lean with more exercise, but ample adiposity is a selective pressure at the level of the species.

I found a second fascinating purpose of the wrens' fat cells, but it was outside the scope of my question. And the danger of pursuing distractions was the most important lesson I learned from my previous attempt at publication. So I set those observations aside and focused on my central hypothesis: how skeletal muscle form is a product of function, and function is a product of environment.

As Cyn and I discussed the three species, and the principles of contextual fitness and ancestral adaptation, she had numerous insights that would have been profitable while I was doing the initial research.

Perhaps in a distant future, that can be another paper we publish together. Maybe. As we continue to read and discuss my old work, I worry the roster of potential projects she and I vow to undertake may grow long.

But the hour has already grown late. It's past my bedtime.

Tomorrow is our last day at home. We leave Nyros morning. Which means I have packing to do. And if I'm groggy while I pack, I'll forget something.

Plus, my back is a bit tender. Probably because of the fencing. After a week without training. Sometimes my back spasms fitfully, twitching like an eyelid after a sleepless night. Other times, the tremor is so steady, it's as though the strings of my sinews are playing a note. Screeching and dissonant, but steady.

That's what I'm feeling now. It's the kind of discomfort I'm able to relieve through focus. Like shivering in cold water. When I concentrate, I can find a calm space in the cold.

But a better remedy is a good night's sleep.

So I'm off to confront the doorman at the gates of slumberland.

Fifteen

Fyros, Second Lufoa, Day Fifteen. Morning.

I just woke up from a weird dream. And it's close enough to morning that I'm going to start my day. The sun won't rise for at least another hour, but I spent the last six hours asleep. Which is more than I usually get.

I don't feel like writing about my dream at the moment. Maybe later. Instead, I'm going to write about my tea, which I'm drinking now. As I write this, I'm taking sips between sentences.

When I got out of bed, my back was still a little stiff. Better than it was last night, but it continues to hold some tension. Probably because I'm nervous about our upcoming trip. And I'm unsure what to do with my life afterward. I was hoping my tea would fix all of that. It didn't. Nor did it have any psychoactive properties to lighten my mood. In the dose I got. A huge dose would induce psycho*cessation*. Death. My nettle had a hint of ryndovyn in it. Water poison. I get this flavor rarely. My mother carefully placed all of her medicines in the bowl. And she knew where every single one was.

I imagine it's like my office when I taught at Farhearth. Person-high piles of periodicals everywhere you looked. That may not sound meticulous, but it wasn't chaotic clutter; I knew where everything was. There was a precise geography to my organization. Extracting a book or journal from a pile might have been a challenge, but that doesn't mean it was disorganized. Midwifery requires care and precision too. And nobody argues gestation is a haphazard process or obstetrics is a slapdash practice.

My mother and I were similarly scrupulous. She knew exactly where each plant lived on her "mortar map", as she called it. Hardly different from my father's mapping of the world's roads. The mortar was a microcosm of that; it could probably be transposed on my father's maps with something close to perfect accuracy. Where on Gaea did each plant grow? That's where they were ground into her mortar. She knew the location of every root, leaf, and seed across the curved cradle of that wooden bowl.

We all seem to organize different parts of the world. In a sense, we're all trying to understand our environments. And exert some control over them. That's probably the reason I write. Although my writing has felt lifeless these last couple of days. Ever since Rorrik left.

My thoughts are cold and scientific. My words are inert. The emptiness of Rorrik's absence colors practically every page. Especially while I'm writing about anything else. That's when the pages feel dullest.

But let's indulge that dullness and return to the topic of my tea. And describe the compound that accompanied this morning's nettle.

"Ryndovyn", according to the botanist.

"River laurel", according to the townsfolk.

"Water poison", according to the poisoner.

And a dozen other names according to a dozen other cultures.

In the words of Ezryn, "The name is the only pointless part of the plant."

No matter what you call this one, its flavor remains the same: deeply pungent. Even in the most miniscule dose, which mine obviously was. Because my mother wasn't an assassin. She was a medic and medical botanist. And in small doses, ryndovyn has a medical purpose: it enhances immune function by upregulating the body's own natural defense mechanisms.

The ryndovyn plant doesn't have arms to swat away insects. Nor legs to flee from them. So it synthesizes a poison. Woe is the fate of the slugs and grubs that crawl upon its leaf. And woe is the fate of the person who eats a whole leaf in one bite. Eventual woe. It might take a couple of days. Immediate woe belongs to the unfortunate Gaean who eats three leaves in one sitting. Numbness, nausea, a sluggish heart rate, low blood pressure, and respiratory depression are first to arrive. Then, finally, respiratory cessation.

My mother would grind a tenth of a leaf to last a week. One dose each day. A sixtieth of a lethal amount. And her patients surely benefited.

I probably had a tenth of *that* dose. Not enough to be particularly therapeutic; its only effect was to ruin the flavor of my morning tea. And ruin my journal by having me focus on the most mundane topic imaginable.

But now I'm done writing. Because I have run out of time. Morning is going to start crowning any minute. And I have to go watch the sunrise. Have to. To honor Rorrik. His "there's truth in dreams!" stuff.

I'll explain later.

Sixteen

Fyros, Second Lufoa, Day Fifteen. Afternoon.

After finishing my last journal, I went downstairs, refilled my mug with tea, went outside, sat on the bench on my porch, and sipped pensively while watching the sun's grand but gradual arrival.

Estevro has perfect sunrises. The eastern sky is huge. The sun is born low, and its colors have such a long reach. It sets high, though. Behind the towering hills of Thevro to the west. Dusk falls on the flatties well before it touches any hillian's home. In the early hours of the night, their mansions remain gilded and warm while our cottages grow cold and quiet. Darkness paints our walls, wanders across our streets, sneaks through our alleyways. Only after it has enveloped our city does it move on, sprawling up the hill.

Last night, I had a dream that the emerging dusk's shadows got trapped in our streets. Like a traveler passing through town accidentally getting caught in the orbit of Steward Circle. It's the most convoluted road system on Gaea. Not counting Druinham, of course. Most of Estevro makes sense, but those half dozen roads that feed the Circle twist and intersect in disorienting ways, bizarrely leading back into each other. It was apparently designed that way to deter people from cutting through on their way to somewhere else. It was meant to keep the community untrafficked, quiet, quaint. It rather defeats the purpose, however, when the cutters-through simply find themselves stuck. "I was just here!", I've heard a thousand carriage drivers shout in frustration.

When I was young, I used to sit on the lawn inside the Circle and test my skills as a fortuneteller: my friends and I would place bets on which travelers would and would not be captured by Steward's gravity. "A penny says that rider will escape", I'd say about the driver of a cheap carriage exiting on Blackstone. "Two pennies say that rider will be detained", I'd say about the fancy carriage exiting on Moonbone. "One penny against your two and I'll take that bet", a friend might say. And then, two minutes later, we'd see the fancy carriage deposited right back into the Circle. And we'd giggle and trade our pennies. No matter who won the wagers, we all found amusement in the frustrations of those interned by the mazy roads. And we all learned never to risk a coin on anyone exiting on Plainroad. That's the most confusing one of them all. It thwarts nearly every departure.

That is what I dreamed about last night.

Except, instead of watching some visitor's attempt to escape, I was on the lawn watching the shadows venture into the maze. Stretching from the trees. Winding through the streets. Then slithering back to where they came from. They were attempting to leave. Eager to ascend the hill. And finish spreading their dusk. But they couldn't seem to figure out how. And I could see them growing agitated. "I was just here!", they didn't actually scream but somehow still communicated. They kept circling and circling. Racing and racing. More and more frantically. Until the sun finally rose and burned them all away.

And then I woke up.

I wonder if this is me worrying that I'll get trapped in this phase of my life. My six years with Cyn will be over soon. Then what? Where do I go from there? Will I know how to move on to some other ambition?

I don't usually assign much meaning to my dreams, but I did sit on my porch and watch this morning's sunrise. Out of curiosity. To see what it looks like when the shade burns away. Does it look anything like it did in my dream?

No. It does not. The landscape simply lightens. Slowly. There was no panic within the blackness. There was no hissing noise emitted from the friction of an incarcerated shadow quivering against the road.

It just gradually – unspectacularly – became morning.

And then Cyn arrived. And we started our first session. We always do two. Once while the sun is young and once again when it's old. We seldom meet during the true daylight hours. That's when I rest. And write. And stare blankly. Then write some more.

During this morning's session, we finished discussing my second dissertation. Specifically, we talked about human applications. Nowhere in the publication did I mention humans. But there *is* a lot to say on the subject. And it was Cyn who did most of the saying. The theme was: humans lack mastery in all three capacities, but we're versatile. So what does that say about our ancestry? It seems to imply a broad range of stresses served as our selective pressures. Maybe someday, Cyn and I will co-author that paper, too. But making any such commitment now would just overwhelm me.

Today's second study session, which we'll start shortly, will be a brief one. Because I have to start packing. Cyn finished her packing already. She even made a list for me. Which included plenty of unnecessary items, like my lute. But there's other stuff she doesn't know to list. And I should get on that.

I do enjoy trips like this. In part, it's the good company. The *best* company. But in another part, it's the wagon. It once belonged to my father. And it was his father's before. Beyond that, I don't know its history. I think my grandfather built it and my father continued to build and rebuild it. And now it's mine. And I just use it. No further alterations have been made to this four-wheeled, green-roofed, precious heirloom since my inheritance.

The roof is made from grassheart larches. You never see their moss-colored planks anymore. During my grandparents' age, every house in Estevro had a green fence. During my parents' age, the hymogs ate the last of the trees. In my age, there aren't too many green fences left. Whatever green you see is *actual* moss. And I drive the only green-roofed wagon I've ever seen. Not because it's fashionable. Quite the opposite: it's functional. With most wood, the East has a way of corroding it before its time. The alternating rains and suns soften it and then bake it. Then soften it again. And then bake it again. A few years of that and the planks are as white as bone and brittle as a cookie. Not the grassheart larches though. The blazingest of suns and lashingest of rains both seem to sustain the wood, practically rejuvenate it. It's as if Gaea designed those trees with our roofs in mind. And our fences. Unfortunately, half of Estevro's green fences (and all of Thevro's) have been torn down and replaced with more stylish lumber. Which has a lifespan of five or six years. If they aren't first demolished by the fleeting whims of fashion. These days, aesthetic trends seem to be reimagined every season, and the dressings of our lodgings (especially those in Thevro) are changed as often as our wardrobes.

It's funny how submission to style so often weakens us. Like the parachute plumage of a crested argus. Its hundred-eyed train of iridescent feathers flags every potential predator in the area and functions as wind-resistant luggage in a chase. But it's just so darn stylish. And so it's attractive to mates. Human fashion is similar: the less functional it is, the more appealing it seems to be. In consideration of our fences, nature never would have weathered the wood that stood before. And that's my longwinded way of saying: the green roof is my favorite part of my wagon. The rest of it is made from other lumber.

The carriage itself – the walls and floor – are long, slender, soil-brown beams of umbrella pine. Not as impervious to the sun, but it tolerates the rains well. And there is no more pliable wood in all the Eastern acres. The Grass Road isn't without its lumps, but the construction of the carriage using interlocking pine absorbs the jouncing, which makes for a much more comfortable ride.

My father also added retractable grassheart awnings for sunny days. Provided I keep the pine shaded from direct sunlight, it should last another fifty years. Maybe longer.

And the harness for the horse has the best engineering on the whole vehicle. Various woods, various metals, and a clever contraption that can be adjusted to harness an additional horse – of a completely different size – in case the load gets too heavy for one. I've never seen a better system on another cart, carriage, caravan, or wagon (whatever the difference between them is, I still don't know; what I *do* know is no other vehicle is quite like this one).

The wheels though. My father tried every kind of tree in the East and never felt satisfied. "I never found a wood that was meant to be made into a circle", he once told me. To this day, he's convinced a perfect wheel isn't made of wood. He must have fitted the wagon with twenty different sets when I was a kid. Every few months, a new tree would audition, and none of them were given the part. They all had some tiny imperfection that made them utterly unsuitable for the role of... rolling.

Then my father made a trip to Cinderheim. To deliver a shipment of lumber. He did this several times a year. But this time, he returned home with a new set of wheels. "Half a percent of carbon, three and a quarter chromium, and *exactly* 0.28 pounds per cubic inch", I heard him declare so contentedly and often in the following years that I – having no understanding of metallurgy – remember the numbers. (He took an unused chunk of the metal to Farhearth to have it analyzed.) It's been over twenty years and those wheels have never been changed. One almost sympathizes with the road rocks that reside in their path. They'll crack before any of the wheels chip. He had five made on that trip. The spare is hung on the wall at my parents' house like a painting.

Nowhere on any continent's roads will you find a more dependable wagon. The roof shields you from nature's frenziest fits, the bed and sideboards keep you comfortable, and the wheels promise to deliver you all the way home... without ever needing to be changed. Which is vital for me as I would have no idea how to do that.

What I *am* proficient at is packing. It's a type of geometry that comes naturally to me. I look at luggage and instinctively know where it belongs. Although belonging isn't always determined by an object's shape. Sometimes its place is determined by price. The most valuable, and thus thievable, of luggage is stowed in the hidden chambers, of which my father (and his father) built several. Working in transportation, one learns how to safely navigate Gaea's miles with an abundance of coins and cargo on board. And they did it in style. Perhaps not *fashion*. But there's no denying the style.

Abbie just walked into my room.

Seventeen

Fyros, Second Lufoa, Day Fifteen. Night.

As I was finishing my afternoon journal, Abbie walked into my room.

I thought I heard hooves on the staircase. I wondered if it was Cyn moving something hoof-like up the steps one at a time. Because why would Abbie be in the house? And coming up the stairs? And then entering my room? And settling at my feet?

She's always been sensitive to my emotions. As though she understands my feelings in every moment. And if I'm lonely or upset or anxious, she attempts to comfort me. Or at least that's how I interpret her behavior. Maybe it's just a basic survival instinct, being attuned to the moods of other creatures around you. But it seems to be more than that. Like an unspoken language that can pass between human and… goat in this case. But animals in general. Whatever that language is, they're far more fluent in it than we are.

After having this thought, I spent half a minute "listening" to Abbie, trying to understand what she might be trying to communicate as she cuddled with my shins. I would have given her more time, but I was distracted by a ruckus in the kitchen.

I didn't assume it was Cyn this time. I figured it was Gyfur. And I was right.

There wasn't much of a mess. He was mostly just running into the furniture. But I still hustled him back outside. Abbie, too.

Cyn was out there. In the yard. Practicing her fencing footwork. By herself.

Tomorrow morning, we leave for Pendelhall.

It'll be a two-night journey for us. I'm sure we could get there in one day. From my front door to the grand gate of Pendelhall, it's about thirty-three miles, almost entirely along the North Grass Road. But that's a lot of strain for one aging horse hauling a heavy load. So Wylmot (my horse) and I both prefer a slower pace. And I prefer good conversation along the way. If we cover a dozen miles each day, we'll get there well before sundown on Seros.

I've done this trip fifty times before. But I'm still looking at my father's maps.

Not out of fear that we'll wind up on some deer trail five miles off course (which I tend to do on less familiar roads), but to plan our sleeping locations. These maps are detailed. And among those details are Gaea's best campsites. Invisible from the road, perfectly secluded, perfectly sheltered, and perfectly berried. And, most importantly, undiscovered. Except by my father. So we'll be undisturbed.

It should be a hassle-free, comfortable trip. And I think we're fully packed. Possibly overpacked.

We started with Cyn's luggage. Impressively little.

Then we loaded everything on the list she made for me. Which included paper, pen, and ink. Although I packed more of each than she expected. Two pens in case one is lost or damaged. Since that's a common experience on the road, I didn't pack my *good* pens. Only disposables: a quill and a reed. And three large bottles of ink. Which is three times what I suppose I'll need. And then the paper. That's where I really overdid it. Five times what I'll use if I document every thought I have.

When I inherited my father's wagon, I *also* inherited his travel journals. Every trip he ever made is chronicled in them. Every mile's detail fully described. These are as important to our understanding of geography as anything Mundus or Elsiel ever did. The difference: I'm the only one who's ever read my father's contributions to cartography. I must have two hundred of his travel journals. Cloth bound. Fifty pages apiece. Thick pages, though. They don't bleed through, so you can get a hundred pages of writing out of each.

I store them in the attic. Next to the *unused* journals. Just as many of those. Or there *were* just as many. I packed nine of them this evening. In addition to the one that I've been writing in for the last week.

Every time I climb into the attic, it's a nostalgic experience. The only access is through a hidden hatch in the solar, and the people who lived here between my parents and me don't seem to have discovered it. Because there is nothing belonging to them up there. And it is cluttered with my family's belongings. At least three generations' worth. It's like a museum of my family's history. Some of it recently added, much of it abandoned in years past.

After retrieving what I needed from the attic, I grabbed a box and stuffed it with travel trinkets that Cyn wouldn't know to list. Like my pitikos whistle. Which I kept from my time as a Magister's student. And a bottle of black linseed oil for the wagon's axles and springs. And lots of medical supplies.

I packed most of that stuff, along with a sack of coins, in the bench chamber. It's a hidden compartment inside the carriage. At the back. The side nearest the horse. The side benches are over the wheel wells, so they have no storage. Although they have leaves that unfold and interlock to form a level surface over the floor storage. Which makes for a nice bed. But the *secret* chamber is under the back bench. It's just as hidden as the attic in my house. And like my attic, it's locked by levers that must be moved into particular positions. Hidden levers. This is better than having a keyhole. Keyholes serve as signs. They signal to thieves, "There's a compartment here! If you're looking for valuables, look no further!"

Despite being so inconspicuous, the bench chamber is large. It extends under the driver's seat outside of the covered carriage. So it holds a lot of storage. And when it's closed, it seals tightly enough to stay dry in the worst of storms. Which makes it the best place to store my journals.

After Cyn and I had finished packing, we went out to the back terrace to sit, eat, and watch the sunset. As the hues of twilight began to bruise the heavens, right on the threshold of darkness, we were granted a rare sight: a sky squirt. We both saw it at the same time. As though it passed through some liminal door into our world. Neither of us said anything. We both just pointed at it. And watched it flicker in the distance. The last scattered beams of dying light all seemed to gather brightly on its wings, glinting as silver as a falling star.

If there's any wind at all, sky squirts can remain in the air for hours at a time migrating to their final resting place. Cyn and I sat still and watched this one finish its day's flapping and descend toward the ground like a leaf in Elyem rattling down from a high branch. The squirt didn't reach the grass, though. It landed on one of the flowers of my taevamuna, the only Southern plant that grows in my yard. This seemed symbolic to me. Or at least "meaningful" if symbolism is the imagined meaning we affix to coincidence.

I'd only seen a couple of sky squirts before. And this was Cyn's first. She'd seen *sea* squirts. Those are fascinating, too. But they're much more common and far less bizarre. Once it landed, we crept up to it – slowly, silently – until we were a few feet away. Its blossom doubled as a beak, its body resembled a centipede, and it flapped a pair of wings that could have passed for the petals on which it lay.

I was hoping it would take root in my yard. But it didn't look settled. It was breathing and eating holes in the taevamuna. Like a common garden pest. But unlike slugs, mealybugs, and aphids, this was a very, very welcome guest.

I'm sure it will resume its journey tomorrow. Wherever it's headed.

Maybe it will return. Improbable but not impossible. They always embark seeking belonging in the great beyonds, but if they don't find it, they often migrate back to the site of their hatching. The whole voyage is as pointless as a hike.

Almost as fascinating as the creature itself is its paucity in academic literature. It was first characterized centuries ago. The earliest publication I know of is Brieona's. Only as a plant, though; she didn't describe the ambulatory state.

To my knowledge, the only scientist to have studied both phases – flora and fauna – is Abendroth. That's the only reason I know anything about them.

Despite the shortage of peer-reviewed reports, everyone seems to agree on one thing: seeing a sky squirt is a powerful omen. Not an ill omen, necessarily. Nor a good one. But an ambiguous one. A chaotic one. A *powerfully* chaotic omen. So be on the lookout for the unexpected. Goods, bads, weirds. *Something* big awaits around the bend.

Most illogical lore has a nearly logical origin. And this random, high-stakes omen is no exception. And, as it happens, Abendroth wrote about that, too. The mysterious portending of the creature's presence is derived from its breeding traits, which are unlike those of its aquatic cousin, the sea squirt.

Let's start with sea squirts. These are filter feeders that live in the photic zone. They take energy from light, but they also feed on a yolk. Metabolizing the energy from both, they travel for a short time in search of a better home. Often, they find it where the mangroves grow, sometimes upon black coral, or the surface of a stone, or the stony shell of a red reef crab.

During the larval phase, sea squirts exhibit ambition, embarking on a great voyage in search of belonging. But once they decide on a destination, they dock, root, digest their nervous systems, and become simultaneously senile and sessile. Animal transformed to plant.

Farhearth alchemists farm and harvest them for a compound they synthesize. It's used as a treatment for tumors of some sort (I haven't kept current on this research).

Sky squirts share many similarities with their wetter relative. Including their indecisiveness on whether to be flora or fauna. They hatch from plant eggs and depart their flowery kingdom with all the zest of a votary on a holy quest.

Old fables say they're searching for a lost paradise somewhere in the wilds where they can develop into something divine. But invertebrate zoology says their voyage is an unconscious one, in which they are simply responding to environmental stimuli. When and where they dock is entirely determined by climate variables. Sometimes they travel far. Other times they return to where they were born. In the end, however, they always complete the circle of life: from plant to ambulatory adventurer and finally back to plant. Unless the inchoate squirt circle is severed inside of a predator's mouth. Perhaps a frog. Or a sparrow. Or a snake.

Here's where the two squirts differ: the swimmer is capable of asexual reproduction and the flyer is not. Procreation of the sky squirt is considerably stranger. It occurs through interspecies breeding, which appears to result in hybridized offspring. The process is comparable to cross-pollination except it's not just between varieties. There is evidence of it "cross-pollinating" with several unrelated species. *Fertilization mimicry* is the name that was assigned to this phenomenon at Farhearth. But names do not explain mechanisms. Nobody has any idea how this one works. And what happens to every gap in human understanding? Whimsical lore rushes through it to fill the void. Such as: "The sky squirt is the primordial mother of every living creature." Speciation is the fate of *other* creatures. Like horses. And the herds of their forebears. One herd divides into two. Each subherd exclusively reproduces with its own members. With each new generation, modifications accumulate. Eventually, the modifications are too great to permit pairings between herds. The separation is permanent; they can never reunify. While most species split long ago, others were more recent, and they preserve a capacity to interbreed. A horse and a horse makes a horse. A donkey and a donkey makes a donkey. A horse and a donkey makes a mule or a hinny, an in-between species that cannot propagate itself. A horse and horrux makes nothing. Same with stags, hymogs, and oxen: no hybrid will result… no matter how fertile the stallion. Too many modifications have accumulated since those lineages divided. This much is true. But the lore goes further, claiming all of these animals can mate with their ancient-yet-extant common ancestor, the sky squirt. Which means the creature Cyn and I saw on my taevamuna tonight, whom we named Percy, will soon give birth to *something*, but what exactly? There's no way to know. And *that* is the etymology of its chaotic omenship.

But now it's time for bed. We plan to be on the road early. After an even earlier breakfast.

Eighteen

Nyros, Second Lufoa, Day Sixteen. Morning.

We leave this morning. After breakfast. Which we'll have as soon as Cyn gets here. Until then, I'm sitting in my bedchamber, looking at the stones on my windowsill. Stones and other mineral mementos.

One of my earliest memories is going to the Vanishing Isles with my father. We found a pearl. And I kept it. Since then, I've made a lot more trips and taken a lot more souvenirs. A dark green agate from the Hallowed Grove. A crystal from the Salt Road Bridge. A black beach stone from Thorn with calligraphic quartz veining. My first time visiting any meaningful destination, I always take a stone.

Today, there aren't many unvisited destinations left on the map.

In the West, I have yet to visit Adonere, Druinham, and the umbra that lies to its north. Although I have been to the soaring, craggy face of Druinham. And I have been to Mulgotha's mazy outskirts. The *outer* outskirts at least. Where the nokfroscs are. And I have walked the bordering hills of Adonere. But never have I gone inside any of those cities.

In the South, I've never been to Yaga-Goro (which I'm not sure even exists) or Cinderheim (which most certainly exists). But I have been to Baguzu once, Eldergard twice, and Moonkruug more times than I've bothered to count. During my first visit to each, I took a stone to remember that experience by.

When I was younger, I used to add to my windowsill with some regularity. Today, it's been years since I last added a stone to my collection. I suppose I'll be taking one from the hike Cyn and I embark on today.

I guess it's not a hike. It's a trip. There's a difference. There-and-back-again with a purpose is a trip. Without a purpose is a hike. And social fulfilment is not a purpose, it's a reason. Although I don't think hikes are conducive to sociability anyway. *Walks* are the social outings... which I enjoy much more. Because hikes – akin to holidays – are just formal versions of a normal thing. Expanding on that akinity, hikes and holidays are both rife with expectations. We *expect* to derive gratification from them. And so the best outcome is not genuine enjoyment, but fulfillment of a contract.

I wonder if the satisfaction we feel in any experience can be measured as the margin between expectation and actual pleasure. That would account for the disappointment people report after an intensely anticipated experience fails to fully amaze.

According to these mathematics, even if walks are slightly less pleasurable than hikes, they still exceed my expectations. The ceiling may not be raised, but the floor is lowered. So the margin is wider. So I enjoy them more.

That was my long-lettered way of saying: people hold "hikes" in too high a regard. They're just hilly walks that end where they began. We set out on an adventure, arrive, look around, and then mosey back down the mountain… the same way we came.

That seems to be a reliable model for most people's lives: they depart where they arrived. Their younger years are marked by growth, exploration, novelty. They reach the summit. Inspect it a little. Then turn around and descend. Step after step, they shrink toward the familiar. Until eventually, they die in the town where they were born, beset by other survivors of adventure who also returned to the site of their departure, never to depart again. Things are a little different here and there. We've lost a bit along the way. And gained some wisdom in its place. But in the end, we all find our way back home.

I'm no exception. Halfway through my life, I've already returned to the house I grew up in. But that doesn't mean I can't see the futility of a boomerang's journey. I recognize the pointlessness of a hike.

By comparison, a "trip" is pointful. And that's what Cyn's and my adventure is about to be.

We'll be leaving within the hour.

Although Abbie and Gyfur won't be accompanying us. It would be too much trouble to bring them. They'll have no problem taking care of themselves while we're gone. And they'll be delighted to keep each other company.

Also, my neighbor will stop by at least once a day to check on them. Although I could feel her judgment when I asked.

Leaving pets behind is very un-Eastern of me. Once my neighbors settle, nearly all of them adopt inpets. And they never travel again. "What am I supposed to do with Pendrake?", they say whenever they're invited to leave the house.

Animal ownership of this kind imprisons pet and owner alike. The only time the pet is permitted outdoors is to defecate. In a well-fenced region to thwart escape. And if the owner were to leave for a week, they would be greeted by their pet's carcass upon their return. So they're just as confined.

I've never felt inclined to bind myself to another's survival.

Outpets are the ways of the West and South.

Lum has Bug. Rorrik has Gyfur. And I have Abbie. Outpets, all.

One more reason I don't quite belong where I am.

In a thousand ways, I feel trapped between worlds.

But now I hear Cyn downstairs. After all these years we've spent together, it's finally time to begin our trip.

Nineteen

Nyros, Second Lufoa, Day Sixteen. Afternoon.

Cyn and I are taking a break for lunch. A few bites of horrux and a glutton's helping of cookies. For breakfast, we had rainclouds. Whipped egg pancakes. A Busik invention. They're a little bit damp and more than a little bit fluffy. The right food for the road when you don't know how light or heavy to eat. Rainclouds are light enough to be whisked into circulation at the first gust of activity, but heavy enough to drizzle their energy for hours.

After breakfast, we washed our dishes, checked that the house was all closed and locked up, and left out the back door. So we could give Abbie and Gyfur a farewell petting.

We're making good time so far. About five miles north of Estevro, and as many miles west of the Spice Rack, those outskirt houses amid the farmland, interwoven with roads such as Basil, Sage, Rosemary, and Thyme.

That's where my parents moved when I left for Farhearth.

During my first break from school, I returned "home" to a new house.

That was the day I started saving pennies and paupers to eventually buy back my ancestral home.

Technically it's not my *ancestral* ancestral home. But it *is* my childhood home. And it's my mother's childhood home. And her father's. But not *his* father's. He's the one who built it. Or at least built *upon* it. He added half the rooms.

My great grandfather's *childhood* home is somewhere along the southern slope. It's not on one of the "newer" roads, though, cobbled a century or two ago. It's on Burrower's Pass, which was cobbled before centuries were counted.

It would be more accurate to call it Hikers' Path. For several reasons. First, it's a closed loop. It doesn't go all the way into Thevro. Only three roads do. Kingwood takes you through the grand gates. The front entrance. Rosemont is the backdoor. Tantamount to a servant's entrance. And the third road is Slippery Leaf Lane, which is basically a sallyport. A little-known passage from square to square.

Maybe Hikers' Path used to pass from city to city, but today it's just a circle. Which was reclaimed by nature. If you walk that loop, you realize the word "road" is a euphemism for the trail under your feet. It practically has teeth. Good luck driving a carriage over it.

I tried once. I didn't succeed.

I also tried to figure out which house belonged to my ancestors' ancestors. I didn't succeed in that either. I don't even know if it's still standing. There must be a hundred houses on that loop, and half of them are kneeling, their old bones bending and breaking, having carried the burden of gravity for too many centuries. Some of the houses are upright though. And a few of those still have inhabitants… who seem to be as antique as their homes.

There are plenty of old districts in Estevro – mine is among the oldest – but that one is *Thestevro* old.

Once Estevro and Thevro formally divorced, the line of separation sprawled outward from my current neighborhood. West became Thevro, east became Estevro, and the southern slope was forgotten by both.

I live on the Estevro side, bordering the divide, where the Grass Road splits the two towns. Nestled between Rosemont and Kingwood, which sort of keep the towns conjoined.

My house is the oldest on its street. At least a hundred years older than my great grandfather, who added the kitchen, the master bedchamber above it, and an attic beside that bedchamber. He also converted the original kitchen into the solar, replaced every door, and remodeled who knows what else.

I never met him, but as the years go by, I come to know him more and more. Maybe we don't share skills or vocations, but values and aesthetics are traits I clearly inherited. It's as though he built the house specifically for me. I feel a connection with him every time I sit at the kitchen table and drink my tea. Or sit at the inglenook and study. Or sit in my bedchamber and write. Every room is perfect. It's one of few places where I can be productive. Even the yard is perfect. The elderly acres might slow most people down – a landscape too peaceful to inspire bustle – but for me, the stillness eliminates distraction.

Am I feeling homesick already?

Why else would I be writing about my house?

It would be one thing if we had spent the last five weeks journeying across the hot Southern sands. And I was tired and thirsty and missing the comforts of home. But we've only been on the road for five hours. Not nearly enough time to provoke longing.

I think I'm just nervous. And I'm thinking about home to soothe my nerves. I'm worried about life's coming changes. I'm worried about Cyn's audition. And I'm worried about the trip itself. About everything that could go wrong. Which includes the supposed sightings of the menace from Thorn terrorizing other travelers.

All morning, I've been hearing rustling noises in nearby bushes. And it's hard not to imagine the worst. When I see a black snake, I don't mistake it for a snake-shaped shadow. But when I see a long, slender shadow, I think *snake!* Likewise, *Thorn's evil demon!* has been my instinctive thought every time I hear birds or bushmoles scampering through the brambles.

But the trip has been uneventful so far. In a good way.

And now it's time to get moving again.

Twenty

Nyros, Second Lufoa, Day Sixteen. Night.

Our first day of traveling is done. It's made me realize how hermitted I've been lately. The average troglodyte is more community oriented. And has a better tan.

In my previous journal, I mentioned how the trip had been uneventful so far. Half an hour after writing that, we saw a family of black mallards. They were puddle fishing. Probably for tadpillars. About a hundred feet ahead of us. This always looks funny. They flap and flounder all dizzy and disoriented, bump into each other, squawk, dive for food, and come up empty-beaked. If they didn't act that way all the time, I would assume it was a fishing injury. Like maybe they stayed underwater too long and suffered anoxic stress.

When we recognized what the splashy commotion was up ahead, we were far enough away that they didn't notice us. Or they didn't *take* notice, anyway; they probably did see us in the distance. But we widened that distance in passing, driving the wagon well off the road. Slowly. Inconspicuously.

It took thirty minutes, but we managed to stay out of their aggression zone. Get too close and they'll attack. Which isn't scary on its own. Only a tiny, helpless babe would be harmed in the assault. But three or four days later, you'll wish you took the long way around. If the sky squirt is a chaotic omen, the black mallard is a literal ill omen: illness befalls anyone who comes into contact with it. They're vectors for a highly transmissible, highly terrible flu. We'd both survive, but there's no way Cyn could audition; we'd have to wait another year. So we doubled our distance and halved our speed. A bit more cautious than we needed to be.

Once their splashing was far enough behind us, Cyn and I returned to our conversation. For ten minutes. And then Wylmot nearly trampled a lumpy-milk wombat that was sleeping on the road. Which would not have ended happily for Wylmot. After such a smooth morning, we had two dangerous animal encounters in under an hour. Lightning arrives in storms, as they say.

The lumpy-milk wombat is a ubiquitous creature. Their total population is modest, but you can find them everywhere on Gaea. Or at least *mostly*where. I don't know how far north or south they go. In the middle belt, though, they ooze their belligerence from coast to coast, attacking anything that lives.

It may be Gaea's most aggressive aggressor, but it's only threatening if you don't have a long, sharp thing to stab it with. Wylmot has no such sharp thing, but I do. I have a sword. Not the wooden ones Cyn and I practice with, but my real, somewhat pointy, metal sword.

We were twenty feet past it when it woke up, came to its incensed senses, and charged. They aren't especially quick, so I had time get into position, standing between the back of the wagon and the wombat. And then I had time to doubt my ability. And time enough for that doubt to become worry. "I don't remember the last time I dispatched a threat with a sword", I thought. "Maybe this won't go well", my thinking continued. But I stood my ground.

It huffed and puffed its way toward me, unaware that fear is a sensation many other animals experience when charging a larger adversary. Who is holding a sharp thing. I stood still. Until it was inside striking distance. Then I struck. And killed it. And felt bad. But not *that* bad since I wasn't the one attacking. I was merely reacting. Still, it was asleep when we came tramping through its territory. Even the gentlest creatures are likely to be volatile in that situation. A knitter gillut might bite if it's frightened enough.

The animals that breed and feed closest to the roads are the only real dangers to the traveling class. Maybe they're defending a litter, or guarding a pile of food, or just plain territorial. I'm sympathetic to these beasts, however beastly their temperament, because we carelessly built our roads right through their homes. We can hardly blame them for retaliating. Or trying to shoo us away with a threatening display of claws or fangs. So I try to respect their authority. Not their *dominance* since I can probably prevail in a fight. If I'm armed with something pointy. But I respect their *dominion*. I'm trespassing on *their* land. If it's possible to retreat peacefully, I will. I'll only kill back if they attempt to kill me first. Like the lumpy-milk wombat did to me, and I did to it.

Now I'm thinking about animals in general. Not just wild, monsterly things, but dogs and cats, goats and geese, my lybax, Rorrik's gyfur, Lum's orkyt. None of these require furnishings to achieve comfort. That's what makes us a feeble species. By comparison. We insist on pads, pillows, and blankets. Perhaps a fire. And walls and roofs if it's windy or rainy.

There's no wind tonight. And it's not raining now, but the clouds are bloated. And they're always incontinent here. So we decided to make camp under the umbrella pines. Nature's impermeable roof. We found a perfect site. It's a hundred feet off the road, completely invisible to passersby, barely accessible by horse and cart, and seemingly undiscovered. Except by my father. It was marked on his map. Which explains our discovery.

After we chose our sleeping spots, the first thing I did was unpack our pads, pillows, and blankets. The second thing I did was gather wood for a fire. And the third thing I did was give a speech: "Six years is a long time", I began. Then, while attempting to start the fire, I said a bunch of coherent-ish things that were either congratulatory or sentimental. None of them memorable. Finally, the fire started to glow and smoke, and I ended my speech where it began: "Six years is a long time."

Cyn smiled and, very softly, murmured one of few international clichés her culture has produced and preserved: "Don't wake the winnower."

Being a Heimer, she deployed the expression correctly. But it *does* matter to me, the passage of time. Because I know how many years I've spent unwisely. Or at least unproductively. And these last six have been the most productive of my life. I can think of no wiser use of time than teaching someone who will be far wiser than I could ever be.

After my speech, we made dinner. The wombat I killed earlier. I don't like the killing of an animal to end with the execution. That's just about violence. But if you save and eat its carcass, then it's about sustenance. So we kept it. And cooked it. Along with some wild carrots we collected along the way. The green ones. And a few wild radishes. White ones that look like big teeth. And some wild seasonings. Which came in lots of colors.

There's a chapter in Brieona's *First Botany* called "The Wisdom of Plants". According to my mother, there is no finer a chapter written in any book on any subject. The theme is how plants make choices, and how those choices rule the world. We think we're in control, but we're not. We yield to flora. What would we eat if it weren't for their gifts? Their generosity is the only thing keeping us alive. That chapter was intended to inspire respect for the leafier members of Gaea, but the value I derived from it was in its utility as a recipe book. What plants can we eat raw? Which ones need to be cooked? And what floral horrors should we avoid altogether? That's where I learned how to discriminate the noxious from the delicious. And how to identify the bits of roadside wilderness that are worth plucking as we pass.

Also, while I was harvesting tonight's vegetables, Cyn was apparently stung by a honeyjacket. She didn't say anything. I just saw a big red patch on her forearm while we were eating.

Maybe that was the great surprise promised by the squirt sighting.

I'm losing light. Time to put the journal away.

Twenty-One

Eldos, Second Lufoa, Day Seventeen. Morning.

I never sleep well when I'm away from home. The nights are restless. I feel like the world isn't quite right. And I need it to be at ease to release my mind. Otherwise, I just lie there all night, tangled in thoughts. That's half the reason I bought back my childhood home.

The only time I've ever been able to sleep on the road is when I was young, and my father brought me on his cross-country trips. In this same wagon. Decades before he gave it to me. For half of those miles, I slept peacefully. Not disrespectfully; my imagination wasn't pretending I was somewhere else. It was a matter of trust. I've never been able to fall asleep in transit with anyone else driving. They're going to run the wheels through roots and holes, tip the carriage on a bank, break down in the middle of Bandits' Bend, or get us lost somewhere worse. I couldn't shake the feeling that if I fell asleep – even for a minute – something bad would startle me awake. With my father, though, I always knew we were safe.

But this trip is different. Because I'm the one driving. So there's no rest along the way. And after the day's travel, when I lay on my bedroll, I don't slip easily into slumber. My mind disobeys my wishes. I want it to keep quiet, and the cacophony blares. I request that it sit still, and it goes wandering off in unexpected places.

Even at home, I don't sleep through the night. I do well in the early hours, and okay in the late hours, but in between, I'm usually awake. The middle of the night is when my mind normally decides to be at its most alert. Last night was different though. It took a long time to fall asleep, but when I finally did, a brief and bizarre dream promptly began. And at the end of it, I woke up. And that was all the sleep I got.

I do think dreams can tell us *something* about ourselves… in that they function as a mirror of our thoughts. Our worries and values and perceptions get reflected back to us in the night. And we're given the opportunity to confront them in a risk-free environment. Should we make poor choices, morning will extinguish any remorse like the sun to a shadow. This enables us to attempt creative solutions with impunity. Which can help prepare us if we encounter similar situations in waking life. Seems useful. But I think that's the extent of a dream's utility. Trying to extract further meaning strikes me as foolish.

"And then this happened, and then that happened, and then I squeezed some lemons into my tea, but when I went to fish out the seeds, there were bones in it, and then I woke up! What do you think it means?"

"Nothing", although typically received as an insult, is the only honest answer.

On the subject of meaningless nothingness, here's the dream I had last night: Cyn and I were back in Estevro. *Still* in Estevro. We never left for Pendelhall. It was late in the evening, and we were sitting on the back terrace staring up at a full moon. Lonvaraka had settled on the eastern edge of town. Despite the miles between us, we could hear the music clearly. They were performing the Urdrose. Near the end of the fifth act, Elyem Syofa, the moon suddenly sped from the sky. As though it were a setting sun, except fast and without any of the grandeur. Like a coat falling from its hanger. Cyn and I stopped breathing. So did the wind. And the music ceased, too. We just sat in that stillness and silence, watching the empty horizon where the moon once hung, waiting for something to happen. Every passing second felt like an hour. Three seconds, four seconds, five seconds, six seconds. Breathless and still. Then the sensation came. If you've ever been sledding in Arzox, you know that initial feeling of plunging after cresting a sharp hill. The feeling of being unfastened from gravity that rushes through your chest and head. And then you land, your body reunites with Gaea's pull, and the feeling passes.

When I was young, that was my favorite part of sledding. But in my dream, it was just scary. We were watching the architecture of the universe collapse like rickety scaffolding. One minute, we were sitting on my terrace listening to an Urdrose. And the next, we were thrust into a vast void, hurtling past dark comets and bright worlds encircled by rings. We were standing on a plunging planet with no idea where we were going or when it would end. Still weightless in my head and heart, loved ones began to gather. The people who matter most to me started appearing all around. And then I woke up. And that was all the sleep I got.

I'm sure Rorrik, who was present at the end of my dream, would spend all morning analyzing it, deciphering a dissertation's worth of meaning from the nonsense. And his meaning would have nothing in common with anyone else's. "Your life feels out of control, so you seek stability", or some such. That's not what Rorrik would say. He'd ask all about the gravity in my dream. And about the wind and shadows and colors. A long, spirited interrogation. There are a million reasons why I wish Rorrik was here with Cyn and me, but for this one reason, I'm glad he isn't. As long as he's safe, of course.

But now it's time to start the day's miles.

Twenty-Two

Eldos, Second Lufoa, Day Seventeen. Afternoon.

We just stopped for lunch. Later than expected. Because we traveled farther than expected. About an hour later and half an hour farther. Because we encountered an extremely dangerous animal. We were almost ready to stop when we saw it. It was off in the distance, too far away to tell what it was. Then we saw it at a nearer distance. And then we saw it at an even-nearer-than-that distance. And that's when I realized what it was: the largest land species in the East with a penchant for person meat.

The most lethal feature of the garlok isn't its dagger-sharp teeth and claws, but its seeming lack of threat. The creature wobbles slowly, playfully, deceptively in the direction of its prey. The closer it gets, the more deceptive it becomes. It has what Farhearth zoologists call "paedomorphic features"; in other words, it is adorably childlike. Its face does not resemble that of a fearsome predator. "If garloks are going to attack us, why do they have such cute ears?" was probably the last thought of every person a garlok has killed. That juvenile cuteness is the boobytrap that tricks us into the monster's jaw. It only becomes scary once the mouth opens. Then it's suddenly terrifying. But before then, while its mouth is closed and smiling gleefully, all you notice is its cuddly ears and enormous eyes. Their size is not pointless. If it weren't for the curvature of Gaea, a garlok's field of vision would encompass the entire world, from pole to pole. Unless its line of sight is obstructed, it could probably spot you from the moon. And unless it recently ate to satiety, it will pursue you as steadily and tirelessly as the moon's orbit. There is no respite from the hunt until it is complete. Predation will continue for days if that's what it takes. Garloks aren't particularly fast sprinters, so they can be outrun. For a time. And they aren't particularly quick, so they can be outmaneuvered. For a time. But they aren't susceptible to fatigue or discouragement. So they cannot be outlasted. And so they cannot be escaped. And so, in time, they always succeed.

As I am alive enough to write this, I obviously survived. Here's the story of our encounter:

It's late morning, almost noon. And Cyn and I are walking beside the horse. We don't ride in the caravan every minute of the trip. Sometimes, we need to move, exercise our legs. Especially if we plan to eat soon. We always walk for at least forty-five minutes first. To earn a few of the coming calories.

We were about half an hour into this walk when we saw the big brown blob moving in the far-off distance. Far off to the west. Which is very far east of a garlok's natural habitat. This was an unexpected place to see one. And an equally unexpected time of day. I should know; that was my first dissertation. The unusual hour – during peak pitikos activity – and foreign location are what prevented me from identifying the wobbling blob sooner. Once I did, however, I was much more frightened than I would have otherwise been. Because if the garlok's behavior was as unpredictable as its time and place, Cyn and I would have no chance at survival. Whereas if its behavior was typical of its species, we had *one* chance.

The garlok isn't very widely known. In small part because I never published that dissertation. In much larger part because they aren't widely threatening. They exclusively reside in a confined region of the Birdsong Meadow, where nobody ever goes. Except for *this* garlok, which was east of the River Grey. And that makes it the first of its species to threaten people in the acres that civilization owns. At least the first one I know of.

A garlok will hunt the biggest thing moving within the boundaries of its horizon. And Cyn and I were the second biggest things on the move. Behind only our horse. Wylmot would have certainly been the first victim, but the garlok would have killed all three of us before taking its first bite.

I guess we could have set Wylmot free, hoping the garlok would chase him into the next horizon. But that would have been both cruel and inconvenient. First: Wylmot has been in my family for twenty years. He was born in my grandfather's yard. I'm not inclined to use him as bait. Second: how would we tow the wagon to Pendelhall?

But what other option did we have? This is not a skirmish we could win with a sword. Nor one we had a chance of escaping. A garlok may look sluggish. It may even *be* sluggish. But it can catch and kill any horse.

"Don't move", I said – calmly but assertively – and then I started to slink slowly backward. It probably appeared as though I were offering Cyn up for sacrifice, hiding behind her. But Cyn trusted me. As I knew she would. Obviously, if one of us could be sacrificed to save the other, I would have been slinking *forward*. But I stepped back. And then back again. And maybe five or six more agains. Until I reached the rear door of the wagon. I climbed inside, opened the hidden bench chamber, and pulled out my old-but-intact pitikos whistle. While still hidden from the garlok's line of sight, I began to blow into it. I hadn't tested it in years. So I had no idea if it would work. But it was the only option I could think of to save Cyn, me, *and* Wylmot.

The instant my breath entered the chamber, a shrill screech rang out so loud, I had to plug my ears. But I didn't want to drop the whistle. So I covered one ear with my free hand, and I half-plugged the other by tilting my head into a shrugged shoulder. Good enough. I kept blowing. And blowing.

At first, the wagon was being jostled around violently. I think Wylmot was startled by the sound, and he was romping and bucking in response. But then everything became calm, piercing noise aside. Since I couldn't see what was happening, I had no idea what that calmness meant. So I continued to blow. For a full minute, I hyperventilated into that once-upon-a-pitikos throat.

Finally, dizzily, I peeked outside. And I didn't see the garlok. So I climbed out and joined Cyn, who was standing exactly where I left her. Except she was trying to soothe a startled Wylmot, petting his muzzle and speaking in a relaxed voice. *Sort of* relaxed. There was a slight vibrato in her tone. And her pupils were gigantic, dilated by the panic.

"Inevitable death evited", I said, attempting to coin a phrase. I don't expect that particular coin to do very well in the idiomatic economy, but it's the best I could do in the midst of my own panic.

Cyn charitably ignored my attempt at wit and said, "Is that what I think it is?" She wasn't referring to the hulking monster, but the device that drove it away. Her voice was still quivering from the excess of adrenaline splashing around in circulation, but her curiosity remained unflustered.

"It is", I said while handing her the whistle. Then we both started laughing. Not because anything was funny, but because everything was tense. So much tension that our brains conflated it with humor. Sometimes this can help relieve it. This was one of those times.

After our nervous giggles ended, we started moving again, both of us walking beside Wylmot, eyes fixed on the western horizon. We traveled this way for about forty-five minutes before we felt safe enough to stop. And before we regained our appetites. Which the garlok had scared away.

Our previous plan was to eat some meat and caravan cookies and move on. But after nearly dying, Cyn offered to make a more comforting meal. To help restore our wits. She's been preparing it for as long as I've been writing this. But "preparing" has just become past tense. So now it's time to eat. Then it will be time to go.

I think I'll keep the pitikos whistle in my pocket for the rest of the trip.

Twenty-Three

Eldos, Second Lufoa, Day Seventeen. Night.

We set up camp early tonight. The sun hadn't set yet. Hadn't even started. But we're farther than we planned to be, and there aren't any good campsites in this stretch. If there's any reason to stop at all, my father didn't mark it in his maps. But the weather is perfect. We couldn't ask for a better canopy than the open sky. So we pulled the wagon over. About ten feet off the road. Against the brush line, beside a couple of trees. Then we built a cookfire. Away from the brush and trees. In a flat span of low grass. And we started making dinner.

Just as it began to sizzle, we heard neighing in the distance. A minute later, we saw two horses towing a carriage in our direction. Another minute later, we were met with "ahoy!"s and other common greetings.

All the travelers-by we had seen previously had passed us silently. Not rudely. They just had old-fashioned etiquette: when you see another carriage coming, you move over. And then you nod at one another as you pass. That's the wagoner's way. The earlier and farther you move over, the more courtesy you show. It's completely unnecessary. Between Pendelhall and Farhearth, the Grass Road is broad enough to hold two carriages driving abreast. The generous berth is just about the gesture. It's the lack of necessity that makes it polite. But the entire effort is ruined if you speak. Because then you're insisting on a response. Which is a rude thing to demand of a tired traveler.

Being my father's son, I'm an extremist here. I move over ludicrously early. And far. And my nod is practically a full-bodied bow. And I never speak. Until this evening, anyway. When I was met with some "ahoy!"s... and other common greetings. In total, there were six people. And all of them were insisting on a response.

I didn't have the energy to address each person individually. So I muttered "hi everyone" at the lot of them. And gave half a wave.

"We're looking to hunker down for the night; can we trouble you for a seat at your fire?", the driver asked.... after already pulling off the road.

"Actually, do you mind going somewhere else where we can't see you?" is what I wanted to say. But didn't. Instead, I asked, "Where are you headed?"

"Farhearth. We're submitting our work to the Faire."

"You're researchers?"

"Among other things. We're a motley mix of medics."

Everything about that response – even the tone – sounded rehearsed. Which made it sound dubious. The kind of thing I would expect a bandit to say. But "Are you bandits who killed some researchers and stole their wagon?" didn't seem like the right question to ask. So I asked about their research.

They took turns explaining their projects. With enthusiasm. But that's easy to fake. So I interrogated them with extremely detailed follow-up questions about data collection, methods of analysis, relevant physiological principles, and so on. Believable answers here would be impossible for a bandit to fake. And they passed my test, revealing competence in every response. So I set my suspicion aside and explained that Cyn and I were also going to submit research at Farhearth. "Although not until after the tournament", I specified.

"Are you spectators or competitors?", one of them asked.

I didn't want to admit that Cyn was auditioning to be the Pendelhall Medic. "This one's fixin' to be the most elite clinician in your city!", while pointing at Cyn. A response that uncouth would make honest men commit banditry. But I didn't want to lie either. So I just praised Pendelhall instead. "In part, it's your hometown we're visiting. No better place to be this time of year."

"I agree. But it's different for locals. This is the only time of year we *do* leave. Finals are on the twenty-fifth. We're aiming to get back on the twenty-sixth." And then one of them asked, "Where's local for you?"

I loathe this question. Because when I say Estevro, people always respond, "If you can afford to leave, why would you stay?"

This question makes two false assumptions:

First, that leaving is affordable. I understand this one. My wagon gives an impression of wealth I do not possess. Wealth enough to be a "hillclimber".

Second, that leaving is preferable. By leaving, they mean moving up the hill. And this one I *don't* understand. It's like asking, "Why would you choose to eat a thagimallo if a komallo is available?" I've been asked that before, too. It assumes komallos are *objectively* better than thagimallos, which isn't true.

There's a similar question that science denialists frequently utter at biologists: "If people evolved from gimuts, how come gimuts still exist?" For those who have never been to the Hallowed Grove, a gimut is a diminutive tree ape that dwells exclusively on the center island, sleeps exclusively on Nemusenex's branches, and has been critically endangered since it was discovered.

The "how come gimuts still exist?" question makes two false assumptions:

First, that we evolved from gimuts. We didn't. Gimuts and humans simply share an ancestor. And while our mutual foremother surely resembles gimuts more than she does humans, that's not the same as us evolving *from* them. Rather, we are cousins. *Distant* cousins. Far enough removed that never the twain shall breed. Neither species is sky squirty enough in its capacity to produce progeny, and so our lineages are destined to remain distinct.

Second, that being a human is better than being a gimut. "Why would any gimut opt to remain a gimut?" implies humans are simply upgraded versions of them. But that's not how evolution works. Every species – including humans, gimuts, and lumpy-milk wombats – is a product of its environment. Traits that confer an advantage within that environment are preserved in the succeeding generation, while disadvantageous traits perish with the deceased. Neither species is "better" than the other; our viability is simply tuned to the orchestra in which we play.

But even within a generation, our individual penchants are partly determined by our environments. In the flats, we have an expression for this: "Sauce fosters the turnip." In other words, what you sauté your vegetables in changes the nature of those vegetables. You can rear sourgums to be sweet or figgyplums to be sour. Likewise, the cultural pressures marinading any city's maturing children will change the nature of *those* turnips.

Harthies have a different expression, evidently derived from the old North, which has a similar meaning: "From cloud to ground." Originally, it meant raindrops, snowflakes, and hail pellets are assembled by the environments the water droplets pass through between their birth in the clouds and their death on the ground. Accordingly, hard-as-hail warriors are not born, they're reared into the role. That explains a lot about parenting practices in the old North. But today's version of the expression – the Farhearth interpretation – is much softer: as snow passes from cloud to ground, the shape of the flake is formed. Each one is unique, but no flake is "better" than any other. Every structure is simply a reflection of the environment whence it fell. And just like the clouds above, every culture below has a climate of its own… which rears countless unique individuals… none of whom are "better" than anyone else.

I accept that no Gaean is born better than any other. But I do think Estevro is a better "climate" than Thevro. Because it shapes its flakes with patriotism. And honesty. And a desire for self-betterment. Hillians have no interest in any of these. As for patriotism, the only care they have for their community is in the comparison. It's not enough for a Thevroan to live a lavish life. The lives of their peers must be comparatively less lavish. Envy is the commodity most prized upon that hill. So wealth is often sought at the expense of one's neighbors. Conversely, at the base of the hill, solidarity pools with the rain. Those who reside in a heaven high above the sea are not risen by a rising tide. It's the humble and the meek who help each other succeed. Patriotism is the province of the poor. As for honesty, any day of the week, half the surfaces in Thevro will be coated in wet paint. To cover the stains, the rust, the cracks. Beneath the vibrant sheen, it's a broken city. And the hillians themselves are no more forthright, hiding their diseases and depravity under stylish fabrics. Estevro, by comparison, is honest in its weakness. Its decay. Its utter lack of glamor. It conceals nothing. And I'll take worn-out honesty over elegant secrecy any day. And, lastly, no hillian seeks self-betterment because that would be an admission of imperfection. Just listen to them in conversation. There's no desire for learning; all they care about is winning. Any indication of curiosity is a ruse. If they ask a question, they already know the answer. Or they think they do, anyway. The less they know, the haughtier they are. And the more *you* know, the more muzzling they become.

All things summed: no amount of wealth could induce me to climb that hill. I may not always feel like an Easterner, but Estevro is where I belong.

Did I say all of this (or any of it) to the Pendelian who asked, "Where's local for you?"

No. I simply said, "Estevro." And before he had a chance to respond, I said, "By the way, there's a garlok ahead. Half a day south, west of the road."

While expressions of dismay and disbelief were quietly grappling on his face, I faked a gaping-mouthed yawn and said, "Well, I guess we should pack it in for the night. Fire's all yours." Then Cyn and I took our pan off the fire, went to our wagon, and ate in peace. Or, failing peace, at least we ate alone. The Pendelians are *still* talking about the garlok. But now it's time for sleep.

Waning half-moon tonight. And our last night on the road. At this time tomorrow, we'll already be in Pendelhall.

Twenty-Four

Seros, Second Lufoa, Day Eighteen. Morning.

I remember my dreams better while I'm traveling. Not because I sleep more or better. But because I sleep less and worse. I wake up constantly. To the sound of the wind separating an acorn from its branch. To the sound of a squirrel burying that acorn. To the sound of a mosquito shrieking in my ear. Often, these interruptions yank me from the peak of a dream. So I'm thrust back into the waking world with a vivid image in tow.

That's what happened last night. I was exhausted by the events of the day, so consciousness abandoned me quickly. But not deeply. Nature remained restless, and her noises fragmented my sleep. I got twenty minutes here, thirty minutes there, and each fragment seemed to have a dream of its own. All but one were too dull to describe. And that one I've had a hundred times before: my flying dream.

I'm not flapping and swooping around like a bird. Its closer to floating than flying. I take a breath, squat, leap, and soar about fifty feet above Gaea, as if unhinged from the cords of gravity. And I remain suspended in the upper air for several minutes. Until, eventually, I sink slowly back to the ground. Then I leap again.

Every time I have this dream, I'm trying to escape something. Some wicked creature that's stalking me. But it can't float through the air like I can; it just waits for me below. So I jump out of its reach, coast, land, and jump again. And again. I'll land safely four or five times, but as I begin the next descent, I find myself headed straight for it. Closer and closer. And then I wake up.

If Rorrik happens to be there when I do, he'll dissect the dream, isolate each nonsensical image, reconfigure them into a coherent narrative, and extract a prescription. And it's never what you expect. Like if I had a dream where I was roaming around asking people if they knew where any rabbits were, so I could start a rabbitry (that was one of last night's *other* dreams), Rorrik would insist I fix my posture. Or that I was allergic to that little spot of blood inside of chicken eggs. Or something even more bizarre and impossible to predict.

Like all Westerners, he gets carried away with his interpretations. He thinks everything is prophetic. Dreams most of all. They must "mean" something. Probably because they're free. One cannot purchase them from a merchant.

They simply visit us in our sleep, and there's no entrance fee for that venue. If prophecies discriminate social or financial rank at all, they seem to frequent the dreams of the meek more regularly. Scarcely do they anoint the waking wealthy with their promises of great fates and purposes. The social order of Dreamland is wholly separate from the society we experience outside of bed.

Hillians see prophesy differently. Less humanely. They believe prosperity is a fate chosen by the universe. So every coin held is justly hoarded. By asking the wealthy to share, you are violating the very will of Gaea.

Pretty much every hillian subscribes to that creed. Less common, but more obnoxious, is the hillian newspaperist. Not ordinary journalists who report ordinary stories. Thevro has plenty of them. But the *Chronicle* writers who see *themselves* as prophets. And they boast endlessly if any of their predictions come true. No explicit prediction has ever transpired, though. It's only poetic ambiguities that dubiously come to pass. The flowers in the prose contain the only pollens that fertilize. So, those newspaperists garland tiny facts in beautiful, fragrant gibberish.

For some reason, I still subscribe.

...

I finished that last sentence ten minutes ago.

I planned to write more on the subject, but I needed to relieve my bladder. So I put down my pen, walked twenty feet into the brush, behind some trees, and began to urinate.

Then I heard a footfall. A heavy one.

It was beyond the brush that was collecting my urine.

I stopped peeing. I stopped breathing. I stopped whispering my thoughts aloud, working out the phrasing of the sentences I was going to write when I returned to my journal.

I didn't have my sword. Or any other way to defend myself. Or any idea what I would have to defend myself against.

I just stood there – frozen, silent – staring in the direction of the sound.

And then I saw it: an adult yrtog. No more than twenty feet away.

I couldn't see its belly, so I couldn't tell whether it was a lok or mox – male or female. The yrlok is relatively harmless. But the yrmox is a rampaging monster permanently on the brink of a riot. A single-creature stampede.

I played the role of a statue with a two-thirds full bladder, barely breathing, watching the yrtog munch on a stillpine. It wasn't devouring it whole, like a hymog. It was only eating the sweet, sticky, resin-covered cones that collect and arrest every fleck of pollen that passes by. It's as if each cone's thousand pineal scales are designed to seize anything that moves and send it to sleep. And so the wind itself learns to avoid the stillpines. Or so it seems. And the yrtogi calm themselves by dining on them. Or so it seems.

I stood still, watching it eat, for maybe five minutes. That's how long it took the creature to pluck seven honeycones from the branches. While carefully avoiding the needles.

And then it trampled onward, southward, through the brambles.

Once I could no longer see it, I crept back to the campsite. And wrote this. I didn't want to start driving the wagon immediately and make a big show of motion. That might attract it back.

But it's probably far enough south by now that we can move without being obliterated. And still close enough that we *should* get moving.

We'll skip the formality of a stationary breakfast this morning. But I'll warn the Pendelian researchers before we leave. They might consider delaying their trip. Otherwise, it'll be a dangerous road ahead. A long, lethal gantlet flanked by a garlok to the west and an yrtog to the east.

Twenty-Five

Seros, Second Lufoa, Day Eighteen. Afternoon.

We neither heard nor saw the yrtog again. I think we're safe now.

I hope the same is true for the Pendelians. But I'm less confident. Because every time we crested a hill, I looked behind us. And scanned the horizon. And I never saw a wagon. I take that to mean the researchers are still headed south. Undaunted. Perhaps five hours into their gantlet.

During those five hours, I must have eaten at least fifteen caravan cookies. Whenever I'm this tired, my body confuses sleeplessness with foodlessness. "If I just eat some more, maybe I'll wake up", my body reasons. Even though gluttony has never once resulted in wakefulness.

But I knew I wouldn't be able to sleep, so I sat in the driver's seat all morning. It wasn't bad. Except for the wind. Which was aggressive for the last hour. And not steady. It came in explosive gusts. As though nature were sneezing. Which makes *me* sneeze. Like watching someone else yawn, I find myself involuntarily imitating the action.

I feel like I've met my year's quota of sneezes. And Cyn has met her year's quota of bee stings. She was stung again. Another honeyjacket. That's twice in three days.

I'm all for wildflower reproduction, but the means of pollination – the bees and the breeze – have obvious downsides. My symptoms will go away when the wind relents. Cyn will be itchy for a few days yet.

At least it was only honeyjackets. If I had to be stung by something, and I got to pick what it was, that's the bee I'd choose.

In the south of the North, you're in whitejacket territory. Not a happy place to be for people with an allergy. If you weren't already wheezing from the frigid air, a couple of those stings will rattle your lungs. In the southern East and eastern South, the blackjackets riddle their stingees with edema. And in the northwestern West, the bumblejaws reign. Those striped puff balls that lack stingers. I don't remember what they're actually – apiologically – called. But they almost appear cuddly, buzzing clumsily around a flower. Until you get too close. And they bite. And leave behind pits where flesh used to be.

All four species – the three jackets and the bumblers – make honey. It's one of the great examples of alchemy taught at Farhearth. There are specialized structures in the bees' foregut which have enzymes to convert the ingested nectar into everybody's favorite toast topper. Although bumblejaw honey is nobody's favorite. It stinks like it's made of meat. Which it probably is.

As I write this, Cyn is making lunch. "Want help?", I asked.

"It's okay. Keep writing. I'll let you know when it's ready."

"You sure?"

"You'd just sneeze in it."

I was holding in a sneeze at the time. So I didn't respond.

"By the way, I think I'm done with the cookies", Cyn added. "So the rest are yours." Probably because they're sweetened with honey. From honeyjackets. And, again, Cyn has recently met her year's quota of those critters.

I guess the good news is that her arm has no pit in it. Her lungs aren't rattling. And her legs aren't swollen. She just has some red, itchy spots. And I'm just sneezy. And will continue to be until the wind calms down.

I do wonder how animals perceive the wind. Wylmot doesn't seem fazed. Which I think is weird. Because how would he know what wind is? Or air in general? What does he think he's breathing?

At Farhearth, I learned that invisibility does not imply emptiness. The air is composed of several different molecules. Recently, chemists have managed to divide those invisible constituents, segregate them into separate chambers, and study their properties individually. And they discovered unique features and behaviors of each gas. I also learned – through publications, lectures, and laboratory experimentation – how the air can be heated like a pot of tea. And this heating occurs upon land faster than it does over the sea. The hotter the air, the faster it rises. And as the "kettles" of warm air are lifted, gales of colder air blow in to occupy the would-be-empty space. And blast me with pollens they've picked up along the way. And then I sneeze. Mystery solved: the wind and its effects on my lungs are non-mystical phenomena.

Animals, though. Horses, garloks, yrtogi. They aren't eligible to enroll at Farhearth. So they have no way of learning this. So I wonder: what do they think wind is? A ghost? An invisible apparition eternally tormenting them?

That's what I would think if I were a member of a species without scientists. I would believe Gaea was just a huge, round haunted house. And that would be unsettling. But animals never seem unsettled by the wind. So perhaps they think it's something else. Maybe it's the spirit of their ancestors gently (or gustily) reminding them of their presence. And maybe those breezy spirits are the basis of animal religions. Although if that were true, you'd think all fauna would migrate to the West, where the winds feel alive. So maybe that's not it. Maybe there's more to think about on the subject.

But Cyn is telling me that lunch is ready. So I'm going to put these thoughts away and eat. And then we'll get moving. Last leg of the trip. We'll be in Pendelhall this evening. And sleeping in comfortable beds tonight.

Twenty-Six

Seros, Second Lufoa, Day Eighteen. Night.

In his younger years, Wylmot won a sled pulling contest. Set some sort of record, I'm told. I wasn't there. That was my father's thing. And his father's. And probably his father's. These days, Wylmot is well past his pulling prime, but he's a purebred dragan. Not a drag*on*, the scaly, winged fake thing, but a *dragan*, the uncommon and uncommonly bulky horse breed. And Wylmot is on the brawnier side of that brawniest bloodline.

Despite his stubby legs, which take a full hand off his height, he stands a bit over seventeen hands at the withers. Back in his prime, he weighed two bits over two-thousand pounds. He's lost some since, but not much. And every bit of his bulk is lean. His age is clearly shown in his cloud-colored muzzle, but not in his muscle. Strap him to a stone-sled and he could still outpull all those eager colts and brown-muzzled stallions. But not two days in a row. Wylmot gets tired. Like me. He can't go day after day like he used to. Or as many miles in a day as he used to. He's just as magnificent as he ever was, but he needs more rest. So I was nervous about the day-after-daying he'd have to endure on this trip. But we finally made it. We arrived in Pendelhall. Wylmot took us all the way without showing any sign of strain.

Although, when we were approaching the front gate, maybe half a mile away, he was nearly bit by a naga croc. It was in the road, lying still, warming itself. Those narrow-bodied, slithering reptiles mostly reside in the shallow waters around the Delta. And they warm themselves on the sand. But occasionally, they wander near the road. Or, in this case, onto the road.

Wylmot charged ahead. He didn't even neigh to warn it of our approach.

I was distracted at the time, staring at the regal towers rising in the distance. So I didn't see the croc until it was too late. Too late to do anything but gasp. And Wylmot didn't lose a hoof strike. Didn't hesitate at all. He marched straight at it. As if aiming for it.

When he entered snapping distance, the croc fled. It scrambled off the road. In the direction of the water. And Wylmot marched onward. Proudly. Looking half a hand taller. Clearly perceiving himself invincible.

Then we arrived at the gates.

Pendelhall is the most inspiring city anywhere on Gaea. Visitation functions as a remedy for lethargy. All you have to do is look up. And see the pennants lining the ramparts, endlessly snapping in the Eldsyn wind. They never fall slack. And the people beneath those pennants exhibit the same vigor. One cannot walk the streets and lack for luster.

Being here musters a feeling of sentimentality. Which animates my ambition. It makes me eager to fence. Maybe I could enter the competition once more. Or maybe even apply for the Pendelhall Medic position after Cyn has finished her first term. Then my imagination slips off its leash: if I were appointed, the two of us could take turns serving in the Operating and Incumbent roles. I could build a second career – a much more important and exciting one – in the natural gaps between Cyn's service. We'd have unlimited resources to pursue our research. We could lead medicine into frontiers of our choosing. Why tend my garden between naps when I could create a meaningful legacy?

Then I stop looking up. And I reason myself out of those foolish thoughts. Inspiration of this kind is a form of lust. It's chased in the heat of passion, and it seldom ends happily.

There is an earlier age that we remember with such affection. In our quiet moments, we look over our shoulders and reminisce, longing for its return. It was an age of loyalty and honesty. An age of bravery and achievement. An age that never *really* existed at all. But we think it did. And we remember it so fondly. And what else would we defend so strongly? Or endeavor to revive so ardently?

The reality is: my life is good at the moment. That's not to say I don't lament the loss of earlier moments. I can dig complaints out of any soil. But I can also recognize the beauty that grows there. And I don't want to yank out the flowers for the sake of adventure. Plus, I need to focus on the present goal: Cyn's audition. Although the fencing tournament doesn't begin for five days, Pendelhall is already crowded.

We're staying at an inn in Billets, the oldest district outside the fortress itself. We didn't get the inn I wanted. Eldsyn Tower. I don't know if it's my *favorite*, but it's the nicest. And it's close to the rings. Instead, I got us adjacent rooms in Pygil's. Which has… charm. It's different from the rest. Even the name itself. It's a misspelling of a breed of cat. You'd think the woodworker who created the sign would have noticed the proprietor's error before carving its elaborate heraldry. It's like the inn isn't from here. It's in a district of its own. That exists in an older world. One that's more fitting to Cyn and me, I guess. And close enough to the fencing. So that's where we're staying.

The crowds, which crowded us out of Eldsyn Tower, are partly here for the wrestling, boxing, and regnavus championships. Those begin the day after tomorrow, the day after that, and the day after that.

The annual Colloquium of Mayors is also going on now. And lasts all week. But only mayoral staff are here for that. And I'm sure they're staying inside the Keep itself.

There's likely to be *some* daily turnover in Eldsyn Tower, so I'll check for vacancy on occasion, but I suspect most people are here for the fencing. Early arrival, early registration, and a week of rest to recover from the travel, scope out the competition, and train.

If you're an aspiring anything – medic, fighter, military strategist, whatever – you'll be here. Either competing or in the crowd.

Or, in Cyn's case, under the mending tent.

It's funny how celebrated the Pendelhall Tournament is. In all three sports, the winner is glorified as the best in all of Gaea. Unanimously. Indisputably. For a single year. The "world champion" title is not susceptible to change until the next Pendelhall Tournament. No matter what happens in between.

What I find funny is how many other championships occur throughout the year in which most of the top athletes compete. The winner of the Pendelhall Tournament often loses in a different championship during the same season. But no spectator sees it, no paper reports on it, and no crown changes heads. To most Gaeans, the Pendelhall Tournament is the only contest that matters.

Registration opens in the morning for both fencers and auditioning medics. And I'll be anxious until Cyn's station at the mending tent is formalized. Then I'll be anxious until the winner is announced. I'm confident Cyn will be appointed, but getting an audition at all is a career highlight.

The committee spends months reading reference letters. My letter for Cyn was the only time I've ever written a recommendation for anything exceeding a page. It exceeded ten. And it was one of perhaps a thousand other letters they received.

From that deep pool of applicants, the committee selects five candidates and two contingents. The contingents are eligible to be called up if a candidate withdraws. Cyn was the first contingent, and there was one withdrawal. So, she was invited to occupy the vacated seat.

That means Cyn is right on the edge.

And that gives me anxiety.

Which we could remedy with a trip to the apothecary.

And then we could go explore the wider city. To harvest my old nostalgia and plant some new seeds.

But not tonight. After being on the road for three days and barely sleeping, a long rest in a soft bed, not beset by nature, is too inviting to leave waiting.

We'll start early tomorrow.

It's Opening Ceremonies, but there isn't anything we need to be present for. Registration aside.

Twenty-Seven

Aldos, Second Lufoa, Day Nineteen. Morning.

Last night, I finished my journal, took a warm bath, then went straight to bed. This morning, I woke up disheveled and didn't bother to address it. Or eat. Or write. I just got dressed, went to the room next door, and woke up Cyn. Then we went to Citadel Square to register. Fencing starts in four days.

We got to the registration table *really* early. Not even the sun was willing to be there at that hour. And the workers weren't going to beat the sun to work. We assumed if it was still dark out when we arrived, there would be no line. So we would only have to wait for forty-five minutes, an hour at the most. Whereas if we showed up *after* registration opened, we were at risk of waiting all day. Because it's a single line that everyone uses to register for everything. Contestants in wrestling, boxing, regnavus, and fencing, and the personnel serving each one. Everyone gets in the same line. And by showing up early, we could find a spot in front.

We waited for three hours. Because the line was already long. And we were among the least disheveled people in it. The people ahead of us appeared to have slept in their positions.

By the time we got to the front, the line behind us was substantially longer than one we started behind. So it was worth showing up when we did. Also, we got to see the procession of mayors pass us, headed to the Colloquium. About fifteen minutes before the registration staff came, they paraded by, two by two, bickering politely. Mischaracterizations of each other's interests, so articulate. Patronizing complements, so eloquent. I can only imagine what the conversations sound like once they're inside the war chamber.

Every year, most of Gaea's cities are represented. All of them are invited. And they're all urged to attend. But only some of them do the attending. From the East, it's all of them. Provided you don't count the Gaea Whalers as a mayorally represented unit. They have no interest in the politics of the "noakraska" (the rivalry between those seafarers and their landfaring cousins is comparable to the enmity between the hillians and flatties). In the West, the mayors of Lir, Laberyn, and Midrodor never miss a Colloquium. Given the recent attack in Laberyn, I had wondered if this year would be different. But then I saw a Labero among the ranks. Sauntering in unmistakable attire. They put considerable effort into having their garments appear free of effort.

Lir and Midrodor are comparably recognizable in their fashions, but for very different reasons. I saw both of those mayors in this morning's procession as well. I did not see an Adonian. It would have been unexpected if I had; Adonere almost never sends a delegate. *Exactly* never has any Druinite or Mulgothan attended. And that tradition was upheld with this Colloquium. In the South, Baguzu, Moonkruug, and Eldergard are represented every year. Cinderheim: no years. Not for a lack of invitations, or insistence that they accept those invitations, or extravagant convoys sent to their gates. Heimers simply prioritize work and can't be bothered with frivolous wastages of time. Such as political meetings. And, of course, Yaga-Goro receives no invitation. Because where would one send it? No one knows if that city is even real. The Nameless Isle is real, but its inhabitants are snubbed. Because they don't reside within the Connected Continents. So they aren't granted a voice in its governance.

All cities summed, there are thirteen mayors who do the determining of our global politics. And I saw all thirteen this morning, each of them wearing their nation's colors. But there was one more figure in attendance this year. A fourteenth "mayor": Bonstan. He was wearing *all* the nations' colors.

Bonstan, who has never served any public office, was leading the procession. Not by himself, but in the ceremonial two-by-twoing, he was paired with Pendelhall's mayor. In the front of the line. Behind them strode the mayors of Eldergard and Midrodor, the foreign capitals. And they were followed by everyone else.

Bonstan is not one to waste time and resources *pretending* to serve. If he's in the line, he'll sit at the table… where the most important decisions affecting all Gaeans are made. The conflicts of interest here are troubling. Giving a merchant legislative authority cannot possibly result in fair economic policy.

And of course, Bonstan wasn't alone. His wife and son were with him in line. I wouldn't have known who they were, but the woman was holding Bonstan's hand, and the child was holding hers. So who else would they be? Who else would accompany Bonstan in his front-of-the-line position?

None of the actual mayors had the privilege of bringing a date to the venue. Not even a scribe or administrative assistant. But there's Bonstan, treating the Colloquium like a family vacation. Clearly, he's the most powerful person in attendance. The mayors probably answer to him. So, whose interests are being represented during this week's deliberations?

The ludicrously wealthy, I suspect. As a flatty, this is discouraging.

Hoarding wealth is such a selfish ingestion. It's consumption necessarily denies nutrition to others. And Bonstan, I've always thought, is the biggest glutton on the continents. I've long regarded him as a pox upon civilization. A malignant merchant from Baguzu whose insatiable greed inflicts disease. And as of this morning, he appears to be spreading into new cities.

We cannot thrive – as a species – if we don't share. Consider biology. When a single cell or confined tissue begins to consume more than its fair ration, its growth will escape regulation. For a brief time, it will flourish relative to the flesh around it. Until it finally destroys the body it inhabits. Every time.

The same fate awaits any culture that lacks regulation of its rations. A single extreme surplus breeds a thousand deficits. As greater and greater wealth is amassed by the individual, graver and graver poverty metastasizes through the many. Until, eventually, the population collapses. Every time.

Without the equitable allocation of resources, the host always dies. So how will Gaeans survive the uncontrolled growth and spread of Bonstan?

If I have to credit him for something, it seems wealth *is* culture. The men and women of banks are those who build our stages and theaters, print the pages that fill our libraries, and decorate our cities with art and architectural wonders. And those entertainments become our culture. In turn, reactions among the downtrodden serve as the inspiration for counterculture.

But this seems to occur with *reasonable* accumulations of wealth. Bonstan's fortune is several standard deviations beyond the range of reason. That's why Bonstan's position in this morning's procession was concerning.

Fifteen minutes after they passed, the registration staff arrived, and the line ahead of us began to shorten. Slowly.

As it did, Cyn and I listened to our line mates bicker about contestant rank.

"Unless you revive a corpse or two from the Champions' Quarter, Tauro has no challenger", a man said.

"*Maybe*, momma", a woman said to a man. "He'll do better than you think."

Before I had time to make sense of that exchange, some other woman said to some other man, "I'm telling you, Tumyn, this will be the tournament that Zelig out-mugogs the swan."

"It'll all come down to Bolgwin and Alnuk", another pair's squabble began. "And my copper's on Alnuk this year."

"Oh, please. He's never even faced a real fencer. He may be a star back home, but Pendelhall's got a whole other sky. And the stars here burn brighter."

"When was the last time you watched one of his bouts?"

"I don't know. Last Elyem, probably."

"Then you wouldn't know. He's got a spark you don't see in anyone else."

"He'll need a lot more than a *spark* to win *here*. If he makes it to the top eight, he'll realize he can't hold a tallow candle to Bolgwin's lich fire."

"That might'a been true when Bolgwin was in his prime, but he's a greyin' ancient these days."

"And you think *that* matters?"

"Of course age matters. Alnuk must be thirty-five years Bolgwin's junior. He's quicker. Hungrier. And he'll *definitely* last longer. *Especially* if he makes it to the top eight."

"Bolgwin's smarter."

"Alnuk doesn't need smarts when he's got the whole of Farhearth workin' for him. Every pound'a plannin's taken care of."

The prattle went on. Until we finally we stood at the desk. And we got Cyn registered.

She was the first of the five medics to register. I looked at the roster of her yet-to-arrive peers: the four candidates ranked ahead of her and the one remaining contingent.

One is a Pendelian, and former Pendelhall Medic. Not an Emeritus Medic, having served once upon a time, but the Incumbent Medic, the second term of the two-term role. The first year – "Operating Medic" – is a public position involving learning and service, while the second year – "Incumbent Medic" – is served in private. The minor role of the Incumbent is mentorship of the Operating Medic while the principal expectation is scholarly contribution. While the Operating Medic cannot audition, the Incumbent can. And is.

That's Cyn's primary competition. Everyone else, including the contingent, is from Farhearth. And, of course, all five – including the contingent – are certified. With the Bonstan Medical Certification. Which I find ridiculous.

In Baguzu, one needs a license – granted by the mayoral office – to work as a merchant. So Bonstan didn't establish certifications for that. Even though that's a trade he understands. Instead, he established certifications in fields in which he has no business proctoring, influencing businesses he has no business influencing. Such as medicine. Aspiring medics pay a substantial fee to take an exam that any mediocre student can pass. And upon passing, they receive formal approval by Bonstan's certifying body. It's such a scam. He might as well take over the Farhearth curriculum.

Being the only uncertified applicant to make the tent says something about Cyn's capacity. Tantamount to matriculating at Farhearth without a primary education.

Every fencer who goes to Cyn's tent will know she isn't certified. And they'll know she was the first alternate. Because her lanyard looks different from the rest. Hers is green, the color of alternates, rather than the standard red. *And* it lacks Bonstan's stamp.

This shouldn't matter for the judging though – for the selection of the next Pendelhall Medic – because the judges shouldn't know. It should be blind. The committee has no idea whose medical journal is whose.

Part of the reason the Operating Medic can't reapply during the active year of public service is because they're one of the judges of that year's auditions. But they *can* reaudition the following year. As the Incumbent. Any Emeritus Medic can reaudition as well. But few do. Some retire. Some are curators for the state Archives and Apothecary. And some work independently. But most work in the Citadel Hospital. Which makes it the best hospital in the world. For the majority of conditions, anyway. The Commons Hospital at Farhearth is better for others.

Here's where I harbor *some* concern about this year's process: the Incumbent doesn't seem eager to retire or contribute to the public workforce. So he is reapplying. He was the current Operating Medic's mentor, and presumably voted that person in. *And* his handwriting is sure to be recognizable by his mentee, who will be judging his journal. If the tiniest hint of compensation is expected, we'll have a biased medic selection process. Historically though, the appointment has been fair. Or at least that's its reputation.

I was granted an audition twice. Two years in a row. Not because I was the best medic, but because I was a tournament winner myself. *And* I had a Magister's Degree in a related field. *And* I was a legacy: my mother had been a Pendelhall Medic. Once. For the two-year appointment. Then she left the profession – in a formal sense – to focus on her garden in Estevro. I may be the only applicant ever who could check all three of those boxes. So it was reasonable to extend me both auditions. But it was just as reasonable not to grant me the position. Back then, at least. And probably still today, as I continue to be impressively unskilled at diagnosing by sight or palpation. Even the most obvious injuries escape my detection.

People show me a swollen appendage and say, "Look how swollen this is!" I look. Then I look at the contralateral limb. Then back to the injured one. And I don't see it. I can't tell the difference. Not beyond the margin of error that contains the power of suggestion. Do I see what *might* be swelling? Sure. But only because I was told it was there. So I'm trying to see signs of it. If I was told it was the other side that was swollen, I'd be trying to see *those* signs. And I would be just as likely to find them. Swelling must be catastrophically pronounced for me to detect it on my own. The same applies to the range of a joint's motion. A few degrees on a goniometer isn't discernable to me. I'm a little better with discolorations – the changing hues of bruising – but in most situations, an injury has to be extreme before I can diagnose it. And in cases that extreme, there are too many disrupted tissues for a simple diagnosis to suffice. So I'm useless in that setting. Applied physiology has never been a strength. *Philosophical* physiology is where I shine. But that's not particularly therapeutic to anyone. Unless it's their curiosity that needs curing.

Cyn can do both. She can see the subtlest changes brought about by injury. A barely tensed muscle, a minor shift in posture, the slightest hint of swelling. She sees it all. But she can also recite volumes of scientific understanding about each. That's why she's the best candidate. Better than I could ever be. And as of this morning, she is officially registered.

While she was going through the registration process, and I was just standing beside her, I was snooping at the other lists. I looked at the fencers' names and destinations of origin. I didn't recognize any of them. Bolgwin aside. But I haven't paid attention in years. So I may well have been skimming over famous names.

As for the locations, I saw very few Westerners. There were some, but not many. And the few Westerners who *were* registered were all from Midrodor. There's so little violence west of the thickets. With the exception of Rorrik. He's a Westerner, and he won the Pendelhall Tournament twice. Years ago.

I won once. More years ago. Mizjak is the winningest. Even more years ago. Fifteen in a row. Every tournament he entered.

That's a record will never be surpassed. Or matched. Or even threatened. *My* record – youngest tournament winner ever – was broken in three years. By a Westerner, actually. Holmgrin. I've never formally met him – so I can't say whether I like him – but I hold no bitterness. Because the world held a lot of bitterness for me when I set that record. The reputation haunted me for a time. And that time ended as soon as Holmgrin won at a younger age.

I do think I started fencing too early. And trained too intensely too quickly. Because today, my body is a menagerie of pains and problems, lingering relics of the race to triumph. As I write this, my weary back (stiff from standing in line all morning) is resting in a chair at the eatery. Cyn ordered us breakfast while I sat here, scribbling unsociably. For a long time. Because it's *so* busy. Everyone who was in the registration line before us seems to have come here. Before we did. And every other waking Pendelian seems to have joined them.

But the food should be here any minute now. Elk. When in Pendelhall…

I'm done writing.

Twenty-Eight

Aldos, Second Lufoa, Day Nineteen. Afternoon.

After breakfast, Cyn and I went exploring. She's been here before – twice – but on those trips, we just watched the fights and talked about the injuries. This year, we're adding a tour to our visit. If she's going to be moving here, a better orientation of the city will be helpful. The first attraction on this morning's tour was the akira pits. I've never understood why it's called "pits" when there's only one of them. A single subterranean kennel of arena lions. Plus, it's getting opulent down there. Either way, that was our first stop.

When I was young, and my mother was the Pendelhall Medic, she took me to see the cats. I remember them looking like flame incarnate. In part, it was the way they moved. But even lying still, they seemed to mimic an active fire. Their bodies were grotesquely lean with straw-colored fur so short and sleek you could see intricate webs of vasculature streaked across their haunches. And from the top of every head to the tip of every tail blazed the fire stripe, a path of fur that was six inches wide and as crimson as spilled blood.

When Cyn and I saw them today, they looked more docile than I remember. They're still incarnations of flame, but more like candles rather than wildfires. Not driving threats away but drawing them near. According to the Guard, the *summoning* of peril has always been their purpose. Since the first akira was captured. They were never meant to repel war. This never made sense to me. Unless we're talking about the kittens. Those are adorable.

No one knows what they were like in the wild; the last akira was captured before the first book was published. And in the intervening generations, they were selectively bred to be fiercely loyal and somewhat fiercely fierce.

Docile as today's pit pets appeared to be, I still wouldn't want to fight one. That was the original trial – the rite of combat – Pendelians had to undertake, and survive, to be appointed to the Champions' Guard.

Beyond the pit is the Forbidden Quarter, where the guards themselves reside. And train. And dine. And ultimately die. Not even the mayor is permitted to enter. That's how forbidden it is. As I write this, even *Bonstan* is barred from entry.

Inside that mysterious, inaccessible metropolis, the Guard has no monarch.

Today, there is a single-year, limited-authority, elected-from-within position called the First Knight. The last real monarch – called the Morning Sword – was Velox. The role was retired after his tenure.

Velox wasn't his actual name. No one knows what it was. Members of the Champions' Guard are assigned new names as an effort to erase their past. As though they were born into the role. This tradition was established after Velox's time, but the history of the Guard is written by the Guard, and it's revised regularly. They rewrite the past and pretend it was always that way.

I don't know if this is a uniquely Eastern trait – the Book of Druin is said to undergo generational amendment as well – but Easterners are *notorious* for it. Most of the Morning Swords are just fable fodder. Myths intended to glorify Eastern annals. And hometown heroes aren't the only figures invented here. Just play a game of regnavus. Velox leads his regiment against the legions of Brontus, Bellator, and Regnatrix. Those are exactly the kind of names one would expect an Easterner to invent. To contrive a more exciting past.

Eastern school children, in the early grades, are taught these fictions as facts. I thought all of it was true until I read Gundric's *Life of Mizjak*. The first volume, with all those annotated begats. Terribly tedious, but also important.

Cyn and I talked about all of this as we looked at the cats. Which weren't doing anything interesting. They sleep all day to save up the energy to sleep all night. But they look elegant as they do it. Like fireballs taking a nap.

Then we walked to the Champions' Quarter – half a mile away – where rows of granite monuments, which look like giant tombstones, are engraved with the names of every tournament winner from the past. Not just in fencing, but regnavus, wrestling, and boxing, too. And other competitions, from the East and abroad. There are granite slabs that chronicle the victors of the Salt and Stone Circle, horse and rider alike, even though it's a Southern contest. Other slabs are chiseled with achievements in rowanoki. And every record in running and throwing sports. And swimming and boating. And it's not just athletics with headstones on that hill. Academic advancements have rows of their own. Every mayor is memorialized. Hundreds of inventors, writers, and war heroes have great histories immortalized there. And thousands more. Countless monuments with dead people's names inscribed beside extensive epitaphs of their accomplishments. There aren't any *bodies* in the Champions' Quarter – it's not a cemetery – there are only stones of remembrance. Which register everyone's deeds in enough detail that they can be compared to the deeds of others. That's rather the point. The hill is held sacred, but it's also the bedrock of the ranking structures that remain so rampant in the East.

The most pathetic and abundant ranking quarrel of all is political tabulation. How many seats am I from the mayor's chair? Am I two seats away? Ten? A thousand seats from the throne? "If these eighty-two people died, I would be declared mayor!" I find it creepy that so many Easterners know their precise political rank. And I find it creepier that they conflate it with societal importance.

The mayors themselves are not exempt from the rankings. But they rank their feats against each other's. Which mayor was the youngest to be elected? The longest serving? Whose reign oversaw the greatest economic expansion? Who was the best martial tactician? The most pious, most just, or the wisest? And a hundred other metrics the still-living mayors identify themselves by. So they can know their place among their peers, living and dead, dating all the way back to Urfeo, the first mayor of Thestevro. The first official mayor anywhere on the continents. He lived on the southern slope. Somewhere. Where the oldest houses are. "House" is a euphemism for most of those old hovels embedded in the hill. When I was young, I went inside one of them. The last descendant of a family had died, so it was on the market. And my parents would occasionally spend Seros afternoons touring homes for sale. All I remember about this one is how tiny it was. There was a bedroom that doubled as a sitting room, a kitchen that doubled as a dining room, and no bathroom. I assume the same is true for every other house that's rooted into the slope: they're as modest on the inside as they are on the outside. Which means Urfeo was probably a modest mayor. Despite this – and because there is no record of what he accomplished or what became of him or his family – he now has all the mythos of a regnavus character. And so every mayor since is ranked against him.

I don't think hierarchies of this kind became prevalent until recently. Today, however, it's the great pathology of the East. People can barely shake hands without descending into a childish thumb war. At the very minimum, it's a squeeze contest. It's not a handshake but a ranking of masculinity against one's opposer. Pathetic, really. When I'm forced to engage palms, I often relax my hand completely. I just find the whole practice weird, so I try to be as creepy as possible every time a handshake is thrust upon me. Limp hand, wriggling a little, hoping people will never again attempt to snatch it from the end of my arm.

I'm just not competitive in these kinds of engagements. Petty, infantile ones. But I do enjoy touring the Champions' Quarter and wondering who would win in a duel: Mizjak or Velox. Gundric or Gewyn. Rorrik or Rinalt. Me at twenty or Holmgrin at nineteen. Or either of us against Erluk, whose original youngest-ever record we both surpassed.

Outside of duels, I can appreciate ranking contestants in general. That's the whole point of participating in a competition. But competing in things like music or food seems pointless. These are pleasurable enough on their own; they don't need our attention augmented by gambling and ranking structures. Although I do love the annual Cookery Banquet, I recognize the absurdity.

As I get older, I emancipate myself more and more from this culture. Perhaps because I can see the day in which I'll no longer be able to *out*compete others. It's not today. But it *is* coming. And if my self-worth is measured by my station in the hierarchy, the emotional blow will be both devastating and inevitable. It's like defining one's dignity by what's reflected in the mirror. I've watched plenty of attractive people, whose identities were based entirely on attractiveness, descend into sadness when their beauty began to atrophy into ordinariness. And then came madness once ugliness claimed their flesh. But this happens to us all. That's how life progresses. Beauty always expires. So it can't be an identity we hold dear.

Although mirrors have never contributed to my sense of self, winning has. Lately, I've been more mindful of this. And I've been pruning those Eastern instincts whenever I notice their overgrowth. That way, I'll be ready for the day in which winning is no longer an option, and I have to find satisfaction living outside of the hierarchies.

Cyn and I talked about all of this as we looked at the rows of monuments.

"Your name will be on this hill soon", I said.

She gave me a curious look.

Then I took her to the spot where every Pendelhall Medic is immortalized. But we didn't stay long. Because even there, it's all about rankings. Who was the greatest among them? The second greatest? Third? Fourth? Worst? Cyn doesn't need to get caught up in this nonsense. But I did want her to see how revered the role is. To be appointed at all is to earn immortality on that sacred hill.

Then we returned to Pygil's. So we could rest. And eat. And I could write. But now Cyn wants to explore some more. So we're heading back out.

Twenty-Nine

Aldos, Second Lufoa, Day Nineteen. Night.

After lunch, Cyn and I did some more exploring. Our first destination was the library. Not the public one, near the fencing rings. But the private library. The Archives. About a mile away. In a far less trafficked area. The building is beautifully constructed, meticulously maintained, and vigilantly guarded. To enter, one must either be a Pendelhall Medic (Operating, Incumbent, or Emeritus) or one of the five lanyard-wearing candidates of the current event. Or be actively accompanied by one of those people. Cyn's lanyard grants her access. And so it granted me access as her guest. It was my first time inside since I was one of the five.

The Archives is where they preserve every journal from every tournament. Each year, the five auditioning medics maintain a diary of their diagnoses, treatments, and justifications. And when their audition is over, they submit it for evaluation. That's the whole interview. The process is overseen by the Operating Pendelhall Medic. She'll wander the rings, from tent to tent, observing, listening, judging. But she doesn't have the exclusive authority to appoint her replacement. She's one of six committee members. She's the Chair of the committee – and the only member with two votes – but there are five others. The curator of the Archives also casts a vote. So does the most recently elected member of the Champions' Guard… for some reason. And then some physicians from the Citadel Hospital. After the tournament is over, there's a whole day without any public activity. This is when the committee convenes, discusses, votes, and decides.

Once that decision is made, all five of the journals are moved to the library. Forever. And if you're not selected as the new Pendelhall Medic, the last time you see your work is likely to be during its ceremonial placement on the shelf. After that, the lanyard is just a keepsake. Or really clunky jewelry. Its wearer receives no special permissions. The temporary access – for the duration of the tournament – is a just a courtesy extended to the candidates in exchange for their contributions to the library. At no point do they hold any rights to their work. It is the property of Pendelhall. To recite or replicate one's own words would be plagiarism. That's part of the agreement. When you sign up to audition, you sign over ownership of every word you write.

They've been collecting five journals every year for so long that the collection would take a year to read. A year of doing nothing else. My two are in there.

I saw them. And showed them to Cyn. We skimmed some pages together. And I realized how much I've grown since then. In my understanding of the sciences, in my control of language, and in my ability to discern what's worth writing. Cyn is way ahead of where I was when I auditioned. Assuming she is appointed the next Pendelhall Medic, and is granted permanent access to the Archives, I'm sure she'll read my work in full. And the work of everyone else who came before her.

There are some missing journals. Mostly from my mother's year. All five of those are absent from the shelf. As though the tournament wasn't even held. I noticed that the first time I auditioned. When I asked my mother about it, she told me every candidate submitted as usual, and their work must have gone missing later. Excepting that one year, the annals are nearly complete. It must be the most comprehensive bank of medical knowledge in any room. Not comprehensive enough to *fill* the room though. Because it's enormous. The building is comically larger than it needs to be. The builders knew the collected works would ultimately outgrow any room designed to collect them. So they made it fit to last a millennium. A single shelf long enough to hold five thousand journals.

While Cyn browsed the more recent entries, I went to where the shelf began and carefully extracted an antique volume. Before reading, I gently fanned its pages and inhaled the air the book breathed out. To Westerners, this is the aroma of ancestry. Of history. There is a scent that stately volumes have. It's not mildew. Or any other variety of contamination. It's more like the pheromones of a mature tome. Easterners don't do this; they never smell their books prior to reading. It's considered poor manners. As unseemly as sniffing someone's worn garments when no one is looking. But to me, and to Westerners, it's not a sleazy practice at all. It's just getting to know a book before rushing into its sentences. If anything, it's respectful. Or at least that's how I see it. And so I always do it. But being as I am currently in the East, I did my sniffing surreptitiously. Right as I finished inhaling this ancient journal's pheromones, I looked up and saw Cyn giving me a knowing smile. She saw me. But she now sniffs books too. She understands. Still, I felt like I was caught. So I put the book back. And we both went to the other side of the room.

Both walls – eastern and western – contain a single shelf. Whereas the west side is lined with every candidate's auditioning journal, the eastern shelf holds the truly treasured works: the annual contribution of every Incumbent Medic. At the end of their term, they submit their "okin-gast", which means "journey inside the mind" in Rivervalan. It's the equivalent of a dissertation. Written by the most qualified medic anywhere on Gaea.

The ceremony to place the okin-gast on its shelf is same ceremony that places the five auditioning journals on their shelf. Which is the same ceremony that announces the next Pendelhall Medic appointment. So Cyn and I will be in attendance this year. Regardless of whether she is appointed to the position, we'll watch her works enter that sacred room. It's not *religiously* sacred, but it's the secular equivalent of the Druinham Library, where the most treasured works are kept. If anything happened to Druinham, civilization would lose a hundred pseudo-prophetic poems, of which scant few are known outside of the catacombs. By comparison, if anything happened to the Archives, civilization would lose half of its understanding of health and medicine. Which continues to advance every year. With the addition of five candidate journals and one okin-gast.

Once the six works are placed, none of them will ever leave the Archives. Other than the shelving of each year's new works, no paper of any kind can come into or out of the library at all. If Cyn and I had access to this room before now, we would have done a lot of our studying in it. The number of reading tables in the room exceeds the number of people permitted to enter. I cannot imagine a better location for scholarship.

After the Archives, we visited the Pendelhall Apothecary. It has everything. To provide optimal care, the Pendelhall Medic requires access to every single root, stalk, seed, and leaf Gaea offers. And every mushroom. And mineral. And ground-up animal part. If it can be bottled, it can be bought here. To remedy any ailment that might ail the world's militia.

The building is nearly as restricted as the Archives, though. I wasn't allowed inside. But Cyn was. So I had her buy some caligoroot, solarosales seeds, and spiroleaf. To help me sleep, temper my anxiety, and relieve my on-the-road sneezing and wheezing. Respectively. It's almost impossible to find any of these anywhere else in the world. There's just too much processing. And if it's done incorrectly, they're all dangerous. The last time I had any of them, this is where they came from. Back when I was a lanyard-wearing candidate, I purchased years' worth. And I ran out of all three years ago. Cyn picked up some products of her own. Medications she expects to need in her audition.

After leaving the apothecary with some large bags of drugs, we went to the Citadel Hospital. This is where competitors go who sustain injuries that are too catastrophic to be treated at the mending tent. Quick tour.

Then we went through the Smith's Quarter – to the Royal Row – where I showed Cyn the contest weapons. Fencers don't get to duel with any weapon they want; they have to use sanctioned swords, which are all smithed here.

There are six different models available. Collectively, they don't encompass every possible use of swords, but they represent a fair range. There are some for cutting, others for thrusting. Some are light and nimble, others are heavy and formidable. There are various lengths for reach, different shapes of the blades, although every blade is dull. There's enough variety that one of the six should be a good fit for any fighter. Or at least a reasonably good fit for any contestant who is dueling on foot. Swords have other purposes, too. But nobody in the tournament will be mowing through mobs of enemies from horseback. Nor will they be sheathing and unsheathing their swords as they alternate between martial tasks. All that matters is dueling. And the six models suffice for that. Each one is numbered. One through six. They also have nicknames, but mostly they're known by their number.

Number one is tiny. It's closer to a machete than a fencing sword. Were it not dulled for competition, it would be better for trimming through untamed wilderness and well-tamed sugarcane than dueling an opponent. The blade is about twenty-five inches long and it weighs next to nothing. It neither has the range nor the heft to inflict any harm. Some contestants choose it – those who conflate fencing with dancing – but they shouldn't. Because fencing is not dancing. The number one is for acrobatics, not winning.

Numbers two and three are the most common swords. Perhaps a third of contestants choose number two, and number three is even more popular.

Two is for those trying to win on quickness alone. The blade is short – about twenty-eight inches – and slightly curved, which reduces its length by half an inch or more. This is the closest option to a saber among the sanctioned six. And while I enjoy hack-and-slash fencing, I don't like curved blades. To me, that shape seems best for beginners who swipe frantically at their opponents. During battle, the instinct that gets animated among the untrained is frenzied slashes wrought from fear. And sabers do this well. Berserk cuts may inflict more harm than articulate pokes, depending where they strike and how deep they go, but for veterans who can control their panic, saber is short on reach and weak on defense. Unless you're fencing at grappling distance – which I seldom do – it's an inferior weapon. But it's an inferior weapon that's been used by numerous tournament winners. So it continues to be chosen.

Number three is the biggest sword that's reasonable to swing with one hand. For most people, anyway. At about thirty-three inches, it's not quite a calvary officer's sword. And it's slightly too long and heavy to be an arming sword. And too short and nimble to be a longsword. But in many ways, it offers the best of all available blades. It can press and parry, cut and thrust. It's sturdy but quick, graceful but brutish. It's the choice for most tournament winners.

Among the two-handed weapons, number six is a massive greatsword, swung only by the massivest of contestants. Its colloquial name is the "oar sword", as its dimensions – length and breadth – would make it serviceable in a boat. With a blade over sixty inches and a weight over six pounds, it's unwieldy for any wielder without Arfig proportions. The reach is great, but good luck hitting anyone with it. A few tournament winners have managed to do so, but just a few.

Number five is the more common of the two greatswords. Swung by most two-handed fencers, this is the third most frequently chosen sword overall. It's longer than a standard claymore. The blade is almost forty-four inches. Looking at it, the sheer volume gives the impression of a cumbersome tool for agricultural use. But holding it, you find it to be extremely well balanced and surprisingly sprightly for its size. Much lighter than you'd expect it to be. It wouldn't be ideal in compound battles – it's the least durable of the six and even the longest-limbed user would struggle to draw it from a scabbard – but it's a strong sword in tournament dueling.

Lastly, there's the sword that is never chosen: number four. It's an ungainly, in-between blade that can't decide which type of weapon it wants to be, so it attempts to be all of them. And fails to be any of them. It's too big to swing one-handed, too small to swing with two. Even if you wanted to use both, the grip isn't long enough to fit two palms. Maybe it was intended to be a single-handed longsword, but it accidently overdid the bulk. Or it was meant to be greatsword, but it was born as a malformed runt of its litter. If you add half a hand, it's manageable. Which explains its names, the "hand-and-a-half" or "bastard" sword. Or the name I detest: "peasants' plow". The blade is about thirty-seven inches, and it's heavier than you'd expect that length to be. In all my years of watching competitors, I've never once seen anyone choose the number four. And, after surveying every monument in the Champions' Quarter, I know of only one tournament winner who has ever used it: me.

I meant to talk with Cyn about the types of injuries that pair more frequently with each weapon, both striker and stricken. But we ended up discussing smithing instead. Royal Row has the best smiths in the East. But to Cyn, who hails from Cinderheim, everything looked like the work of an apprentice.

If I had any energy left, we would have gone to the competition rings next. But I didn't have any energy left. So, we didn't go to the competition rings. Or even talk about the weapons from a perspective other than metalworking.

We'll do that tomorrow. And we'll go to the pits to watch wrestling.

I was way too exhausted to prolong this evening's outing with *any* activity.

Including eating.

"Do you mind if we skip dinner tonight and double up on breakfast instead?", I asked Cyn as we were leaving Royal Row.

"I don't mind", she said. And her amenability seemed honest.

But on our way back to the inn, we saw a food vendor. At first, we *smelled* the vendor. And then we saw him. He was grilling seafood in a battered pan beneath an old, shabby umbrella. I could tell the color used to be luminous, but it has since faded to a pale yellow. The entire scene – cook and equipment both – were clearly weathered by hard years.

Also, he wasn't a local. That much was obvious. He was there for the crowds. I doubt he even had a permit. Which means any food purchased from him was contraband.

"Fresh scallops, live and local!", the cook under the yellow umbrella yelled as he stirred and tossed the contents of his pan… which was so dented, I assume he uses it as a weapon when he's not cooking with it.

I looked at Cyn. And she looked at me. The look each of us gave the other said, "I don't know what those are, but they're definitely *not* local scallops… because that would mean this transient sidewalk chef is the first person ever to open a live Delta Reef scallop."

Whatever it was, we ate it. Because the location was so convenient. And the smell was so appetizing. And I was too tired to play culinary detective, so I didn't try to figure it out what I was chewing.

But now I'm back at the inn. And it's time to sleep. Otherwise, I won't have the energy to make it through tomorrow's plans.

Thirty

Lyros, Second Lufoa, Day Twenty. Morning.

Yesterday was exhausting. For me. Not for Cyn. She already went out this morning. And returned with breakfast. For both of us. I'm not sure what it would take to deplete her energy. Or her curiosity. She's so eager to explore the city, and learn all of its streets and quarters, its history, resources, secrets. Her interest is insatiable. And it shows. By comparison, mine has been sated by decades of prior visitation. And that shows, too. I'm sure it's apparent to anyone who sees us walking together that I've been here too many times to be astonished by my surroundings. It's in the way we walk. In our posture. And our expressions. There's almost an aura; you could probably smell it if you sniffed hard enough.

Wherever you are, you can identify the tourists in tour by their dilated pupils and animated gait. But as we grow accustomed to our commutes, we stop marveling at our environments. We begin traveling by habit. We depart and arrive without paying much mind.

Over breakfast, I expressed my thoughts on this to Cyn. "There are three classes of people present at this tournament", I said. "And it's not a matter of wealth or nationality. It's attention. You can distinguish them by the angle of their necks."

I went on to explain that the posture of the residents has been bent into canes. Their eyes are fixed on the ground before their feet. The cracks in the cobble, puddles in the path, maybe a rooster or polecat or pachyshrew strutting past. The sights above – the grand, spiraling towers – are too familiar to entertain. Catching a glimpse is not worth the risk of tripping. So the residents mosey cane-ly along. The next class is tourists. Their necks are kinked backwards, gazing up at the rooflines, marveling at every majestic gable, golden belfry, and soaring spire. Their faces are garbed in ecstasy and their gait is clumsy. And then there is the final class: the sentimentalists. Former Pendelians who have recently returned with remembrance in full bloom. Their attention is as keen as the tourists, but their necks are not crooked. They're scanning the streets and storefronts, the houses and yards, searching for familiar sights, attempting to revive the past by revisiting its destinations and reenacting its behaviors. Treating youth like a lost belonging. Where did you see it last? If you retrace your steps, maybe you'll find it there again. Accordingly, they pace Pendelhall's streets radiating both joy and desperation.

None of these classes is more or less dignified than any other. They're just characterizations of people's attention. Where is it aimed? What enlivens it? And what does it overlook?

Before Cyn and I left Estevro, I had a thought, which I wrote in my journal, that if we know this much about people – if we know the objects of their keenest attention – we can understand them pretty deeply. I was referring to friends, family, and other familiar folk, but I suppose the principle applies to strangers, too. In the present case, a hundred thousand Pendelians and at least as many visitors. Likewise, those residents and guests can observe Cyn and me – the dilation of our pupils, the angles of our necks, the spryness in our step – and categorize us into the same classes.

I don't know that I fit neatly into any of the three, but if I had to place myself, it would be the third. Cyn is definitely the second. And if Rorrik were here, he'd be in the first. All purpose and action, no leisure or distraction.

When I finished describing my three-tier civilian class theory to Cyn, she said, "A similar phenomenon exists with muscle actions. We all begin as frenetic tourists, but through repeated exposure we adapt into efficient residents."

She followed this with an explanation that the more skill we develop at mechanical actions, such as swimming or dancing or playing an instrument, the less cognition we assign to them. Novel tasks require considerable focus. But the more we rehearse, the less it takes. Until, finally, it becomes a habit, hardly requiring a brain at all. "Concentration is crucial for growth, but not maintenance", she concluded.

"I wonder if that's how we all go through life", I said. "From youth to death, we assign less and less attention to everything. Cats certainly behave that way. The skittish kitten springs into a wild panic with the tiniest hint of a stimulus, while the old cat will sleep through a felling crack."

Then I excused myself from breakfast so I could write my morning's journal. And now that I'm reflecting on our conversation, I wonder if we're all feline in our aging. That's why, as we get older, growth slows and time accelerates. The clocks don't actually quicken; it's how we *perceive* the passing hours that varies with attention. While experiencing the alarm of a kitten, time dilates like a pupil in the night. Which explains why a one-minute fencing bout can feel like a whole afternoon. And why a whole afternoon spent like a listless old cat has the opposite effect. "Where did all the time go?", people wonder. And "It feels like only yesterday", they say about old memories. I do it, too. I've been working with Cyn for nearly six years, but it feels like we just started.

I know it doesn't feel that way for her.

And to Rorrik, whose inextinguishable zeal would make the sprightliest kitten envious, yesterday must feel like a lifetime ago.

But to me, six years flew by.

And now it's time to stop writing. Because Cyn is eager to start the day.

It's going to be difficult to keep up with her. But I'll try.

We're off to the rings first. Then the pits.

Thirty-One

Lyros, Second Lufoa, Day Twenty. Afternoon.

After breakfast, Cyn and I left for the rings. We'd been there before – in the past, we've watched the tournament together – but we hadn't been to the rings while they were unoccupied. Both of our previous visits were brief and purely academic. We watched some matches, discussed injuries and physiology, and then left before it got too crowded. We never even stayed for the final day. During the last fifteen bouts, the venue is too teeming and loud to see or hear anything worth seeing and hearing. So we watched pools and the first day of direct elimination. And talked about the matches all the way home. What we *didn't* do – aside from watching the end of the tournament – is a proper tour of the facilities. Since it is the environment Cyn will be working in this year, that's what we did this morning.

There are five outer rings. And one inner ring. Cyn won't be working that sixth ring though. She'll work the outer five. One at a time. The Operating Pendelhall Medic, who was selected in the previous tournament, provides all medical supervision for the final fifteen bouts. Cyn has no responsibility that day. Only in the direst of circumstances would a substitute be called to serve. And that substitute would not be an auditioning medic.

The five outer rings are positioned in the shape of a star. The region within the star is called the Sanctum. During the tournament, only staff and athletes are allowed inside of it. No spectators. While no tournament is being held, no one is allowed inside of it.

In the center of the Sanctum is the sixth ring. The only one without a name. Without a *formal* name, anyway. It must have a hundred colloquial names: the nydel ring, the night ring, the silent ring, the Seros ring, or simply "Melas", which is treated like a proper name. Rorrik told me it's an Old Adonian word that means either gravity or, perhaps more applicable here, the ring of a bell. But not the *auditory* ring. It's the shape of it. The circle itself. And not while that circle is ringing, but while it's still and silent. I find it bizarre that any language has a word for that. Although *every* language has a word for dragon. A fake creature. At least melas, as a noun, describes something real. And it's a fitting name for the center ring. Which is where the final match occurs. And *only* the final match occurs there. It's far too sacred for any other use. Entry is strictly forbidden to those who have not "mastered the five rings".

The outer five rings have a white surface. The surface of the sixth is black. But not in the way that darkness is black. It has all the vibrancy of a spark, but none of the light. Like a spark's station in the color wheel was inverted. Instead of emitting a glow, it absorbs it. I've seen a lot of minerals in my life. My windowsill has a large collection of stones, many with peculiar features. But I've never seen anything like the black ring. It seems to be mostly clay... of some kind. Mixed with charcoal... of some kind. Could be Lichland ash or shadow frost or something. Not even Farhearth alchemists can tell you its composition. No one alive today was alive when it was made, and it's too sacred to be studied. Unless you've "mastered the five rings", you'll be seized before you manage to touch it. And incarcerated to prevent further attempt.

I've touched it. Once. During the final bout of the tournament. In the only year I competed. I didn't touch it with my *hand*, but I stood on it. And could feel enough. It's not just the least noticeable entity I've ever tried to notice; it also provides the perfect footing. It was like I was standing on a weightless ether that captured all light and sound, casting no reflections, no distractions. All that existed was my opponent and me. In a consecrated space of both reverence and violence.

The black ring does have one colloquial name that most people believe to be official: Lamenting. It's believable because the other five rings are named after the other five seasons. Although Lamenting isn't technically a "season". It's the *resolution* of the seasons. A period marking the death of the previous year and the birth of the next. But it *is* the sixth distinct phase of the calendar, and there *are* six rings, and the other five are named after the five other phases. So how could the sixth ring *not* be called Lamenting? It's better than Melas. But it's not official. Only the outer rings have complete birth certificates. In order: Arzox, Lylir, Rynoa, Lufoa, and Elyem.

That order matters. Just as the hands on a clock make precise and predictable revolutions, and Gaea makes its annual, calculable orbit around the sun, the outer five rings revolve around the inner sixth, signifying the passage of time. Each ring is about three hundred feet from its neighbors. Arzox, is located at the far eastern side, such that it's the first one touched by the sun. At the southeastern point is Lylir, the second ring. Then Rynoa is in the southwest. Lufoa is in the far west. And Elyem, the final ring, is at the northern peak.

Despite their proximity, each of the rings also resides in a surprisingly unique environment. Touring them almost feels like the turning of seasons, each has a climate of its own. In Arzox, you'll be oppressed by the smell of pig feces. To be more specific: truffle hog feces. East of town are the sniffing groves. And the pens are close enough to Arzox that the smell can be overwhelming.

Moving to Lylir, you're suddenly surrounded by taverns and their tavernites. It's the ring where contestants can drink after their successes, but they never do if they want to keep succeeding. It's also where contestants can drink off the disappointment of their losses, and they generally do. Especially those who previously drank to their success. For some reason, there are no other taverns anywhere near the rings. Every one of them is just southeast of Lylir.

Southwest of the rings, there's a stage where musicians play. You might be able to hear a few distant, muffled notes from Lylir and Lufoa, but in Rynoa, it thumps and bellows. And people fence and fight differently because of it. They insist on being more heroic. I don't much care for the style of music. It's mostly Harthies playing the instruments of patriotism: a bunch of horns with the timbre of a goose. But it inspires valor in the pyloe and mettle in the pouzo. And that makes Rynoa the most enjoyable ring to watch.

At the far west side, Lufoa is the quietest of the five rings. The songs blaring from Rynoa are subtle enough to sound almost soothing. And directly behind the ring is the front entrance to the public library. Here, contestants are more focused in their fencing, and spectators are more attentive in their viewing.

Lastly, at the far north, you'll find the eateries. All of them. Elyem is where everybody gets their food. There's an aroma that's unique to this ring. There's a bustle here. And there's the incessant sound of full-mouthed conversation. Everyone is a commentator, and no one talks between bites. "Are you having difficulty understanding me through half chewed food? I'll just talk louder!" That seems to be the rule around Elyem.

Beyond the rings, the whole area is encircled by elevated concentric steps. Like an amphitheater, except the gradations are small and the steps are long. Cyn and I walked along the lowest step, discussing the environment she'll be working in at each ring. When we finished our orbit, it was time for lunch. So we sat down to eat by the Elyem ring. That's where I've been writing this. While taking an occasional bite of a thick tomato-flavored paste. I'll explain later. For now, we should get to the pits. To watch what's left of wrestling.

Thirty-Two

Lyros, Second Lufoa, Day Twenty. Night.

We finally watched some wrestling. We missed the first half. Those matches happened while we were wandering the fencing rings. But the wrestling lasts all day. For this one day. And we watched well into the evening.

There weren't many wrestlers competing this year. It used to be a much more prominent sport at the tournament. A hundred years ago, the wrestlers were as famous as the fencers. A few hundred years ago, it was the most popular sport in the East. Then boxing surpassed it. Then fencing surpassed boxing. For a time, though, all three events had enormous rosters of competitors and even enormouser hordes of fans.

In those years, the triple crown was sought. Nobody managed to achieve it, but countless contestants tried. If *The Handbook of Gentlemen's Sports* can be trusted, there were years in which every Easterner who registered for any of the three sports registered for all three. Until Mizjak. Who had no interest in wrestling or boxing. Once he entered his first tournament, fencing became the only sport that mattered. No one ever cared about the triple crown again. They just wanted to be the next Mizjak. And that's still true today. Wrestling and boxing combined have about a quarter as many contestants as fencing. In this year's tournament, there are only thirty wrestlers listed on the bracket.

It's double elimination, so there are fifty-nine possible matches, and each one lasts a maximum of nine minutes… if it goes all the way to the judge's ruling. But I think most bouts end with submissions. The tournament was about half over when we arrived. And more than half crowded.

There are two pits. One for each bracket. The undefeated-so-far wrestlers square off in the Pyloe Pit, and the Pouzo Pit is where the pouzos grapple.

We went to watch the pyloes first. I don't know why. I don't know enough about wrestling to recognize impressive feats or talk about strategies or even enjoy what I'm watching. And I *definitely* don't know enough to appraise the performers and their performances. If the worst and best wrestlers in the brackets were pitted together, I wouldn't be able to tell who was more skilled until the judge declared it. So there was no benefit to Cyn and me watching the undefeated tier. The already-once-defeated wrestlers would have been just as useful to inspire our discussion on injury, healing, and performance.

We also had a difficult time getting pitside amid the pyloes, so we could hardly see the action. We were trapped in a crowd of spectators, which was behind another crowd, which was behind another. And another. From our position, we couldn't see much more than our neighbors. And they didn't seem very interested in the wrestling itself. Instead, they were quarreling over rankings. "Tauro is top ten of all time; I would rank him at number six." "I'd say fifth." "Definitely top three." "No way he's higher than seventh." And on and on the debate went, each debater articulating his or her reason for the ranking. And then providing a roster of historic wrestlers who were better than Tauro. In order. With comprehensive justifications for each rank. Clearly, this was a crowd of Easterners. Who else would care?

Cyn and I withstood this prattle for a few minutes. Until we couldn't take it anymore. Then we went to the other pit, where we could actually see the wrestlers. But it was just as prattley. And all the prattle was still about rank. Albeit lower rankings. But there were three with "top hundred" standing: Weiss, Rance, and someone named Mamma, whose rank nobody agreed on. I assume this was one of the few women competing. Because the arguments on behalf of Mamma, as well as those opposing that behalf, had an intensity of animosity we generally reserve for political disputes.

If you're standing next to a raging fire, you can't help but feel the heat. And if you're standing in the eruption radius of a raging argument, you can't escape the bludgeoning from both sides. Collateral damage of a kind. Here are some of the facts I was inadvertently bludgeoned with: Mamma has wrestled in the past thirteen tournaments held at Pendelhall – counting a couple of the minor events – and hasn't won a single time. The thirteenth was the worst outcome of all: eliminated in two matches.

Thirteen strikes me as a reasonable number to give up on, having thoroughly tested the bounds of defeat. If you haven't succeeded by then, the fourteenth effort is unlikely to be a "charm". But Mamma is still at it. And I must admit: I admire the persistence.

Cyn and I stayed for a few bouts at that pit but didn't see any of the wrestlers who were so hotly debated by the crowd. Eventually, we stopped watching and went behind the corral of coaches and trainers. Since there are no official medic tents like there are with fencing, each contestant can bring an assistant. The same is true with boxing. The athletes are allowed to bring a trainer of some kind. With both sports, every one of those helpers is a former athlete. Most are former tournament winners – from the past fifty years – who now earn their living training the current generation of contestants on matters of technique, conditioning, and contest strategy. Each of these is rife with lore.

Cyn and I couldn't see – the corral blocked our view – but listening to the lore gave us more to talk about. There were lots of topics. General preparation, warmups, care of injuries, and so on. But the most frequent and unscientific of them all was how to best recuperate between bouts. Stretches, exercises, nutrition, hydration. Each prescription was stated with a degree of certainty that only ignorance can uphold. So eavesdropping provided plenty of fodder for Cyn's and my afternoon discussion.

And then we left. Without even seeing the finals. We don't know who won.

During our walk back to Pygil's, Cyn and I talked about the Eastern zeal for rankings. And my envy of the zealots. Having grown up in the grasslands, I share some of those tendencies, but I lack the fervency of my fellow grazers. And I'm slightly jealous of anyone who can summon *that* much passion about mundane matters. Such as, "Who is the best wrestler of all time?" Questions like this seem so pointless, yet Easterners will squabble over the answer. Vehemently. For hours. And I find myself wishing I could be that passionate in life. About anything.

"Is there any *top ten* topic you'd invest that much emotion in?", Cyn asked.

"Sure", I said. "But it would have to be conceptual. Not a top ten mayor or wrestler or whatever, but something that could only be ranked by an almighty, omniscient deity who, for some inexplicable reason, cared about top tens." Then I gave some examples. The ten paintings I would find most inspiring if I saw them. Or the ten books I would find most engrossing if I read them. Or the ten songs that would conjure the deepest emotion if I heard them. Or the ten foods I would find most delicious if I tasted them. Or the ten facts I would be most fascinated by if I learned them. Or the ten people who I would feel most connected to if I met them. And then I wondered: have I seen any of the paintings, read any of the books, heard any of the songs, tasted any of the foods, learned any of the facts, or met any of the people?

Books, for example. Perhaps my fondness of Rothrick's work would dwindle if I were exposed to fonder texts. I can't imagine better sentences or stories, but I can imagine the *possibility* of their existence. And on the topic of food, is there any culinary entity better than a perfect omelet? Some undiscovered nut or fruit so delicious that, by comparison, all other groceries would taste like tea fannings? And what about people? That's difficult to even consider. Cyn is certainly in my top ten. Abendroth, too. But there are over a million Gaeans… who will produce another Gaeling before I finish this sentence. Am I really so lucky that I've met all of my favorites? I wonder if everything I love would be supplanted if I simply encountered my deity-chosen top ten.

The concept was worth contemplating. For a minute. Which is roughly the duration that Cyn and I gave it. Then we changed the subject. To biology's top ten. The largest or longest living or fastest or most intelligent or deadliest creatures that have ever existed. Are they flora? Fauna? Squirt-like hybrids? Are they extinct? If so, were any features of their inheritance preserved in extant species? Have they been discovered in either living for fossil form? Are they present in our textbooks? What can we learn from them?

This topic held our attention for longer. But eventually, it began to feel as futile as the conversations one hears around the wrestling pits. Or around the boxing wreathes, which is where we'll be tomorrow.

Thirty-Three

Fyros, Second Lufoa, Day Twenty-One. Morning.

It's early. But Cyn has already gone out. To explore Pendelhall some more by herself. And just like yesterday, she returned with breakfast for both of us. Traditional dishes. I haven't had these in years. One is made from beans, and you expect it to have a savory flavor, but it's as sweet as honey. And the other is a pastry that you expect to be sweet, but it's as savory as dried meat. As we ate, Cyn told me what she learned while she was out:

Yesterday's wrestling tournament is being celebrated as the greatest in the sport's history. According to some people. According to others, "It was in the top ten, sure, but not the top five."

"What made it so special?", I asked.

"Triumph from below", Cyn said, quoting Mizjak. Well, technically quoting Gundric, who was quoting Mizjak.

"A pouzo beat the almighty Tauro?", I asked.

"A pouzo who was sent to that pit after the first round. By Tauro himself. One more loss would have meant elimination. But he refused to lose again. Bout after bout, he battled his way to the end. Until, eventually, he earned his rematch against Tauro. And he won. So it went to the fifty-ninth match. The final bout. Where he won again."

"Did you catch his name?"

"Rugyn."

That's not a wrestler Cyn and I heard ranked by any crowd member. So he must not have been in anyone's top hundred. So it must have been an upset of staggering surprise. Rugyn spent the entire tournament grappling in the Pouzo Pit, only to beat everyone's favorite in the finals.

Cyn and I both know what Mizjak's opinion would be on the matter, but he's not here to express it. So I took the burden upon myself to deliverer the necessary diatribe: "Cheering on a pouzo is usually unprofitable, and if those cheers are rewarded, it's often cruel", I said.

Cyn didn't respond. She just nodded. And smiled. Which I interpreted as an invitation to continue… with a huge, uninterruptible monologue:

"The reason we root for pouzos is that we perceive ourselves in their place. We, too, reside in life's lower brackets, scraping by, day after day, desperately clinging to the hope that luck will someday come to our aid. If we can just hang on a little longer, it will be our turn to be rescued by luck's random grace. Hope of this kind grows heavy, though. If it goes unrequited long enough, we'll lose our grip. And the last spark of our optimism will be extinguished. That's the reason, when we see a pouzo triumph, a part of us feels restored. And that's what we're *really* cheering for. Not some stranger in a wrestling pit, but the preservation of our hope. So I understand the reason most people would regard this tournament as the greatest in the history of the sport."

"Mizjak couldn't have said it better", Cyn replied. "Or as harshly", she added.

"But was it as harsh as *Mayor's Mercy*?", I asked.

"Not *that* merciless. I would place it in the middle of Mizjak and the Mayor. It would have fit nicely in *The Soldier and the Smithy*."

I wonder how many people here are familiar with these references. I doubt any contestant has ever heard of the Southern fable, but how many would even know where "triumph from below" comes from? I'm sure the older demographic would. But no one from Cyn's generation – excepting Cyn – has read Gundric's work. Which is precisely why they harbor such strident opinions. As is usually the case, the ignorant are the most outspoken class. "Gundric didn't deserve the gift Mizjak gave her", they growl. "Society is just giving her what she *does* deserve!", they blast their audience with a torrent of acidic spittle. According to those righteous spittlers, what Gundric deserves is a life of exile. And possibly death within that exile. Nobody knows if she's still alive. What people *do* know – *without a doubt!* – is that Gundric's behavior and emotional temperament at the end of her time with Mizjak resulted in his downfall.

People who have never read *Life of Mizjak* allege that Gundric ruined Mizjak's reputation in her final chapters. The veracity of his background, his loyalty to the East, his general valor. She called it all into question. Upon release, her work kindled little controversy. But after a few years, the consequence of Gundric's publication became something of an urban fable: "In an effort to extinguish those rumors, Mizjak met that mooncursed minion of the devil out in the open. With no men at his side. Just his sword, his wit, and his duty pitted against the corruptor of Thorn in single combat!"

Apparently, Mizjak fought Rorrik's eternal nemesis – "the filler of morgues, the sculptor of perdition!" – by himself in the fields southwest of Pendelhall. A long time ago. My mother was auditioning for the Pendelhall Medic role at the time.

I've never read a first-hand report of the events. What *is* first-hand reported from that time, however, is Mizjak's reputation in the East. His impeccable honor, which Gundric supposedly spoiled, was not beyond the reproach of common journalists. According to some papers I've seen, Mizjak was hardly popular among Easterners. Because he was an expatriate living in the South. To leave the grasslands for less green acres is practically a form of apostacy. And Mizjak left early in his life. Years before his first tournament appearance.

He was always revered by his fellow fencers. Who had never seen his equal. And he was beloved by young aspirants everywhere. Who fancied themselves Mizjaks in training. But most Easterners seemed to regard him with a scowl. Gundric, by comparison, is still beloved by a *few*, including Cyn, me, and the old guards of Midrodor and Pendelhall. But she's beloathed by the many. And her books have been all but burned at Farhearth.

When Cyn finished reading them for the first time, she had an interesting analysis. "He was foolish", she said. I tilted my head and blinked a couple of times. So she explained how Mizjak talked about humility, and the futility of "hunting monsters", but then he marched off to duel the king of monsters. "If there isn't more to that story, then he must have been a fool", she finished.

I was in a daze, thinking about Cyn's and my first year together – the year she read *Life of Mizjak* – when she interrupted me, and returned me to the present: "By the way", she said, "Tauro was from Thevro, and Rugyn from Estevro." She said it with a smile, knowing I would immediately change my perspective, and my prejudice would be obvious. And I did, and it was. No longer was this a story of the hard-working failing to receive their hard-won reward. Suddenly, it became a story of the penniless challenging the prosperous. The downtrodden trodding upwards by grit alone. No one to carry the luggage or rake the road ahead. With every obstacle in his path, Rugyn still prevailed! That's how I reframed the story in my mind. With hypocrisy acknowledged. I just wish we had stayed to watch the final. The final *two* bouts. Aside from Cyn's audition, that would have been the most exciting experience of our trip. Worthy of a top-ten-ever ranking. As far as tournament experiences go.

And with that, we're off to watch boxing, the most brutal of the three "noble arts of combat".

Thirty-Four

Fyros, Second Lufoa, Day Twenty-One. Afternoon.

Cyn and I are back at the inn. We're taking a long lunch break. Because it was a long morning.

We made it to Wreathes in time to watch the opening ceremony. Wreathes is an old district of Pendelhall. It's where most of the craft laborers work. The *old* crafts: cobblers, carpenters, wheelwrights, weavers, tanners, thatchers, and so on. The district is named for boxing, but it's no longer defined by it. The crowds tend to be there for commerce. Except for this one day of the year, when it is overrun by spectators eager to watch men punch other men professionally.

In the center of the district lie the three "wreathes", pentagons encircled by three thick ropes of braided willow vines. Each one resembles a huge wreath, sixty feet in circumference. With wrestling and fencing, there is no boundary keeping the competitors enclosed. If you step out of the pit or ring, you lose a point, step back in, and begin again. For boxers, there is no stepping out. This is where the expression "vines across the back" comes from. It's not about being whipped; it means there's no escape. You either abandon all hesitation and thrust yourself into the ruckus like a frenzied mugog, or you preserve your dread, scrunch up like a pillbug, and attempt to withstand the unwithstandable bludgeoning until the bell's ring.

What makes this *particular* boxing event interesting is the variety of strategies. The most frequently used ones have animal names corresponding to them (the mugog and pillbug being two such names). These strategies aren't as obvious at any other event. Because a boxer typically fights one or two bouts per season. But here, it's a single-elimination bracket which can take all day to get through. If you're going to survive clear to the end, you need a plan.

I checked the roster this morning. I didn't want to make the same mistake I did with wrestling and miss the most spectacular event of the tournament. There was one contestant I recognized: Lanko. He's famous enough to be known by boxing enthusiasts and disenthusiasts alike. He was the only one I recognized. But often, famous competitors will register under pseudonyms. If they don't, crowds can form, and hassles can arise. The most notorious hassle occurred about thirty years ago. The top boxers all fell ill on the day of the tournament. And no one else did. Not one townie, not one spectator.

Not even one middle-of-the-pack boxer. But every boxer that any gambler had placed a bet on suddenly became a fitful fountain of vomit and diarrhea. Ever since then, athletes in all three events have been permitted to register under a pseudonym. It muddles the gambling, but it keeps contestants safe. What you can't do is list a pseudo-*city*. You must either report the actual city you represent or declare yourself unaffiliated. Out of hometown pride, and sometimes municipal sponsorships, hardly anyone enters without affiliation.

As I scanned the roster for familiar names, I also looked for any Estevroans I could root for. There were three. Out of forty-two registered contestants. Which makes forty-one total fights. Which means, in the final bout, the two boxers will be in their sixth match of the day. *Two* in a day is brutal if anyone punches you in the first. Or if the first one lasts all three rounds. The first two rounds are three minutes, the final round is six. And sometimes boxers finish that six-minute round and start a new match within as many minutes. Minor differences in leg conditioning start to become apparent early.

By the championship match, no contestant is in any condition to be fighting. So that bout doesn't really determine who the best boxer is, but who the best strategist is. And that's the fascinating part. Are you going to try to knock your opponent out in the first minute to minimize the amount of time on your feet and maximize the duration between bouts? Or are you going to play defensively and try to take no hits, maintaining your wits at the cost of your legs, and advance to the next round by judge's decision?

After watching the first round of fights, you can start to make predictions about how the next round of pairings will end. The mugog and the pillbug. The pillbug and the snake. The snake and the mugog. It's like a game of Natural Order. Except there are so many more animals to choose from. Lanko's animal, the swan, is the only one that bores me. Not the bird itself, in real, ornithological life, but the fighting style it represents in the wreathes.

It seems like the tournament should be over in a relatively short duration. Each bout lasts twelve minutes if it ends by decision. With forty-one fights divided between the three wreathes, you'd think it'd be over in a few hours. But it never is. Mostly because one medic works the whole event. And that person is beset by a horde of helpless interns wearing Farhearth uniforms. Their institutional affiliation is identifiable from half a mile away. And so is their incompetence. They get worse every year. Twenty years ago, they were probably useful. Ten years ago, they were benign. Now they're just a burden. Only fencing has enough contestants (and diverse enough injuries) to require a team of medics. For wrestling and boxing, the Operating Medic oversees all diagnosis and care. So if all goes right, this will be Cyn's burden next year.

The oversight isn't particularly challenging from an intellectual perspective. Among wrestlers, there are only a couple of injuries a year, and they're easy to predict. Every injury occurs in the Pouzo Pit, never in the early rounds, and they always belong to an Easterner. When a joint insists on submission, its owner may refuse, sacrificing that joint in exchange for one tier higher in the rankings. There's no way they can win the next round... unless their next opponent *also* has a newly sprained appendage dangling from its tattered ligamentous harness. But if the current bout is even close, and it goes to decision, the owner of the pop! will almost surely advance. And it's always an Easterner. Because who else would care enough about rank to make that trade? There are only four or five matches each year where this *might* occur. And those are the only matches the medic has to watch.

Boxing is different. To an extent, every athlete gets injured. But every injury is the same: a concussion. So the medic sits at a clearance station. After each round, every boxer must be cleared prior to participation in the next. There are a few disqualifications every year. And, of course, this sparks accusations that the medic was "bought" by the next opponent. I doubt it. For many reasons. I've seen some of the disqualifications. They can't name the mayor. They don't know what day it is. Or where they are. A gust of wind could have knocked them out in the next bout. And yet the judge's decision will still be contested. No matter how obvious it is. Because it is the boxer's nature to argue *everything*. So I just feel sorry for the medic here.

Most years, the medic spends the entire day working in the clearance station. There's a restroom, a storehouse for medical supplies, and beds in case the boxers need them. The responsibility tends to be constant, so the medic can't watch any of the matches. That job belongs to the interns. They're supposed to describe the relevant details of the fights and report any symptoms they witness outside of the clearance station. It's the clinician's equivalent of being a squire. I interned once. Back when I was a Farhearth student. It's where I learned that medical theory and medical practice seldom sing in harmony. "Make do with what you have" is the clinician's rule that horrifies academics. In part, it's about resources. But it's also about getting athletes in the pit, the wreath, or the ring in time for their match. "Bouts and rounds don't wait for bodies to heal; tissues must accommodate the tournament structure, and not the other way around", I was told.

I learned a great deal from the experience. But I also *contributed* a great deal. I took my role seriously. And back then, the interns still provided some value. Anymore, it's not mutually beneficial. The interns are just fleas riding a host. Maybe they can transport water. Or rake the wreathes. But usually they're told, "Just sit and observe. And try to stay out of my way."

There would be no point in having Cyn intern. Better to watch. And discuss. And maybe gamble. Boxing, more than any other sport, is a gambler's game. The odds of which can be influenced by the medics' decisions. For example, if a boxer advances to the third round but his next scheduled opponent is made ineligible by a "technical forfeiture" (concussion), he will advance to the fourth round without a third fight. Resting – rather than being punched in the face – makes a huge difference in subsequent performance. And it's one of many variables that influence people's wagers.

Cyn and I will probably place some bets tonight. But we stayed away from the bookmakers this morning. We just enjoyed all the pomp and punching. Boxing, more than any other sport, is defined by mythos. Great, legendary figures, many of whom are actively legending today. Colorful recitation of their deific deeds is a defining feature of the sport. Each boxer's assistant also serves as promotor, and their most important role (even more important than training them) is introducing them to the crowd. Not with real career achievements, but with wild stories that portray them as demideities.

Here's my favorite pair of pre-match introductions from this morning:

"In the black post, hailing from the hills of Midrodor, stands Jerich, the Builder. A direct descendant of Arfig, Jerich builds without tools, hammering architectural spikes into framing timber with his bare fists!"

The crowd cheers. Then the next introduction:

"Standing in the white post is Zelig, the Lumberman, who fells trees with his bare fists. Whether in the wreath or the pub, he has never lost a fight nor a contest of pints!"

Again, the crowd cheers. Then the bell rings.

Other boxers had just as spectacular of introductions, but these two seemed an ideal match, right down to their day jobs: they both work with lumber. And they both boasted of bare-fisted miracles on the jobsite.

Zelig advanced. But not without taking some hard hits. It'll be difficult for him to preserve his undefeated record in the next bout. Although I doubt it's even true. Half the boxers' introductions claimed they were undefeated. Have none of them ever faced each other before?

In the final match, the speeches aren't limited to half a minute. They'll drag on for several. Probably in the traditional style: rhyming couplets.

I'm sure I'll have to hear Lanko's. I skipped it this morning. It was easy to avoid his wreath. But I did hear him singing his *own* praise when he wasn't quarantined in the vines.

He's far and away the most famous boxer today. But, if I had to report my personal ranking, he would be my least favorite. Because he neither receives nor delivers any punches. He just dances for the judges, winning every match on technical decision. King of the swans.

I have no interest in watching that in the wreath. Grace is a misrepresentation of the sport. There isn't supposed to be blood in ballet, but there is in boxing. The brutality of a mugog is a much better representation. But no matter what animal they channel in the bout, they always bicker when it ends. Especially if it ends in decision. No matter who wins, or how obvious the decision is, "The match was fixed! What a hoax! It was decided before the first punch!"

All right, lunch is over. It's time to get back out to the wreathes. For more punches and arguments and gambling.

Thirty-Five

Fyros, Second Lufoa, Day Twenty-One. Night.

After lunch, Cyn and I watched the rest of the boxing matches. The further into the event it gets, the more boring the bouts become. Each boxer grows more and more sluggish, less and less alert. By the end, I feel like I, with no formal training in boxing, could get in the wreath and contend. Because my legs aren't wobbling, and I don't have two purple, swollen eyes that can barely make sense of a wobbling opponent. Surely those physical advantages would offset the disparity in skill.

This afternoon's bouts led to some good physiological discussions, though. In the last round of the first fight, Cyn and I saw Zelig "the Lumberman" take a really hard hit. Guard down, like he didn't even know he was boxing. After he was hit, he *definitely* didn't know he was boxing. He took a brief nap, long enough to lose the bout, got up, staggered out of the wreath, and was escorted to the medic. Not for clearance, but for evaluation. We followed him there.

The Pendelhall Medic suggested Zelig use the beds. Not to sleep, but to rest. She told one of the Farhearth interns to stay with him. "And keep him awake. Monitor him for changes to his status. Behavior, alertness, responsiveness. If anything changes, report it to me."

Then the Pendelhall Medic returned to her own duties.

Then Zelig started vomiting.

"Ohhhh", the intern said in three singsong tones. The exact three I would have expected her to intone upon witnessing an adorable puppy bump its head on a cabinet. "Ohhhh", beginning on a high note, dipping into a lower register, then sliding back up, nearly to the original note. After trilling her three-tone song, she asked the vomiting man, "Are you okay?" Even if the concussion hadn't knocked the wits out of him, he was incapable of expelling a response in tandem with the fluids. So how was he supposed to answer? When no answer came, the intern just sat there.

"Are you going to let the medic know?", Cyn asked. She had hoped the question would be understood as a suggestion. It wasn't. "What would I even say?", the intern asked in a reluctant tone.

I stared blankly for a moment. Quietly seething but concealing it with a smile. Cyn interpreted my expression correctly. I was about to say something sharp. Deservedly, I think. If this intern isn't going to take her duty seriously, she has no business working in any health discipline. Or with anything that lives. As I opened my mouth to say that, Cyn interrupted: "I would tell the medic about his status."

"That he's having stomach problems?"

"Tummy aches… tell her it's tummy aches", Cyn said.

The intern left Zelig's bed, headed in the direction of the Pendelhall Medic.

That was way better than what I was going to say. The message conveys two meanings: 1) The patient needs additional attention, and 2) I am too useless to provide it; you would be wise to rescind any trust you may have had in my abilities, or optimism concerning my future, and you should never write me a letter of recommendation.

I looked at Cyn with a gesture of approval. And then said, "Tell me what you know here."

Cyn explained all of the probabilities. And then the possibilities. And I could identify no error in her explanation. Then she said, "Look at his breathing." Zelig had an elevated ventilatory rate. So Cyn explained the "Gogan reflex" (named after Gogan, the boxer, who famously died after exhibiting these symptoms). "It's a multistage cardiovascular phenomenon", Cyn began, as though answering on a formal exam. "First, swelling causes an elevation in intracranial pressure. When the pressure of the cerebrospinal fluid exceeds the mean arterial pressure, the arterioles in the cerebrum are compressed, resulting in a reduction in brain blood flow." She paused to take Zelig's pulse. Then continued: "That cerebral ischemia affects the exchange of blood gases, so the partial pressures of those gases begin to change. This is followed by vasoconstriction and an elevation in cardiac output, attempting to force more blood into the brain. The elevated pressure induces a baroreceptor response, which results in the tenth cranial nerve slowing the heart." She took his pulse again. "And the breathing?", I asked. "A consequence of carbon dioxide tension. Part of the cluster of responses meant to stabilize the gases. Typical presentation of the Gogan reflex."

As Cyn finished her explanation, the Pendelhall Medic arrived. Cyn told her about Zelig's symptoms. Then we got out of her way. If you're not providing an active service, the most useful and compassionate thing you can do is leave.

Our hearts are with Zelig. But it's unlikely he'll ever return to the wreathes. I hope he really does have a secondary career as a lumberman.

While Cyn and I walked to the nearest wreath, I told her, "You're ready." And I meant it. Nobody has ever been readier to be a Pendelhall Medic.

Then we watched some more bouts.

And when it was down to the last four boxers – the semi-finals – Cyn and I joined the gambling. Barely. We each placed a bet for the minimum amount. An amount that was wagered by no other adult. Just Cyn, me, and the local kids gambling their chore coins.

This year, the bookmakers modeled their structure after the Salt and Stone configuration: in addition to selecting a winner, you can choose a boxer who *won't* win. Neither of us knows anything about boxing, so our choices were just guesses. But we agreed not to pick Lanko as the winner. I picked the broadest, muscliest of the four because at this stage, all that really matters is how much of a beating you can endure and still keep your knees. Plus, he looks familiar. But I can't place him in my memory. So maybe he's famous. And fame tends to belong to winners. Cyn's choice was a sinewy Southerner. Whom I did not recognize. When I asked why she chose him, she said he's taken the fewest punches so far, excepting Lanko. I assume the real reason we picked the boxers we did is that we see ourselves in them. And we want to see our likenesses win. We're not immune to the pouzo complex.

Cyn and I agreed on the boxer who wouldn't win. But I felt bad for him, so I changed my bet to Lanko. Wishful gambling. Cyn stayed true to her prediction: the guy having the visible panic attack. The guy I would have chosen if I weren't gambling wishfully, spitefully, and ultimately incorrectly. He was the youngest in the group. Quick and nimble, but this was clearly his first time in the tournament. And his nervousness was invading his heart. He kept checking his pulse, then standing erect with his hands on his head, fingers interlocked, elbows flared out like elephant ears, breathing deeply and deliberately. The Pendelhall Medic came to speak with him. And encouraged him to control his breathing. Which he was already trying to do. So it wasn't that helpful. "It's my heart", he kept telling her. "Breathe with me", she kept saying in response.

I looked at Cyn with the expression of a question (head nodded downward, eyes aimed upward to meet her gaze, brow maximally creased). Cyn's speech went something like this:

"Slowing his heart would go a long way to calming his nerves. And since it's nerves that do the slowing—the tenth cranial nerve in particular: *the wanderer*—that's what I would work with. In *addition* to his breathing. Plenty of options. The gag response works for some people, but it's hardly a calming experience. There's the oculocardiac reflex — applying pressure to the corneal surface — but perhaps pressing on his eyeballs before and after being punched in them is not ideal. I suspect this method is better suited to settings without facial trauma. He could try closing his glottis and blowing out against the closure, increasing intrathoracic pressure, thus stimulating a baroreceptor response. But temporarily heightening his panic to elicit a cure may not be ideal either. He could dunk his face in ice water for about ten seconds; the combination of apnea and the cold stimulus can activate the tenth nerve. But where would he get a bucket of ice water? If I were the Pendelhall Medic, I would have him continue to focus on his breathing, but at the same time, I would perform a carotid sinus massage. In a gentle, non-threatening way. One side at a time. Five seconds or so. Then switch sides. Back and forth. While saying calming things in a calming voice. Given the circumstances, that's probably the best way to seduce the wanderer into cooperation."

Cyn said something like that. But better. And I decided: not only is she ready to become the next Pendelhall Medic, but she's better than the current one. And she's from Cinderheim. She can do this without fatigue or distraction sixteen hours a day.

After our medical discussion, Cyn and I watched the end of the tournament. We also *heard* the end of the tournament. Since the last match determines who "wears the wreath", it garners the most attention. And the most volume. Every year, the final bout in boxing is the single loudest event of the entire tournament. A school of screeching torrent otters would be envious of the collective holler resounding from the crowd.

Cyn's chosen winner didn't win. Neither did mine. Tyfir, the brawny one. Although Tyfir did make it to the final. Against Lanko… who beat him by decision after neither boxer landed a hit on the other. At least Tyfir tried. Lanko never even threw a punch. I can't imagine a more boring match. But that wasn't the worst part. The worst part was Lanko's introduction speech. "The strategist", his bellower called him. And then went on for five minutes about how Lanko can defeat any enemy by movement alone; he can topple entire armies by strategizing *their* movements. "He can win unwinnable wars; against the prince of grace, no nation stands a chance. Tonight's bout is but a taste, a glimpse, a dance." This was followed by a series of comparisons, which went on for at least a full minute. Like this:

"Ugly is the sunlight dancing upon the fountain waters of Thevro; clumsy is the wind dancing through the flowers of Lir; and pitiable is the challenger who chances the wreathes of Pendelhall."

The pronunciations of Lir and Pendelhall nearly rhymed. Somehow.

It was at this unbearable moment of the generally unbearable speech that Cyn turned to me and said, "Lanko is among the top five braggarts of all time… indisputably!" She was imitating the culture we were surrounded by.

I laughed. Lanko won. Then we returned to the inn.

Regnavus is tomorrow.

Bedtime is now.

Thirty-Six

Nyros, Second Lufoa, Day Twenty-Two. Morning.

I'm so glad Cyn didn't go to Farhearth.

That's what I was thinking about when I woke up this morning. I constantly worry it was the wrong decision to discourage her enrollment. But days like yesterday put those worries to rest.

Farhearth only sends their best to the Pendelhall tournament. Their absolute best are the graduates who will be auditioning for the Pendelhall Medic role. But their best *current* students are the interns. And the interns we watched yesterday were spectacularly incompetent. Full of institutional pride though. Their uniforms looked like repurposed Farhearth flags, wrapped around and secured with Farhearth pins.

The reality is, Farhearth is not a student-centered institution. Or a student-care-the-tiniest-bit institution. It used to be. But today, the only priorities are wealth and reputation. Not education. Any unbiased appraisal will come to that conclusion. So what do its administrators do when confronted with this truth? Do they reexamine their priorities with student interests in mind? Of course not. Instead, they invent a shield against the we-only-care-about-money criticism: "school spirit". It's the academic equivalent of patriotism. If you question your government's questionable ethics, you risk deportation. Or it's the equivalent of piety. If you question your religion's tenets, you risk excommunication. One must never question. One must exhibit obedience at all times. With deaf and blind patriotism. With deaf and blind piety. With deaf and blind school spirit. Any institution that teaches loyalty of this kind is one to be distrusted. I think.

Even at its best, a Farhearth classroom functions as a flowerpot: a container meant to fertilize curiosity in its budding state. Mastery never grows there. Maturation beyond mere competence requires a much larger container.

I did learn a lot while I was there. But it was mostly outside of the classroom. Experiences, discussions, and reading the me-sized pile of academic books annually discarded by faculty members. Many of those volumes still reside on my shelf at home. The students who have a childlike zeal for their field – eager to read every word ever written on the subject – could still benefit from Farhearth's nearly infinite resources. But few do. Maybe none.

I tried to create an environment for Cyn that was similarly rich in resources. Nowhere near the scale of Farhearth, with its endless troves of ancient tomes and laboratories of machinery the rest of Gaeans would believe to be magic. But I created abundant enough resources to sate the hungriest learner I have ever met. There was never a night without options of great volumes available to her. Someday soon, I'm sure she *will* manage to consume every word ever written in her field. Or at least every word worth reading. And plenty more, which may not be worth the time, but she'll still glean uncountable profound insights from the effort. Among those unworthy works, I would categorize my old journals. That thousand-page pile of my own insights is back at home, wrapped, waiting to be given to Cyn as a congratulation present.

It seems like a pompous gift: my writing. "I bequeath my genius unto thee!" But that's not my intention. She can read it – nearly twenty years of work – in a matter of weeks to sweep up whatever scraps of a Farhearth education we missed along the way. So it has some utility. But much more than that, it's a matter of sentimentality. When I met Cyn, I was still chronicling every lesson I learned, aspiring to create the most comprehensive compendium of physiology and medicine ever published. So my scientific voice might live on after I've died. But over time, the bulk of my entries became more narrative. I found myself describing Cyn's progress and the joy of our studies together. So, after Cyn gets through every scientific observation I deemed important enough to document, she'll find a portrait of her own life from an earlier time. And a daily account of her journey. And an absurd amount of praise. Which she has never seen or heard. From that perspective, it feels like the right gift. But giving it is just as much about me.

The only way to truly be immortalized is through the words you leave behind. I've always felt like Mizjak didn't really die. Because so many of his thoughts were so well preserved that his mentality can still be constructed. His mind remains long after his body is gone. I harbor a similar motivation. By giving Cyn those pages, I hope to preserve myself in her memory. How we met, how our mentorship began, and the years we spent together.

Also, Cyn will write the greatest okin-gast of all time. And when she does, I'll get to feel – in some small part – like a coauthor.

Now that I think about it, this gift more selfish than I thought. It puts the burden on her to do all the work, while I nap at home. And yet I still expect her to loiter in sentimentality, basking me in a fond and positive light.

That's an expectation I will always keep. And cherish.

Writing the okin-gast is contingent on her audition. Which starts tomorrow. Regnavus is today. Normally, regnavus is the first event of the tournament. Then wrestling, then boxing, then fencing. The smallest crowd to the largest. And that increasing crowd moves clockwise around the city. But this year, it's different. Wrestling was first. Then boxing, then regnavus, then fencing. According to official statements made by the organizers of the tournament, the day off between combat games is reported to exist so that wrestlers and boxers can ready themselves to compete in fencing. To my understanding, there are exactly zero two-sport competitors. Like every other "reported to", the truth is the opposite of the report. Unless you're contradicting obvious facts, official statements are seldom necessary.

In this case, putting regnavus third maximizes its audience. When it's the first event, no one watches it. Because it's a board game. There's so little thrill in seeing a pair of sedentary players move around some small hunks of wood. If regnavus is scheduled after fencing, everyone will have gone home already. If it occurs on the same day as another event, the regnavus players themselves won't even be there. There's no possible position in the sequence that would result in more spectators than creating a pocket between boxing and fencing. So successful is its timing that Cyn and I are planning to watch.

It takes place in Warhale, a massive chamber that otherwise hosts "fests" of feasts and drinking. And dancing to seriously aggressive fiddle music. That's what happens in this hall when regnavus players aren't insisting on silence.

And with that, Cyn and I are off to whisper back and forth while watching sedentary people think really hard.

Thirty-Seven

Nyros, Second Lufoa, Day Twenty-Two. Afternoon.

Cyn and I watched regnavus this morning. On the way to Warhale, I was fortifying my soul to endure a long, dull affair, followed by an afternoon respite with nothing to write about. And then I saw Bonstan take the stage. I've never seen the hall so full. Not even during fiddle and liquor holidays. And when Bonstan began to speak, I had never heard the hall so hushed. Especially during fiddle and liquor holidays.

To the best of my memory – and the quickness of my penmanship; I always come prepared for such an occasion – his ceremonial speech went something like this:

> Today, each of you will challenge your opponents in a battle of wit. A game of brutal incursion, of swift evasion, of military cohesion and cunning tactics. Seeking to topple the tyrant that seeks to topple us. Our success protects the three estates of our realm: the mayoral court, the nobility, and the commoner. But even after victory, we continue warring among ourselves. For there is a fourth estate: the starving, the suffering, the impoverished. Collectively, we call them criminals. And we have long been their oppressors.

> We think ourselves just as we condemn the thief who steals our bread, revile the beggar who spoils our walkways, and revere the martyr who succumbs to his poverty in silence. They all come from the same class, but only the martyr is celebrated. In children's stories, it is honorable for the destitute to remain invisible, and the leper's sores are worn as jewels of dignity. It is time we admit: veneration of this variety is cruel. It is how we pardon ourselves from blame, and simultaneously ensure their misery continues. And it is time we acknowledge that oppression of the poor bears predictable consequences. Segregating them from society promises a revolt from within, as we learned from Milas and Malus. And exiling them from the realm promises a war from without, as we learned from Sinnistyr, upon whom Bellator is based.

> We have a great enemy today – all of us – whom we do not discuss. And it is not some tormentor from Thorn that strikes us so rarely. Fixating on that creature only gives cover to the monster that haunts us daily.

> To address this enemy, we must unite. No longer can every continent be torn in a dozen directions. Imagine a regnavus game in which every piece was controlled by a different player enacting a different strategy. How could that possibly end in victory? Now imagine the governing forces of humanity operating with as many discordant aims. There are dangers in such diverse democracy. Only united can we confront our true enemy.
>
> I propose we begin by building unity into our maps. With bridges that link our nations directly. No longer would the Connected Continents be connected only by the roads of Thorn. No longer would we dwell in distant cities. Or pursue disparate priorities. We would be united. As one Gaea. One people. One family.

Something like that. I know my phrasing is off here and there. And I'm sure I missed a few lines entirely. Bonstan spoke slowly, and I wrote frantically, but it was impossible to keep up. That said, I know I captured the spirit of his message faithfully. And when that message concluded, applause erupted. As loud as any moment yesterday in Wreathes.

I have two reflections:

First, listening to Bonstan portray the plight of poverty is tantamount to me describing the suffering of sea anemones. How could he possibly understand abject privation in his fellow Gaean any more than I understand the despair of reef disruption from a marine invertebrate perspective?

Second, it sounded like Bonstan was calling for the consolidation of power. And what could be more dangerous than that?

Nevertheless, upon his climactic incantation of "one family", the captivated crowd roared its approval.

And then the games began.

I haven't watched regnavus in years. I forgot how funny the first round is.

There were several hundred players. Young and old, masters and novices. Even though I'm not particularly skilled at the game, it's easy to distinguish the professionals from the amateurs. The amateurs are the ones who can be heard blaming their cards. Especially when they lose; that's when they launch into a fervent explanation about how they were going to win – the next eight moves they planned to make – if the cards didn't thwart their brilliant strategy.

Despite vehement claims to the contrary, no one has ever lost because of the randomness of the stack. If you're truly talented, you should be able to hand the deck to your opponent before the game and have them put it in any order they want. And it shouldn't affect the outcome. The same can be said in wrestling, boxing, and fencing, where points are tallied and violations to the rules are enforced. If you can't win when the calls aren't made in your favor, you don't deserve to win.

A reasonable definition of an amateur is someone who requires advantages to be competitive. Thus, whenever a referee's call fails to show favoritism, they argue. They have to. There's no other way to win. The professional, by comparison, interprets overt antagonism as a compliment. Even the most egregious call is received with a smile, understanding it to be a sign of respect. Especially when the intention is otherwise. Recognizing the disparity in skill, the referee is contorting the rules to flatten the imbalance, even the odds. The more obscene the referee's behavior, the greater the respect shown. That's why talented players never contest calls. And whenever an opponent begins to argue, the professional quickly cedes. And exhibits generosity at every opportunity. As if saying, "How about I spot you another five points to make this match more interesting?" Without having to say it.

During my fencing days, my training and technique were both unorthodox. To a degree that seemed to insult traditionalists. This was not my intention; I was merely being true to my nature. I was incorporating my understanding of physiology and honoring my personal tendencies, akin to a singer finding his or her unique timbre. But many referees did not like my "singing voice", so to speak. And it often resulted in unfair calls. And I always felt flattered. Because they wouldn't have risked bending the rules in my opponents' favor if they thought those opponents had a chance at winning on their own merit. The flattery was obvious. So obviously everyone in the audience saw it, too. Which would make it pointless for me to point it out. The only dignified response was to feel grateful for the challenge. If you can't win when the conditions aren't perfect, you're not a winner.

This was never much of a problem for me at Pendelhall. They care deeply about convention... until it impedes achievement. Then they discard those conventions. "To the victor belongs the victory", as they say. It's Harthies who serve as custodians of tradition at the expense of excellence. They do it in academics, too. Although I would argue that actually *facilitates* excellence. Credulity is the enemy of science. All ideas need to be criticized, scrutinized, picked apart and every piece analyzed. Only ideas that can withstand the pummeling of skepticism are permitted to endure. That's how progress is made. Vitriol is a valuable component of the scientific method.

Similarly, if you're completing a Magister's Degree, you want enemies on your committee. Otherwise, you'll never learn to defend your claims. Accordingly, every couple of weeks, I would spend a day lambasting Cyn's every sentence. In time, she learned to parry each attack with perfect grace and riposte with perfect precision. That's the path all heroes take to heroism. I think. You don't hear them complaining when life insists on persecution. Everyone can already see the unfairness in their circumstances. It doesn't need a barker to spread the news. That's why those who complain, even when they're right, are perceived as petty and desperate.

Although I don't believe anyone should practice martyrdom. On this matter, I actually agree with Bonstan. And I assume everyone else does too. Unless they hail porklarks as heroes among birds.

Before the Nameless claimed their Nameless Isle, it was apparently covered in fat, adorable, flightless birds. They wore the coloring of elder crows – the black beaks and tree-moss capes – but their bodies were at least three times the size, and their wings were no bigger than a common lark's. I doubt they were born from the acorns of some deific tree, so their ancestors must have arrived by flight. Having discovered a land where berries were abundant and predators were absent, they settled. And the rest is a tale of evolution that's told in every biology book on a Farhearth shelf. Wings were a metabolically expensive luxury, ample energy stores became a possibility, and worry never served any purpose. So each new generation clipped its wings a little more, pruned its predisposition to panic, and grew in rotundity. Until, finally, the birds were entirely flightless, utterly fearless, and deliciously bulbous.

That's when the Nameless arrived. And ate every single porklark on the isle. Because what could be easier to capture and kill than a creature without fear? A juicy martyr that sits unflinchingly as its predator draws near. Unless it can exterminate that predator in the process, protecting its flock by self-sacrifice, that's not heroism, it's gullibility. The porklark was killed for its belief that life is always fair. And the tamest birds were celebrated by their predators, revered for their silent sacrifice. Or at least that's what anthropologists say.

Someday, oppression of the "fourth estate" may well bear the consequences Bonstan promised. But until that day comes, victory belongs to the victor. And it's won by action. And Cyn is all action. She's no martyr, no porklark; she's a pyloe through and through. If the cards are stacked against her, she'll smile, accept the compliment, express gratitude for the challenge, and win.

But that's tomorrow. When her audition begins. Now it's lunchtime.

Thirty-Eight

Nyros, Second Lufoa, Day Twenty-Two. Night.

After lunch, Cyn and I watched the second half of the regnavus tournament. Only the talented players remained. The players who know every defense, every attack, and the probabilities of every opening board position pairing. And, most importantly, they don't make excuses. Because they know better.

When regnavus is played well, it *is* entertaining. So calculated, subtle, graceful, and sneaky. And the most calculating, subtle, graceful, and sneaky players are always regarded as geniuses. Even if they can do nothing else. Some of them are barely literate, yet they're still lauded as demigods of scholarship. Just consult the portraits of past winners. Each one is sitting in what looks like a sorcerer's laboratory beside a pile of books, wearing reading glasses, thinking deeply behind a furrowed brow. Sometimes a heavy head is resting on the back of a hand. Other times, the hands are making a contemplative gesture of their own. "What a burden it is to know everything about everything", the figure seems to be communicating.

The reputation of regnavus as a contest of extraordinary intellect has led to ludicrous comparisons.

Such as: "Political negotiation is like a game of regnavus."

Or: "Medical diagnosis is like a game of regnavus."

Or, as I'll hear a hundred times tomorrow: "A fencing match is like a game of regnavus." I'll roll my eyes each time I hear it. Finding eyes insufficient, I'll roll my ears and nostrils and any other facial features I can conscript to contribute to my scoff.

Fencing and regnavus have nothing in common. Regnavus has fifteen pieces that players set up in calculated ways to protect and advance their flagbearer while simultaneously attempting to seize their opponent's flagbearer. That's the boardgame equivalent of rowanoki, which no one compares to regnavus. Because it's considered a sport for commoners. And so it's practically a form of a form of blasphemy to liken the two. But they really are the same game.

In rowanoki, two teams of fifteen players – the ryki – attempt to protect their captain – the ryndar – as they advance him to the victory region – the kavagar.

How is that different from regnavus? Excepting physicality, the two contests are nearly identical. And the attention I assign to each is similar: very little. Not for any high-minded reason, but because attention is a finite resource. There are only so many things I can care about. And my roster is already full. Physiology, fencing, music, writing, and a little bit of gardening and cooking. That doesn't leave much room for regnavus or rowanoki.

But I always enjoy watching talented people exhibit their talents. In anything. So, I was entertained by the final regnavus matches.

In the end, someone named Lydria won.

At the instant of her victory, Bonstan took the stage. Again.

And the crowd went quiet – again – as Bonstan began to speak.

After some compulsory "congratulations to all" remarks, he introduced the two finalists, and rewarded the winner, Lydria, with her winnings. Out of his own purse. Apparently, the whole event was funded by Bonstan this year. At least regnavus was. I doubt the other contests were. I can't imagine the Pendelians would lease their authority over the "noble arts" to any outsider no matter the price.

Bonstan then invited Lydria to give a speech of her own. Which she did. And she used the word "humbled" a lot. Why does that word now appear in everybody's victory speech? Have they forgotten what the word means? "I am humbled to receive this distinguished award", people say while they're being applauded by admirers and decorated with plaques and medallions.

My facial anatomy did some more rolling. Then it was Bonstan's turn again. To conclude the event with one more speech promoting the consolidation of power. "Through unity, an even *greater* leap can take flight", he enunciated like a Lonvarakan in training. He was obviously referencing the Great Leap, the advent of intercontinental cooperation that occurred during the age of regnavus. And, of course, everyone cheered wildly. And, just as of course, the cheers continued when Bonstan announced a bridge being built between Charwarg and Baguzu. Entirely funded by him. "Not a flip penny from any other purse", as he phrased it. "On the eighteenth day of Third Lufoa, Gaea will have its first intercontinental bridge, uniting the grasses and the sands. On that day, we will officially open trade between the East and the South. We'll exchange our coins and cultures, and, most importantly, we will merge our families." Deafening cheers erupted as Bonstan waved and left the stage.

If our nations do ultimately merge, I hope political authority doesn't go to anyone who wants it. Those who desire power should never be allowed to wield it. In the age of regnavus, it was the Northerners who were desperate to rule. And desperation seldom begets empathy; it's much more likely to breed tyranny. Just as it did with Sinnistyr (or "Bellator" in regnavus terms).

Today, there is no North. But there are still countless power-cravers waiting to be crowned tyrant. In this group, I would include Bonstan. And anyone else whose wealth inflicts poverty on others. There are only so many pennies, paupers, coppers, nobles, and crowns to go around. One person's abundance is another's dearth. And a tiny fraction of Bonstan's fortune amassed by one is sufficient to impoverish the many.

I would also veto anyone who knows their position in line for a mayoral seat. Which eliminates most Easterners. It may be antipatriotic for me to say, but they would be dangerous leaders. I wouldn't trust me as a monarch either, though. Flatties would flourish under my leadership. In long-overdue ways. But Thevroans? The crumbs of their crumbling empire would go tumbling down the hill. In long-overdue ways. I think. But I'm biased. And bias has no business in governance. So I would veto myself. Rorrik? Too ambitious. Lum? Maybe. Cyn? Sure. Although Lum and Cyn are both Southerners. As is Bonstan, although I think his ancestry is Western. He was at least born *of* the West if not *in* it. And Westerners don't typically aspire to sit in thrones. But Bonstan seems to be vying for the role of intercontinental king anyway.

To his credit, he has coffers deep enough to serve ten terms without a single coin of taxation. But there's no way Bonstan would empty his bank for the public's prosperity. No one ever has and I suspect no one ever will.

That's enough political talk.

Of much greater personal importance: fencing begins tomorrow. And it lasts three days.

It begins with pools – seven fencers in each pool – to determine seeding. How those seeds matriculate into the brackets, I still don't know. During my competitive years, I just followed instructions, went where I was told to go. Once the brackets have been planted with the seedlings, it's single elimination to the end. Those are called the "direct elimination" bouts or "DEs", and bout by bout, they whittle away the fencers. Until only the finalists remain. And the sixth ring finally opens. For this one moment. For the last match. For the climax of the six-day, four-event tournament.

On our way home this evening, Cyn and I passed by the registration booth. We hoped to look at the roster, but we couldn't get near it. Because there was still a line of registrants. There must be five hundred fencers this year. Maybe more. Probably double the amount who registered during the year I competed. But I doubt it'll be any more difficult than my year. Just longer. The total number of registrants does not reflect the head count of serious contenders. That number tends to be consistent from year to year.

Now it's time for Cyn and me to sleep. Or at least try. I may be too nervous to succeed. But I'll spend the night supine anyway.

I told Cyn that I would collect her in the morning. "Even if you can't sleep, just lie in bed and rest. Mediate, reflect, mentally prepare. I'll bring breakfast when the hour comes."

That hour suddenly feels so… sudden. After almost six years, it somehow seems thrust upon us too soon. But at the same time, I know she's ready. Much more than ready. No one has ever been more deserving.

Thirty-Nine

Eldos, Second Lufoa, Day Twenty-Three. Morning.

I'm awake. I rolled around in bed all night. Too anxious to sleep.

The fencing tournament begins today. Which means my legacy auditions. And there's nothing I can do to aid its success. Anything I could have done is done already. All I can do is wait. And watch. And listen to people scream. That's the worst part. The screaming. Not by injured people. But by fencers who just scored a point. For some reason, all of them – male, female, young, and old – scream after every touch. It's creepy. Imagine if regnavus players did that. Any time they claim one of their opponents' pieces, they bellow like a bison in labor. Fists clenched. Mouth gaping. Howling in the general direction of their opponent.

The display makes them appear fragile to me. Like a frightened cat fluffing its fur. Or a counterfeit currency. Trying to pass for the language of violence. "If my roar is loud enough, people won't hear my fear squealing beneath it", they seem to reason. "If my fists are clenched tightly enough, they won't see the hands trembling within."

Whenever this display rears, all I can see is a terrified child. An imposter. A crook trying to push a counterfeit coin across my table. Needless to say, I was a silent fencer. So was Rorrik. Even though he has the most powerful voice of any living fencer, he lets the whistle of the blade serve as a substitute for screaming. "The warrior's roar", I once coined it. Then Lum truncated it to: "the roarier".

Both of us will be labored in our breathing if the battle goes on long enough, and if it *keeps* going on, our huffing can grow loud. But neither of us grunts. Or stomps around in tantrum or triumph. Victory without subtlety is like gluttony without satiety. It's as gross as it is pointless. Very few people seem to agree, though. Very few people see the screamers as thunder without any lightning, all that rumbling absent the tiniest flash.

The only dignified situation in which a mouth should gape that wide is while dental work is being done. Or while you're issuing a magnificent yawn, assuming it's well deserved. Not because your sword poked someone three seconds ago. That's not merely bad-mannered; it's an indulgence that ruins one's subsequent performance.

Our neurochemicals are not limitless. They function in exhaustible systems. And the compounds that accompany celebration are critical for focus. And focus is critical for success. Which means success favors those who temper excitement rather than indulge it. Screamers energize the present moment by syphoning their chemical reserves, borrowing from their futures. This is something they would know – on a practical level – had they read Gundric's work. But they were too busy practicing their postures. Those are homes with well used mirrors.

I should stop writing. The sun will start its rise before long. It's time for me to go find breakfast. For Cyn and me. I'd like to be at the rings plenty early. Leave in an hour. Hour and a half, maybe. Two at the latest. Okay, I'm off to fetch breakfast.

Forty

Eldos, Second Lufoa, Day Twenty-Three. Still morning.

It's still morning. It hasn't been more than thirty minutes since I put my pen down. When I stepped outside to get Cyn and me breakfast, her window was open, and her lamp was lit.

"I thought you were going to stay in until it was time to go", I said through her window.

"I was up." Then she pointed at a cleanly cut cube of breakfast cake and said, "Got you this."

I came into her room and inspected the cake. It looked like it would be light and fluffy. But I know the sort of sustenance the Pendelhall bakers serve: impressively stodgy and packed with calories. When I poked it to confirm, it had the texture and density of flesh. Like I was poking firmly flexed glutes.

As we ate, Cyn told me she checked registration this morning. She said there were more than seven hundred contestants in all. The West and South were well represented. The youngest contestant was ten, which is the minimum age of eligibility (no one that young ever makes it out of pools). The oldest was seventy-one (I doubt he'll make it out of pools either). And close to half of all contestants were female, many of whom will win their respective pools.

Fencing is the only truly diverse sport there is. But it wasn't always that way. It used to be predominantly populated by Eastern men aged twenty to fifty. Wrestling and boxing are *still* teeming with males in their twenties and thirties from a limited number of cities. But in fencing, men and women across the lifespan representing nearly every culture now participate.

Credit for this rightfully goes to Gundric. Quite wrongfully, none of it does. Everyone assumes it was mere coincidence that female representation at the games multiplied twenty-fold with Gundric's victory. Before she competed, the roster of female competitors was a single digit number. Three or four, five would be a lot, six unusual. The year after Gundric won, there must have been eighty women. And many ended in respectable positions. To this day, however, Gundric is assigned no credit. And worse than being denied her due praise, she's assigned undue scorn.

That's one more reason I've long felt a connection with her: she competed once. And won once. And when she did, she was denounced by the public. I can relate on some level. Although for different reasons. And on a smaller scale. *Much* smaller; it's almost vulgar to compare my situation to hers. After the tournament, she was never seen in the East again. Flung so far into exile that nobody even knows where to find her today. Or whether she's findable at all. Maybe she died. No one knows that either. My experience was minor by comparison. Also, mine didn't defy the systematic oppression of an entire sex in both sport and military. And topple it, cobbling the road for all future women to travel. *That* is a martyrdom I can revere. My life has no such sacrifice in it. Only scorn. Which is what nourishes my kinship with Gundric.

Cyn listened patiently as I blathered on about my favorite fencer. And when I had finished, she said, "I have *more* news… maybe."

I stared at her for several seconds. Blankly. Then I replaced the blankness on my face with an expression that Cyn correctly interpreted to mean, "What news?"

"I think Rorrik is here", she said.

"What makes you think that?", I asked. Using actual words.

"The final name on the fencing roster was Olryn. Representing Laberyn."

If Cyn is right – if Rorrik is competing – this will be his fourth tournament. I entered once. And won every bout. Even in pools. Which means my undefeated streak remains intact. To this day, I have never lost at Pendelhall. So how hard can it be? That's the exact sentence I used to say to Rorrik all the time. To coax him into participation. "I won at twenty, so how hard can it be?" It never coaxed him. Instead, he'd say, "If you're going to recite a poem, you should just learn to sing." By this, he meant: why *pretend* to fight when you could do the real thing?

It took a few years, but I did finally persuade him to compete. With beer. Not just any beer, though. It was a hard-to-come-by Moonkruug ale, which I came by easily through Lum, who came by it the hard way. I had six bottles. And Rorrik agreed to compete if I gave him three. I did. So Rorrik entered. And won every bout. Even in pools. After the final, we each drank a bottle. To celebrate. In many ways, he was in his prime back then. No fencer had ever been more imaginative. So uninhibited by the constraints of classical technique. Watching him fence was like witnessing the birth of an art form. Like the first brush strokes of impressionism decorating a canvas.

The victory had an inflating effect on Rorrik's self-assurance, though. Which emptied him of any motivation to continue training. Instead, he spent every spare minute playing his lute and singing, surrounded by admirers, whose constant flattery functioned like bellows, keeping Rorrik's ego distended.

The following year, Rorrik entered the tournament again. With no coaxing from me. And no preparation at all. And he failed to make the top eight. He *just* missed; I think he ended in ninth place, which is a respectable rank for anyone else. But not for Rorrik. It ruptured his pride and simultaneously ingrained in him a ferocious discipline. And he's never been the same since. During the year leading up to the next tournament, I doubt anyone has ever trained as hard as Rorrik did. He even gave up beer. For a few years a least. He would have turned down Moonkruug's finest ale if offered. So when the next tournament finally came, nobody stood a chance. In many *new* ways, Rorrik was in his prime. He had sacrificed some of his imagination, but more than made up for it with classical mastery. Mizjak himself might have found him a worthy adversary. And again, he won handedly. From pools to finals, I don't think a single sword touched him. That was the last year he competed. Until now. If he is, in fact, "Olryn".

Time to put the journal away. Cyn has a date with the mending tent. Fencing doesn't start until 9:00, but she has to be there an hour early for orientation, which means we'll be arriving an hour earlier than that, which means it's time to leave.

Forty-One

Eldos, Second Lufoa, Day Twenty-Three. Afternoon.

I just finished eating. At the food court by the Elyem ring. Alone. Because I'm too nervous to watch. All morning, I felt the anxiety beating in my heart, churning in my stomach. So I'm going to sit here for a while and distract myself with writing. Until my insides unclench.

The games are currently on midday break. For another ten or fifteen minutes. But the medics don't have open breaks. They have to stay at the rings until the day is done. It's not as bad as it sounds. Food is available during every ring change, and each tent has its own restroom in case bladders grow so full the sphincteric levees can no longer hold. Most auditioning medics dehydrate themselves before the event. And those who don't tend to be too distracted with duty to notice the urgency accumulating within. Or at least that was true for me during my audition. When I finally excused myself to urinate, it must have taken ten minutes.

Cyn didn't bother dehydrating this morning. Probably because the breakfast cake was impossible to swallow dry. With no syrup to irrigate the parched flour clod, every bite had to be followed by a swig of water.

After we finished eating, we left for the rings. Early enough that Cyn was the first medic on site. By half an hour. Eventually, everyone else arrived and orientation began. The Operating Medic gave them a tour of the rings and explained their duties over the next two days. And violations to those duties, which were brief and simple: do not leave your tent, do not consult anyone, and do not lose or forget to submit your journal at the end of each shift.

If this were Farhearth, the explanation of violations would take half the day. And the other half would be used up by safety precautions. Obvious things that shouldn't need to be said. Don't put other people's blood in my mouth? Okay. Got it. Here, the explanation of all responsibilities – and breaches of those responsibilities – lasted about three minutes.

At the end of orientation, Cyn was given her journal. Today and tomorrow, it will be issued to her at the beginning of her shift, and when the shift ends, it must be relinquished. During all active hours of the tournament, Cyn must document every diagnosis and treatment, and record every pertinent detail about each.

This is how each auditioning medic will demonstrate their understanding of physiology and medicine and prove themselves capable of distinguishing the extraneous from the germane.

Bodies don't fib. But the patients themselves often do. They can generally be trusted to report temporal patterns and aggravating and alleviating factors truthfully. But the onset and duration of their injuries are seldom described accurately. Because honesty precludes care. The auditioning medics provide free service to all contestants, but there is a clause in the contracts that the fencers must sign, which prohibits "soliciting diagnosis or treatment for any condition unrelated to the contest". This doesn't stop anyone from seeking care. It just stops them from telling the truth about how their ailment came to be. Half of all fencers who visit the mending tents on the first day have injuries that were sustained prior to pools, but none admit it. And as long as they *say* it's a new injury, the medics are required to diagnose and treat.

This is an important part of the interview process. What the auditioning medics write about these patients is given considerable weight in selecting the Pendelhall Medic. Because it's an effective way of demonstrating biological literacy. If you can read body language fluently – not just postures and facial expressions, but the deep grammar – you can discriminate facts from fibs. And those who can do that are shown favoritism. Subjective favoritism. *Objective* favoritism is shown by one's starting place.

Cyn was assigned the Rynoa ring as her first station. As I write this, she has finished that shift and is moving to Lufoa. Those are the two best rings. Which means she was assigned the worst starting position. I suspected that would be the case. Being the alternate who made it into the tents, she was given the last seat.

Rynoa is enriched with music. The fencers try harder here. Their ambition is magnified, pain sensitivity minimized. This is where the most spectacular matches happen. But it's wasted on the opening rounds of pools, where the talented attempt to conserve energy and the untalented are too nervous to notice. Then there's Lufoa, the quietest of the five. Where focus is sharpest in fencer and medic alike. Also wasted on pools. This is where you want to end. And it's where the favored medics and fencers both do.

Tomorrow, there will be three shifts. Cyn will start early at Elyem, transition midmorning to Arzox, the stinky ring, and conclude the day – and her role in the tournament – at Lylir, distracted by the drunkards. The closer it gets to the finals, the drunker those drunkards become. They grow louder and more belligerent by the hour. Which makes Lylir the worst place to end.

The favored medic always starts today in Elyem. Before the whole crowd has filled out. And the spectators who *are* present have far more interest in food than fencing. Pools are just getting started. Nothing has happened yet. So there's nothing to talk about. So they eat their breakfasts quietly. So the usual hubbub is muted. This is the one instance Elyem is as quiet as Lufoa. By the time the bustle begins, this medic will already be moving to Arzox. And for tomorrow's rotation, they start in Lylir, while the drunkards are still hungover in their beds. They move to Rynoa before the first drink is served. And then they finish the day in Lufoa. They work every ring at the ideal time.

I looked to see who started in Elyem this morning. It's the Incumbent Medic. Whenever a previous medic auditions, if there's only one of them auditioning, they *always* get that ring. And they *almost* always deserve it. Pendelhall Medics learn an enormous amount while serving the role. Part of what makes the year of service so fruitful is their access to the historical works. The Archives are open to them twenty-four hours a day. Interminably. If Cyn isn't hired, her access ends when the games do. When she returns her inferior-looking lanyard, she can no longer enter. But a Pendelhall Medic's access is for life. And the good ones make use of it. That's why medicine is so much more advanced here. Not for diseases of disuse, what the elderly and the sedentary develop, but the afflictions of the exerting class. Nowhere in the world are soldiers and athletes better understood, or better treated.

The earliest works in the library are scarcely useful for their therapeutic recommendations, but they had great descriptions of the injuries themselves. In the more recent journals, sound recuperative medicine accompanies the characterizations of injuries.

Even better than the auditioning medics' journals, however, is the shelf on the opposite wall. Which contains the okin-gast of every Pendelhall Medic who has ever served. Those are the best works on health ever written. And, a year from now, I hope Cyn will begin writing her own.

To do that, she'll have to beat out all four medics positioned ahead of her. I spent more time watching them than I did Cyn. I rarely glanced in Cyn's direction. These days are hers, not mine. So I didn't want to hover. Instead, I wandered around the other rings. And hovered around the other medics. Spectators aren't allowed inside the tents. They're roped off from the public. But you can get near enough to see and listen. If you loiter at the boundary. Which I did. And I heard more than therapy being discussed. There *was* talk of tissue restoration and injury prevention, but I also heard theories about nutrition and hydration. And advice on stretching and warming up, and lots of other blanket lore, all of which ignored the individuality of individuals.

Dehydration was a common theme, and rehydration was a common panacea. Are your muscles unusually sore? Or your throat? Are you feeling dizzy? Anxious? Do your legs feel heavy? Does your head hurt? Or stomach ache? Has your appetite abandoned you? Are you experiencing bowel problems? Elevated heart rate? Lingering fatigue? Just drink this glass of water. And by the greenest grace of Adon, put down that coffee! Or tea. Or hot chocolate. Or any other drink with the tiniest trace of methylxanthines.

I heard one medic prescribe abstinence from these beverages for the duration of the tournament. "Water must be consumed in the form of water lest you gradually transform into a stoneman", she said to a middle-aged male who complained about cramps between bouts.

"I hope she writes that down", I mumbled from my lurking place.

Ingesting pure caffeine powder, isolated by a skilled alchemist, may exert a diuretic effect. But if a small amount is dissolved in a large amount of water, as it is with teas and coffees, one need not worry about bodily petrification. Especially among routine drinkers, who develop a tolerance to the effect on urinary volume. *Also* especially in a male who exercises following ingestion. Attenuating factors, both. I would be more concerned with the consequences of changing an athlete's established routine. Eliminating a compound one is accustomed to will probably impair performance rather than enhance it.

When I was done disparaging this medic, I wandered to a different ring, which was clearly occupied by a Harthy-hillian. Someone who was "raised in Thevro to raze abroad", as we say in the flats. Thevro has a few useful exports, such as the Ryn River birch (which means river river birch... which they named). This is the wood all paper is made from. Meaning every page of my journal began its life in Thevro. As a nutlet on a catkin. So I hold gratitude for some of Thevro's contributions to the world. But the Thevroans themselves are a terrible export. And those who are exported to Farhearth are the worst kind. The kind of person who stands two inches taller than they are just to look down on their peers. The kind of person who wears jewelry they purchased themselves just to flaunt their wealth. The kind of person who is incapable of discerning talent from style, or merit from edginess. Here is the edginess I heard from this bejeweled young hillian: "Alcohol *is* a diuretic, but in your case, it may be of some benefit." That piqued my antagonism – my need to find faults in Cyn's competition – so I listened to his reasoning.

"If morning's chill settles into your tissues, it'll renew old injuries", he said. "Alcohol can keep you warm, though. And a warm fencer is a limber fencer. And a limber fencer is less susceptible to strain. *Further* strain, in your case."

He kept saying "in your case" to the fencer, pretending to be individualized in his generalities. Which was his way of pretending to be smarter and better than his competition.

"In your case", the medic continued, "A drink or two will curb the pain you're currently feeling while simultaneously settling your nerves."

The fencer replied, but he wasn't facing me. So I couldn't hear what he said or see his expression. Both must have conveyed some reluctance, though, given the medic's response: "What you lose in acuity will be made up for in creativity, twice over. The only pressing concern is impaired muscle control. Fortunately, that's a problem we can manage."

Now I was *really* listening.

"Strychnine is a potent inhibitor of an inhibitory compound", he explained. "A facilitator, so to speak. A small dose, which I have here, can set you right. You'll be warm and limber, aggressive and creative. Primed to beat every opponent made sluggish by the chill and foolish by nervousness."

The fencer succumbed.

The fact that the medic had both alcohol and strychnine on hand means he expected to prescribe them. The fact that he deployed several well-rehearsed sentences in his prescription tells me many *more* fencers will be competing in a frenetic fuddle in this medic's ring. And I'm sure each of them will be an "in your case" scenario.

Some of what he said is true, but for every pound of merit, there's a full stone of edginess. Wild fictions built upon modest truths, which aren't nearly broad enough to support them.

A couple of modest truths here. First, alcohol *is* a diuretic, unlike many of the other tavern potions indicted on the charge (no one has ever dehydrated oneself with tea). It inhibits vasopressin, which serves as the chemical jailor of our pee. The percentage of alcohol must be rather high for that inhibition to offset the volume of fluid ingested, though. The average ale isn't potent enough to provoke a jailbreak. Wine and spirits are the bladder brews.

The second truth: strychnine is a competitive inhibitor of the glycine receptor, and glycine is the primary inhibitory chemical messenger in some neuronal areas responsible for locomotion. This pathway was discovered very recently, and it continues to be a topic of considerable attention at the Farhearth Faire.

Now, let's get into the wild fictions. Beginning with the hearth fire effect of alcohol. In hot environments, cutaneous blood flow increases to unload heat. In cold environments, the opposite effect happens: we minimize heat loss by diverting blood from our shells to our cores, thus increasing the temperature gradient between our organs (which *need* heat) and our skin (which *wants* heat). A scalp may stay relatively warm, but fingers transform into icicles. We can't let our shells suffer the frost without respite forever, though. Lucky for us, the muscles inside the walls of our peripheral vessels – which are responsible for constricting away the blood – become paralyzed when their temperature gets low enough. This forces their relaxation. And when they relax, all the blood that's been huddling around our organs pulses to the periphery, which warms it up. Once those vessels are warm, they re-squeeze. And the blood scutters back to the core like roaches fleeing the light. We tend to oscillate in cycles of fifteen to thirty minutes. Unless alcohol is consumed. Downing a mug of spirits will disrupt this regulation. The previously cowering blood boldly rushes to the surface, flushing our skin. Just like it would if we were standing under the Southern sun. In the cold, the heat loss is rapid, but while we're risking life for limb, the cold receptors in our skin give us that hearth fire feeling. Thus, "Alcohol can keep you warm". Nonsense.

As for the benefit of strychnine, less glycine binding *does* mean less inhibition, but, "in your case", if you're hoping for something better than spasms and convulsions, your hopes are likely to be counted among the dashed. And you might spasm yourself into asphyxiation if you take enough.

In *any* case, this medic is unlikely to be hired. Pendelhall would never risk negligence of this kind. Some Farhearth clinic maybe, but not Pendelhall.

I listened to the other medics, too. The Incumbent and a Rivervalan Harthy. I stood at the perimeter of their tents like an angler fishing for mistakes. For an hour. But I didn't catch any. Disappointed, I watched fencing instead.

Some of the fencers seemed talented, but they were too impetuous, and they were beaten by obvious pouzos. Clearly, they never studied Gundric's books. Other fencers appeared even more talented and might have been contenders for the top sixteen if they hadn't cut so much weight. Whenever I endeavor a feat of athleticism, I prefer to err on the side of auctionable livestock: overfed and waterlogged. But most people take the opposite tack. For two reasons. The *stated* reason is always "to be nimbler". As though nimbleness automatically accompanies lighter form. But the *unstated* reason is probably the real motivator: people think preliminary seeding – placement in pools – is based on weight classes. Because a few anthropometric measurements are collected at registration. And "those values *must* determine athlete allocation!"

They don't. The data are strictly for research. With no bearing on the games. But since the competitors have no idea how pools get populated, theories get invented. Mostly about bodyweight or height-to-weight index. The athletes prepare according to those theories, often depleting all vitality in the process. Then every lucky assignment corroborates their belief while every unlucky assignment is attributed to a conspiracy.

I also saw some injuries. The usual. Mostly blunt trauma. And two breaks. After each injury, I watched how the fencers were treated. Both medics tried to "set" the breaks, as though every problem is a disjointed thing that merely needs rejointing. The damage can be undone by simply snapping some bits back where they belong. Then the fencer is ready to go in the next round!

That's not really how it works.

And the blunt trauma wasn't treated much better. Whether there was any external bleeding, there was definitely internal. And yet I watched the medics rubbing the wounds, assuming massage – *deep* massage – was a useful therapy. On ten-minute-old injuries. Even if they were few-day-old injuries, massage seems contraindicated. If you see a damaged scaffold, you don't kick it and shake it to fix it. The structure that remains intact is vulnerable to collapse. Otherwise, a raging stampede of mugogi would be an architectural repair-all. Similarly, intact fabric is difficult to rip, but fabric that has a small tear in it is easy to cleave. Our tissues are similar. Penetrative rubbing isn't helpful.

"Why would anyone do that?", I whispered to myself in a condescending tone as I watched the Harthy-hillian brutally rub an arm that was bashed numb by the pommel of a sword. As if he heard me, he explained his reason: "I'm increasing your blood flow." He said that – to a wincing athlete – in a tone that was far more confident than mine was condescending. So I released an even *more* condescending sigh. Because blood flow is already increased. Why else would his arm be so red? Did he get a focal sunburn between impact and treatment? Even if that weren't true, metabolism determines blood flow. So the masseuse's hands experience the greatest increase. Consider the horse and carriage. Perhaps the rider gets jostled a bit in the seat. And maybe the jarring results in a slight augmentation of circulation. But the horse hearts are doing the real beating, and the horse muscles are doing the real receiving. Metabolism is the foundation of medicine. Fortunately for Cyn (though not the patients), any medic who expresses ignorance for this won't be hired at Pendelhall. Fortunately for the patients (though not for Cyn), the Incumbent Medic and Rivervalan Harthy displayed no such ignorance. Every sentence was sound, every treatment perfect, nothing they did was foolish.

The other two were worse than foolish. They conducted themselves with equal parts ignorance and confidence. And that combination is dangerous. Assuming they document half of that danger in their journals, they won't be in the running. Only three auditioning medics are eligible for appointment. One of which is Cyn.

I didn't intend to watch Cyn during any point of her audition. But my eyes disobeyed my will on occasion. On each of those occasions, she was either treating attentively or scribbling frantically. The most focused medic there. The most qualified. The most deserving.

While I was accidentally staring in Cyn's direction, Olryn's name was called. Along with six other names. They were being summoned to the Rynoa ring. Cyn's ring. That's where their pool would be held.

I waited. Curiously.

Six people arrived immediately. Most of them looked anxious. None of them I recognized.

A minute or two passed.

Then, just as the bouts were about to begin, I saw him. Olyrn. It must be. He was walking toward Rynoa casually.

From a distance, he looked remarkably like Rorrik. And walked like Rorrik. He was carrying two swords. His competition sword – a number three – and a personal one.

When he saw me, we exchanged a smile of acknowledgement. Then he said, "Hold this for me while I fight?" Rorrik considers "fence" a euphemism for the crudeness of cutting and stabbing. Boxing, wrestling, fencing. It's all just fighting. "Calling a pig *ham* doesn't trigger transformation", he once said.

Rorrik was holding out his personal sword. "Of course", I said as I took it. Practically every time I see him, he has recently come to possess some old, rare artifact. And I can only imagine how the acquisition transpired. Maybe his smile and charm and renown earn him opportunities that are unavailable to others. One opportunity leads to another. And now he owns this ancient book. Or map. Or material miracle fashioned by a legendary locksmith or woodworker. Or, in the present case, a sword. And the next time I see him, he's traded it away. For some other rare thing. I don't know that this sword is ancient, rare, priceless, or miraculous, but it *is* weird.

While Rorrik stood ringside, waiting to "fight" his pool rivals, I inspected his sword more closely. I couldn't swing it around owing to the crowd. I would end up beheading half a dozen people. But I felt the sharpness of its edges, the smoothness of the metal. It was pristine. The overall dimensions were similar to the number four sanctioned sword. Which is probably the reason it's so pristine: unused swords tend to be unchipped.

While the blade resembled that of a bastard sword, the grip didn't. It had a half-basket hilt with five symmetrical guard bars, only the center one joining the pommel. There was no room for a second hand to help manage its bulk. To compensate for the weight, it had leather straps (which smelled like sweat and grapefruit) to secure one's hand to the grip. If the sword weren't grafted into your anatomy in this way, like an extension of your arm, it would be too unwieldy for the average fencer to wield it.

At the base of the blade there was a short, thick ricasso. Blunt on both sides. Dull and smooth, not embossed. No mark of its maker. Then thirty inches of backsword. Perfect back, perfect edge. And it had a shallow central fuller that continued to the end, where the last five or six inches were double-edged. And hazardously sharp.

As a cutter, it was perfect. Defensively, it seemed perfect, too. The flat back and wide blade would make it easy to brace with your second hand for some half-swording… if I did that sort of thing. And the needle-pointed tip would make it effective at thrusting… if I did *that* sort of thing. Lancing with an actual lance would surely be preferable, but in the absence of pole arms, this sword would work better than most.

But it wasn't normal. Ungainly size aside, what I found most bizarre was the balance. When I first tested it, it was about half a foot from the hilt. Then I held it upright. And moved it back and forth a bit, as though I were tightly alternating between parries four and six. Just to see how the sword moved without stabbing anyone. And something changed. Like it wasn't the same sword in action as it was at rest. In a living creature, blood circulates differently when standing and lying. I don't know how that could be true for a hunk of metal, but I tested the balance again and it seemed to have retracted a few inches. But that's when Rorrik entered the ring. So I slid his sword back into its scabbard and watched.

Rorrik won. Handedly. *Heavy* handedly. And nimble footedly. And quickly. His opponent didn't have a hope of a chance. Then Rorrik won again. The second bout took half a minute. And again. Twenty seconds. After two more agains, each quicker than the last, he finished his pool undefeated.

Rorrik left his ring, made his way to where I was standing, and greeted me properly. As I handed him back his sword, I asked, "Why are you competing? And where have you been? And when did you get here? And are you ready for the tournament? Have you been training?"

He answered every question but one. In the reverse order:

He hasn't been training in a structured way, but he's as conditioned as he needs to be. And no, he isn't ready. "Not yet. But today was just a warmup. I'll be ready tomorrow." He got in early this morning. Hasn't even gotten a room. All he had time to do was register, stable his horse, and get back to the rings. He traveled through the night, which is why he needed a warmup day. "Wasn't sure I would make it in time to compete", he said. "But that's not the reason I'm here." Then he explained the reason: recruitment.

It's not necessarily *me* he's recruiting. The invitation stands, should I change my mind. But along his travels – wherever that was – he's been forming ideas on how to confront the "abomination of Thorn". And upon confrontation, how to kill it. But he can't do that alone. He needs more arms. "Well armed ones", he specified. "No point in recruiting today, though. I don't know a single name in the brackets. Haven't paid attention since I last fought here. After tomorrow, I'll have a smaller sample to scout."

"Sounds like you could use some rest", I said, and offered my room. "I can't rest while that wandering plague still lurks and prowls", he responded. And I took it as hyperbole. Because Rorrik's most restless night of sleep is enviable compared to my best. But I understand the trauma that haunts him. Or at least I understand *that* there is trauma. It's the unpredictable malignancy of the creature that he finds so unsettling. He can't anticipate its attacks, so he can't prepare for them. And if he can't prepare, he has no sense of control. Tavern brawls, no matter how fierce and catastrophic, don't affect us in the same way. Because they're avoidable. We choose to participate; we choose to put ourselves at risk. And we could just as easily choose to avoid that risk. A campfire is every bit as dangerous as an arrow. But you're in control of whether you're singed by the flame. Not knowing if or when the arrow will strike would be a far more anxious environment. So, while I don't share Rorrik's particular trauma, I understand it enough to be sympathetic.

"After the tournament, I'll be back on the road", Rorrik said. And then he invited me to join.

"If I were Rivervalan, I…" "Watercat's worms, I know", Rorrik interrupted, realizing the expression I was about to incant.

I have no idea what the expression *actually* means. "A watercat never changes its worms." I take it to mean the rykub's diet never changes, and a consistent diet begets consistent parasites. Which seems to be a fair characterization of Rorrik. Year after year, he feeds on the same ambition and suffers the same consequences. I envy his perseverance, but his invitation isn't very tempting. I just prefer safer sustenance.

"We see the world in different ways", I said to Rorrik. "It's like we're looking out at the landscape, in different directions, trying to reconcile what we see. You're an adventurer focused on the great beyond, and I'm a sentimentalist savoring the great behind. I can't convince you of the beauty in my direction, and you can't persuade me to go marching blindly into yours."

"You're cutting your own purse", he said.

Then we smiled, embraced, and I told him I was glad he was here.

Say what you want about Rorrik, but he's a man who knows how to make a reunion. No matter what the circumstances are. The more dire the better. Just when you think he's lost or dead, there he is. Bright and spectacular. Usually singing a song. And it's the best song you've heard since his last one.

Somehow, the two of us remain companionable. We meet in every middle. Preservation and sacrifice. Idleness and urgency. Hermit and hero. And we both know there's no amount of heroism that will wheedle this hermit into an adventure. But still he tries.

I should stop writing and get back to the rings. To watch some more bouts. To scrutinize Cyn's competition. I'm sure I'll have more to write later.

Forty-Two

Eldos, Second Lufoa, Day Twenty-Three. Night.

I just took some of the caligoroot I got earlier. It's like the Eastern equivalent of rainbow ruderalis. But less whimsical. The fruit and flower of the ruderalis have compounds that, when inhaled or ingested, inspire artistic productivity. It settles our worries and nourishes our imaginations, making us feel childlike in our attention. By comparison, caligoroot makes us childlike in our sleep. You won't be productive, but you won't be restless either. And that's what I need tonight. There's no way I'd be able to fall asleep without it. And after a poor night's sleep, I'm more susceptible to anxiety. Which makes it difficult to focus. Which makes productivity a challenge. Which makes me even more anxious. Which makes it even harder to focus. Which makes productivity almost impossible, which makes me pathologically anxious… and so on.

Hoping to avoid this spiral, I made a mug of chamomile tea and sprinkled half a serving of caligoroot in it. I haven't had it in years, so that should be a sufficient amount.

It'll be an hour before it takes effect, though. I'll spend that hour writing.

Cyn's first day is done. And so are pools. The bottom fifth will be eliminated. Everyone else advances. More than five hundred fencers begin their direct elimination bouts tomorrow. They'll start early and go all day. However long it takes to get through everyone but the top sixteen. Those final fifteen bouts happen the following day. On Aldos. Then there's a day of nothing. Lyros. Nothing for *us*, anyway. That's the day of judgment for Cyn's committee. From sunup to sundown, the six members will read every journal, praise and criticize each candidate, disagree with one another, argue, and eventually come to a decision. The next day, that decision will be announced. On Fyros. Late morning. Then, that evening, we'll watch the Closing Ceremony, where every champion and reserve champion from all four events will be honored.

During those celebrations, the formal induction into the Champions' Guard will take place. And, much more importantly, the next Pendelhall Medic will be announced. Then, finally, the mayors will deliver the State of the Nations, a formal address in which we, the common folk, are informed of the coming year's Gaea-wide political agenda. Perhaps it's not Gaea's *full* width as places like Mulgotha won't be represented, but most cities will.

Each of the thirteen mayors will give a short speech, and they'll be separated from the audience by the Champions' Guard. Every member, including the latest appointment, will be fully armed and armored, encircling the stage in an intimidating display of authority. This is a formality that gets more formal every year. Not out of necessity. It has nothing to do with security. It's just a theater prop to emphasize authority.

I still think Cyn can win. And *should* win. Despite the Incumbent auditioning.

But even if all goes wrong, we'll stay for the Closing Ceremony. Then we'll head home. For a couple of nights. To sleep in an actual bedroom, to eat garden-grown food, and to brew my own grey nettle tea. And to check on Abbie and Gyfur, assuming I'll be playing host for a while longer as Rorrik resumes his questing. Then it's off to Farhearth. To submit Cyn's abstract to the annual Science Faire.

In the meantime, before any of that happens, there's a lot of tournament left. And this afternoon, I did eventually overcome my anxiety, leave the eateries, and return to the rings.

Between this morning and this afternoon, there were more than a hundred pools in all. Rorrik wasn't the only one who went undefeated, obviously. About a third of the pools had someone match his record. He'll have a good seeding tomorrow, but so will forty other fencers.

Some of the undefeated ones seemed pretty untalented. I would have gladly faced them today. Without warming up. And without a helmet or padding. Others looked a little threatening, and I'd want to double up on the padding. One fencer from that group was more than a little threatening. Terrifying to his opponents. Not much of a "fencer" in terms of his footwork, though. Or his handwork: he was much more of a lumberman than any of the boxers purported to be, swinging his number six sword like an axe, chopping down men and women like trees. Clean strikes to the same spot over and over.

It was in the Lufoa ring. Where Cyn was working. I saw five patients arrive at her tent like felled trees. There would have been one more had there been a seventh fencer.

If the number of contestants isn't divisible by seven, there will be at least one pool with six competitors. And that's what happened here. It was the only pool of six I saw. And this logger of a fencer went undefeated against his five opponents. And each one of them was extremely defeated.

Nothing about it was pretty. His form least of all. The way he used his sword was just as grotesque as the consequence. But I'm not denying his skill.

In his defense, I'm a hack-and-slash fencer too. I've always used my sword as a cudgel. I never poked my opponents; I battered them. It lacks Mizjak's elegance, but it can be effective. In the present case, it was. It kept Cyn very busy. All five of his opponents came to her with injuries. Blunt trauma. Very blunt. And very traumatic.

Cyn did not attempt to remedy the tissue disruption with massage. Or the placebo "setting" of bones and joints into proper alignment. Or any other fantastic lore. She responded with appropriate treatments: immobilization or somewhat mobile compression, an occasional apothecarial intervention, some nutritional fundamentals, and plenty of rest… if possible.

Cyn brought her own apothecarial supply with her. The bag of medications she purchased last Aldos. Every affordable compound she expects to use. She doesn't have an official, lanyarded intern to pick up prescriptions for her, so she needs to arrive fully equipped, prepared for whatever she encounters.

The three Farhearth candidates have access to errand runners: the same inept interns who participated in boxing. Their lanyards allow them to correspond with a designated medic… without that correspondence being regarded as cheating. The only errands they run are back-and-forths to the Elyem eateries and the Pendelhall Apothecary. For food and drugs. They can't enter the apothecary itself; they just hand clerks the prescriptions to be filled. Which can take a while. So the Harthies show up with everything they're *sure* they'll need, but no more than that. This makes their audition cheaper than Cyn's.

The Harthies also have a stack of tomes and a pile of tools to assist their diagnoses and treatments. Cyn's only resources are her mind and her hands. Which more than make up for the lack of other assets.

From what I've seen so far, the minds and hands of the Harthies are bungling and dangerous. They really don't know what they're doing. And yet they're confident in their doings. Because they have had *some* exposure to science. But nothing resembling mastery.

Mastery teaches us modesty. It's only the narrowest exposure – dislodging a *splinter* of our ignorance – that adds boldness to our beliefs. Fierceness to our fallacies. And a tone of certainty in the advice and prescriptions that the Harthies bellowed at their patients. "This works, that doesn't work, always do this, never do that."

In some instances, upon hearing a fallacy delivered from on high, I knew the source. I had read that publication, too. The difference is: I also know the methods of science and the process of dissemination. Which is to say: the limitations of each claim. Understanding the assumptions and mathematics of a study's methods is necessary to comprehend its findings. Without a firm grasp on statistics, for example, all we can interpret from a published report is its headline. Which is always wrong. Because headlines are always bold. And truths are always meek. In the often-quoted-by-me words of Amaral, "Subtlety is the manner of science." In longer-winded words, no single study advances the frontier more than a tiny step. Nor does any study, no matter how bold its headline, escape negation. Truth invites rebuttals. It welcomes fierce efforts to refute it. It does not hide. It does not wear armor for fear of penetrating wounds by those probing its soft spots. To attack truth is to reveal it more completely. So one must never cling to any finding too tightly. Certainty is the fool's mentality, and the Farhearth medics were spectacularly certain in their prescriptions.

Clearly, they never read Amaral's work. Or Gundric's. Even Mizjak, who had no formal education in statistics, had the wisdom to caution Gundric against the boldness of the latest claim. He had a natural insight into the inherent limitations – and limited applications – of every study. And he didn't attend a single semester at Farhearth. What's the excuse of these medics?

As for the fencers, just like every year, no matter how many people register, there are only about fifty who stand a chance. The rest of them don't prepare enough to be competitive. Because they assume life is easier than it is. Every prisoner who entered the akira pit ready to fight a house cat was mauled by a lion. Only those who were ready to face a full-red rykil were exonerated. Preparation is the great divider of the pyloes and pouzos.

And preparation isn't just practice. Or exercise. Or checking the integrity of your equipment. Each of those is necessary, but if you haven't also studied your opponents, you're not ready.

Before I entered the tournament, I stalked all the top fencers. I watched as many bouts as I could. Keenly. And I filled notebooks with my observations.

I wasn't documenting general strengths and weaknesses, such as "fast flèche, but a flimsy first parry position". Notes like that aren't as helpful as people think. The strategies they encourage are highly specific (defend against the former, exploit the latter). If your plan is that precise, it's far too predictable to be of any value.

What I was studying was literal strengths and weaknesses.

For example, "A strong gastrocnemius in the rear leg, but weak pronators and internal rotators in the attacking arm." That tells me everything I need to know about the flèche and parry position, but it also informs me of so much more.

Mizjak emphasized the importance of knowing the mind of one's opponent. If you understand the workings of their attention, you can anticipate their actions. My philosophy was similar: if I understood their bodies, I could anticipate how those actions would be performed.

But this can't be determined at a glance. It requires studying. *Keen* studying. And that takes effort. More than many of today's younger fencers are willing to put in. So, they show up unprepared. If asked about their plan, they'll say, "To win no matter what!", which reveals they've paid no mind to the matters that matter: their opponents. They may have all the aptitude in the world, but when they enter the ring, every fight is a surprise.

According to Mizjak, surprise is the most lethal opponent there is. And most fencers I saw today didn't treat it with enough respect. That's why they aren't counted among the fifty who have a chance at winning. And when they lose, the reason for their loss will elude them.

The year I competed, I didn't win by being a savage with my sword. Despite what the papers reported. I won through preparation.

Although there was one class of fencer I always beat by hard swings: giants. Not gentle giants. Nor mythical giants, like Arfig. But huge, aggressive men who were once huge, aggressive children.

Everyone knows the type. The kind of child who, owing to his innate height and bulk, had no rivals. The kind of child who learned at an early age that it was his birthright to take. From anybody. "That's my toy" may have been his first exhibition of dominance. But it didn't stop there. It gradually grew more and more belligerent. Because nobody fought back. And the biggest cowards of all were those who plied him with ingratiating praise, hoping to save themselves from harm or embarrassment. Which only reinforced the behavior this boy-giant might have otherwise aged out of. Alas, he entered his adult years with the same need to dominate.

But beyond the confines of a schoolyard, he discovered his usual behavior was a criminal offense. So how did he resolve this predicament?

Many of these boys become Farhearth Justiciars so they can continue to persecute with impunity. They used to be called "Civic Managers", which is an even more egregious euphemism than "Conduct and Collection Agents", which is what they were called when I was at Farhearth. But they soon find that professional abuses of power do not produce a flock of sycophants.

So life feels empty. What offers both impunity *and* applause? Combat sports. Perhaps boxing would be the best fit, but fencers garner the most acclaim. So the giants pick up their first sword. And continue their favorite pastime: brutally hacking their way to victory. Until they meet me.

These are the opponents I could always beat by playing their own game: a spectacular collision of swords. In part because they're never as strong as they appear to be. And nowhere near as strong as they believe themselves to be. Because they don't bother to exercise. Because they were born huge. So what's the point in training? This lack of motivation leads to a lack of improvement, which makes them easy to surprise.

But these matches weren't strictly contests of strength. Much more than that, they were about strategy.

My most mathematical fights were against these goons. Because it wasn't just a game of distances – constant vigilance with the opponents' striking range – it was a game of moment arms. If I'm going to hammer away a heavy blade in an even strike, I need a lot of momentum. And a big windup to achieve it would reveal my intentions. So instead, I need to be precise about where our swords collide. The moment arm of the load has to be long for each of us. It can't be ricasso on ricasso. But the moment arm of *my* load must be slightly shorter, and the moment arm of my force a little longer. Then the collision ends – spectacularly – in my favor.

Striking hard is easy. Striking hard and *true* is the challenge.

Like those renowned Laberyn musicians who dress in carefully tailored rags, paying a small fortune to appear tattered, it takes great mental calculation to counterfeit a brute.

On rare occasions, I've encountered an ogre who was simply too strong to be bested this way. The lumberman fencer I saw this morning is probably one such adversary. Even with a wind-up, it may be difficult to out-muscle someone of his stature. The most effective way to disarm him would be a trial of endurance. The biggest, strongest, most explosive muscle fibers, which those true brutes have in abundance, exist on the brink of fatigue.

So, every time I faced a giant among the giants, I would subtly goad them into launching angry, aggressive attacks, which deploy their fiercest ranks of fibers. Then, I would defend carefully but conservatively, withholding any use of my own strongest ranks. Once their second string of troops (in technical terms, their lower threshold fibers) had picked up the charge of forceful contraction, that's when I struck. But I still lured them into a clash, spectacularly besting what they were sure was their best attack. An exhausted ogre is no stronger than a regular bully-goon.

Lastly, there were the old opponents. Too conservative to succumb to a trial of endurance. Too poised to be goaded. Too wise to be beaten by power. To them, fencing is a contest of patience. No overeager attacks or defenses, no wasted steps, no futile movement at all. They've fenced every kind of foe; they've seen weakness expose itself thousands of times. They know what it looks like and where to look for it. So, they wait, playing a game of distances, keeping a hair's diameter from the nearest threat of harm while waiting for their own opportunity to inflict it.

But they *are* old, and a little-known capacity that declines with advancing age is reactive inhibition. Youth can undo the chemistry of their commitments in a way that elders cannot. In all of us, we act only after our neurochemicals have chosen their decision. Only a young fencer can chemically abort those decisions rapidly. This is a capacity we all take for granted… until Time, the sneakiest of all thieves, steals it from under our noses. And we attempt to compensate with superior planning and strategy.

When facing an old, patient master, duplicity is the only reliable way to win. I would feign a weakness. Faintly. Theatrics don't work. They've seen the play too many times. Just like in science, everything bold is a lie. Authenticity is the province of subtlety. If they see a subtle opening, they'll commit to its exploitation. But when the realization of their mistake is made, the action persists for a fraction of a second longer than it should. That's the duration I have to exploit their error. And, of course, I strike hard. Because the fastest fibers produce the most force. And I need to be fast to succeed.

In each of these situations – bully-goon, mighty ogre, and wizened master – I appear to win by force. Really, I win by preparation. Unfortunately for me, that's not how the story of my tournament victory was told in either of the Farhearth newspapers. But that's a tale for another time. The present time is bedtime. When I sat down to write, I was too anxious to be drowsy. Now that the caligoroot has taken effect, my eyes, at least, are ready to rest. And I hope my mind will follow them into sleep.

Forty-Three

Seros, Second Lufoa, Day Twenty-Four. Morning.

The caligoroot worked well enough. I slept better than I thought I would. If I glue together all the fractured moments of sleep – ten minutes here, thirty there – it probably amounts to five hours, which is an average night for me. I'll bet Rorrik was asleep for nine, which is an average night for him. He's the only person I've ever met who loses consciousness the instant his body becomes supine. The transition from frenetic adventure to deep slumber is so quick, it's as though the pillow beheads him.

I cannot possibly overstate the depth of my envy here. It's not merely the duration of sleep that's different between Rorrik and me. My five, his nine. It's also the nature of that sleep. How the brain behaves, what destinations the slumbering mind visits. Rorrik's mind is surely granted access to places the public is not.

At a recent Farhearth Faire, scientists from Apothecarial and Natural Sciences debuted their work on the different stages of sleep we transition through in the night. It was an accidental discovery from their ongoing investigation into the consequences of sleep deprivation on memory consolidation. The researchers seemed to regard this secondary finding as a trivial offshoot from a critical stem of inquiry. Like saying, "I guess we can use this oak gall – make ink out of it or something – but the tree itself is what really matters." But to me, this finding was more fascinating than their primary objective. For over a century, throngs of researchers have spent their lives investigating the waking world, analyzing everything touched by light. And yet the deep, dark world we visit every night remains as mysterious as the depth of the seas.

We don't just die for a while, then revive when morning comes. Or enter a general quiescent state like a wood frog in Arzox. Our bodies experience periods of controlled paralysis – sleeper's palsy, they called it – but our minds remain sprightly. And they journey through several stages in a predictable cycle that repeats every hour and a half, give or take a bit.

What I immediately wondered, upon hearing this presentation, was whether any Westerners were subjects in the study. I asked. And the answer was no. Although that's not how they phrased it.

"We recruited local, healthy, recreationally active young adults", I was told.

That's a euphemism for: "We lured destitute students into participation by offering them free transcript units in exchange for the hassle." The hassle in this case being sleep disruption. The subjects had to sleep in a lab for a while, and they were awoken at various points of the night to be tormented with cognitive testing.

While many Westerners are modest in their means, they assign more value to sleep than transcripts. And Southerners wouldn't even waste their time with an unproductive *real* class, let alone a fake one… on the basis that it's free. That's about as enticing an offer as free lava. "No thanks, it would destroy whatever it touches." "But it's free." "Oh, in that case, pour it over here!"

I'm fascinated by the results of the sleep stage study as it applies to me, but I suspect the conclusions lack a bit in generalizability. Consider how some lineages of people have blood that lacks a clotting factor. In other lineages, the pancreas makes no insulin. Similarly, among Gaeans who lack Western ancestry, it's believable that the chemistry of sleep is different. A key protein that unlocks a deeper stage is missing. For some evolutionary reason. Just like the wood frog, which has evolved to freeze into a solid lump through the long Arzox, Westerners have evolved their own biology that makes use of the long night.

Everyone – Easterners, Westerners, Southerners, the Northerners when they existed, and even the Nameless, I'm sure – will experience periods of dreams and periods without. Likewise, everyone has straddled the waking and slumbering worlds lightly enough to still track the passage of time. Just as everyone has experienced heavy sleep where multiple hours pass in a blink. In addition to those stages, there seems to be another. One that is unavailable to anyone but a Westerner. Forbidden to lineages born beyond their borders.

A week or two ago, I wrote about the cities I've never visited. Cinderheim, Mulgotha, and so on. I'm adding one more destination to that list. Western Dreamland. Or whatever it should be called. That is now top on my list of destinations where I hope to someday play tourist. I will definitely be taking a stone from that world, assuming I could cross the boundary back into my own with the stone still in hand.

But that is neither here nor there. Nor anywhere, really. Much more present and pressing is the day that lies ahead. A nervous one for me. All but the last fifteen of the direct elimination bouts. In which Rorrik and Cyn both compete in their own way. And I'm sure they're both calmer than I am.

I almost never mix anything into my tea on purpose. Other than the nettle.

I let the mortar decide what effect to provide. But I didn't bring the mortar. And it's the last day of Cyn's interview. And I'm nervous. So this morning, I made an anti-anxiety concoction, mixing solarosales seeds into it.

And now it's time to head to Cyn's room for breakfast and our morning plan. The tea should be taking effect by now.

Forty-Four

Seros, Second Lufoa, Day Twenty-Four. Afternoon.

Cyn and I showed up early. Again. Except today, she was more dehydrated than she was yesterday. I accompanied her to her ring, Elyem, where we could hear and smell the sizzling breakfasts. The vendors were getting ready for the morning crowds. Twenty minutes later, those crowds arrived. More bustling than yesterday. Another twenty minutes later, the tournament began.

I wandered and watched the initial DE bouts. Half of these are spectacularly lopsided owing to the method of seeding: the undefeated fencers get paired with the barely-made-its. The rest of the matches are average fencer against average fencer. They're intense, competitive bouts, but you're not watching the pyloes.

Rather than loiter in Cyn's proximity, testing the potency of my solarosales seed tea, I wandered the other rings, distracting myself by feeling invested in the outcomes of the matches. That was easy when I was watching Rorrik. His first round of the day was against a Harthy. Not an independent Harthy. The skilled kind. But an institutional Harthy. They never make it very far. Because their training isn't focused on the sword. In the standard curriculum, each weapon is assigned the same amount of attention. Pikes, flails, sickles, daggers, bows, halberds, and so on. The breadth of their combat literacy is impressive. No matter what they have access to – reliable military weapons, decorative royal weapons, makeshift peasant weapons – they're competent. But they aren't experts at any of them. Because they don't spend more than three weeks on any one weapon. The faculty and coaching staff claim this creates well-rounded warriors. In reality, it creates over-confident amateurs. Whips are given just as much attention as broadswords. What is a whip going to do in combat? If you're simply wearing thick clothes, you're invulnerable. Even if you're naked, just take one hit – it'll probably sting, but it won't strike deeper than the skin – then close in and stab your enemy. With your sword. Because you chose a real weapon. Their only choice at that point is to drop the whip, which is useless in close combat, and defend against your sword with their grappling skills... which aren't good enough because Harthies get three weeks on that, too.

Mizjak talked about all of this, discussing the futility of the flail compared to the sword, for example. But Gundric's books now live in Stables, where no mandatory reading is shelved. It's not even in the canon for fencers anymore.

Despite this, the Farhearth Institute of Warfare was well represented in the morning's DE bouts. One does not need to check the tournament registry to identify them. They're not hard to see. Because they're not hard to hear. If any of their teammates are presently fencing, every member on the team who *isn't* currently fencing must stand ringside and cheer. And before bouts, they do this rally chant, puffing each other up, hollering in unison, arousing a great deal of excitement before sending their teammate into battle. And during the matches, the active contestants bark and yell after every success, no matter how tiny. Did you just land a harmless strike on your opponent's front foot? Release a battle cry! Did you barely brush his arm? Scream again!

None of this is helpful. Every part of it is harmful to everyone involved… with the sole exception being their opponents.

First, they should sit – preferably lie – between matches. Rest as much as they can. Staying afoot will fatigue the lower-threshold muscle fibers, which impairs the function of the whole muscle unit, including the higher-threshold fibers, even though they weren't activated during the ringside loitering. That means when you call upon those muscles, they won't perform at their best. Had you rested between bouts, you might have been able to lunge far enough to land your strike. Or leap explosively enough to evade the strike you were struck by. But since you depleted yourself for the sake of "team spirit", you missed your attack and were struck by your opponent's. In doing so, you let your team down.

This phenomenon should be obvious. Go spend six hours in the market. Afterward, try to exhibit peak athleticism. Sprint and jump as fast and high as you can. At no point in your market outing will you have recruited your high-threshold muscle fibers. And yet any performance that calls upon them will still be compromised.

Additionally, the person being blasted with cheer is not served any better by the ruckus. *Suppressing* excitement is a more appropriate strategy. The event is already too exciting. Pre-competition rallying and mid-bout shouting will just overexpress the neurochemical systems that augment our attention. Perhaps the burst of excitement one gets from a post-touch battle bellow does bestow an advantage. But it's transient. And it's followed by a crash. Sometimes before the end of the bout. Always before the next round.

This, too, should be obvious. Even to a babe with a mouthful of sugar. Every spike is trailed by a lull. But the effect is much more extreme with fervor than it is with food. If you've ever found yourself in tavern brawl, you know what unbreakable concentration feels like. And fencing is similar.

Every second of action seems to linger for a full minute. In these situations, attention dilates like a pupil in the darkness, capturing as much light as it can. Except instead of light, it's information. We're processing more and more, faster and faster, as we make life-or-death decisions, one after another, with limited time to make them. Gaea's rotation seems to slow. Focus narrows. Distractions disappear. External thought fades. Even our sense of self is lost. We just vanish into the moment. But when that moment passes, we crash. It doesn't matter if the physical strain of the fight was minimal, our attention still departs us for a spell. As though the earlier excess was issued as a loan. Which the borrower must pay back. With interest. And the neural bank is a strict creditor. When it calls in its debts, they're due. Immediately. In full. So how much attention did you borrow? If the excitement was extreme and the fight was long, repayment might begin before that fight ends, and you're unlikely to be chemically solvent during the next bout.

Like all things in life, the peak never lasts. It's fleeting the moment it arrives. And if you overshoot it outside of the rings – or off the court or the field – and try to carry its momentum back into play, it won't work. This is what makes those pre-participation rally chants so unhelpful. It's best not to get greedy with stimulation.

Of all places to understand this, you'd think the university would be first among them. Stress Physiology has been taught in Apothecarial and Natural Sciences for decades. Although one need not know the mechanisms to observe the effect. The phenomenon is characterized in Gundric's *Life of Mizjak*, and Mizjak had no background in the sciences, natural or otherwise. But, again, Gundric's work resides in Stables. And members of the Institute of Warfare don't frequent those shelves.

Harthies were the only fencers who were audibly ruining their performance. Everyone else was quieter. And more emotionally stable. Both in and out of the rings. But some of the calmer competitors were foolish in other ways. For example: if you're injured, you don't have to compete. This isn't war. Enlisting here is voluntary. Yet I saw contestants limping on badly sprained ankles and knees, their joints bundled up so tightly they could barely bend. A talented fencer can make it out of pools with both legs encased in a brick, but that doesn't mean they *should*. First, they won't advance very far in DEs. Second, if you're attempting to ward off stress in a joint by wrapping it in a rigid brace, you are warding *on* stresses in the adjacent joints. Not helpful. Eliminate mobility in your ankle and your knee must tolerate the forces that its southern neighbor forfeited. Each joint plays a small part in attenuating the larger load. Thus, removing the contribution of an individual participant is tantamount to removing a load-bearing beam in a house.

Many of our behaviors predispose us to catastrophic injury. And what we blame is seldom accurate. Because we focus on immediate cause and effect. "I drank a glass of water twenty minutes ago and just now my water broke!", cries a hypothetical pregnant woman. A better explanation of the amniotic sac rupture happened nine months ago. And injuries, like babies, often have gestational periods. The spontaneity we tend to credit them tends to be false. "I ne'er once felt a pinch a'pain, then all o' the suddens I heard a pop and felt summin' excruciating!", I heard one competitor cry to his medic this morning after his calcaneal tendon snapped. He blamed it on his landing after a leap.

"Tell me about the impact", the Harthy-hillian medic said as he inked his pen and opened his journal, revealing ignorance of this etiology. If the man were half his own age, I might be curious about this great leap. Because young, healthy tendons are like young, healthy bridges. It requires an extraordinary deforming force to bring about their collapse. But he wasn't half his age. And old tendons are like old bridges. They don't collapse out of nowhere. They've been degrading for a long time. Then one day... *crack!*

Most mechanical injuries arise in the same way. We may experience them as "all o' the suddens", and blame the impact, but it's a gradual development. Which brings us back to the competitors with immobilized ankles and knees. Substantial alterations to joint kinematics are unlikely to benefit the body's bridges. And some of these braces look more like the work of a mason than a medic.

Injury accommodation is one matter. Injury prevention is another. And here, fencers cling to uncountable myths. Observing their pre-participation rituals confirms this. For most, those rituals involve stretching. Holding their limbs in elongated positions for a minute at a time. Attempting to be as elastic as kneaded bread dough when they enter the ring. "If you don't start stretching, you'll get injured!", they scold their teammates. Then they extend their own stretch a tiny bit farther while exhaling loudly. The reality is: *training* reduces the risk of injury. Subjecting our tissues to the potentially injurious stresses we expect to encounter (in sub-injurious magnitudes) stimulates remodeling of those tissues to better withstand similar forces during future exposures. And the stress profile of a prolonged stationary hold has little to do with the ballistic deforming force that causes a strain at the muscle-tendon junction. What static stretching *will* do is ruin the snappiness of your muscle for a while. A long enough while to lose your upcoming match.

"You just don't understand the importance of warming up", I was scolded by the proselytizers of stretching the year I competed... after they noticed that I neglected to beat up my bread dough before each bout.

Stretching results in little warming, though. Heat comes from metabolism. And the metabolic demand of passive tissue lengthening isn't considerable. You're better off loafing in a fur coat. And if you can perform a few heavy exertions during your furry lounging, that seems to help with subsequent recruitment of the activated muscles. That's reasonable preparation exercise if you plan to leap and lunge in the ring. But most pre-participation rituals are pointless. The only benefit is to put the fencer in a particular mindset. Which can help psychologically prepare them for what comes next.

I have my own rituals. Not in fencing, but in life beyond the rings. I use tea to assemble the mindset required to confront the coming day. It's the smell and feeling of the steam. It's the warmth and the taste. And mostly, it's the motions and gestures I make while consuming it. I've rehearsed the action of drinking tea every morning for years. And you can't do anything that many times without developing a style. It's not how long it takes to finish my mug; it's the tempo of a song. And the motions associated with my drinking song have almost become a dance. My morning routine probably looks normal. No different from anyone else's behavior. Nothing pathological to note. But make no mistake: it's a strictly observed, carefully practiced ritual, every bit as sacred as Druinham scripture. And for that reason, I think I can excuse the silly "warm up routines" people do here as a form of contest rites.

After all these years, I still haven't figured out Rorrik's contest rites. He just stands there. Or sits there. Or stands or sits somewhere else until the event staff finally get his attention and inform him that his bout was supposed to have already begun. I guess his rituals are mental. His mind goes wandering through that Western netherworld in search of wisdom and inspiration. And this morning, he seems to have found both. Rorrik won all his bouts.

A few other notable fencers are still in the tournament, too. Bolgwin, who must be sixty years old, is the winningest member of the Champions' Guard. Which isn't saying much, but I think he's won at least five times in the past. Upon his first victory, he accepted his Guard appointment. And he has competed every year since. Guard members don't typically register for the tournament. If they have a respectable performance, it bolsters the Guard's reputation a very small amount. But should they have a poor performance, it will tarnish the reputation by a wider margin. If a member of the most elite army on Gaea loses to a novice, how elite can it be?

I understand this logic. Part of the reason I never competed again is that I didn't want to risk my undefeated streak. A second victory would boost my self-worth a small amount. But if I lost, the reduction in worth would have had a wider margin. So it didn't seem like a wise investment in my well-being.

Rorrik has no such concerns about his well-being. Or his legacy. Or the possibility of catastrophic injury.

Neither has Bolgwin ever been deterred by fear. And that bravery has yet to fail him. He's never finished outside of the top thirty-two, seldom outside of the top sixteen. And he's probably been in the top four at least ten times. He has a good chance. But I don't know if he can beat that giant tree feller. He's still in the tournament, too. And he chopped down a lot more fencers this morning. After one of his bouts, I heard a nearby spectator praise his "axe handling skills", and then describe his tournament performance thus far as "clearcutting a forest". I'm not the only one who sees the resemblance.

Nor am I the only one who recognizes how skilled many of these fencers are. I haven't seen any upsets. Most of the lucky-to-have-made-it-this-far fencers have been eliminated already, and those who remain have earned their rank. Which means it's going to be a competitive road to the end.

My mind has been wandering as I write. I'm letting it roam freely, hoping it won't focus too much on the importance of the present moment. As it just makes me anxious.

This is the final day of Cyn's audition. Her three shifts are Elyem, Arzox, and Lylir. And she's already done the food ring and the stinky ring. All that's left is the tavern ring.

Tomorrow, she and I will discuss everything that's happened, decompress, and watch the last fifteen bouts together. With no obligations. But today, it's all jitters. We've worked together for so long. And now she's entering the final stage of her audition. Which is starting now. And it feels strangely sudden. Like we should still have another month before today happens.

I'm going to watch her. I have just decided. Not so closely and vigilantly that my interests are obvious. But at a casual distance.

As seemingly ordinary, yet intensely meaningful, as drinking my morning tea.

Forty-Five

Seros, Second Lufoa, Day Twenty-Four. Night.

After lunch, I watched the rest of the day's DEs. All but the last fifteen bouts. Those happen tomorrow.

I didn't roam around the rings, though. I stayed at Lylir the entire time, beset by rowdy drunkards. I hope Cyn managed to maintain her focus. I didn't. But I did see some good bouts. Especially later in the evening. During the first half of Cyn's shift, the ring was populated by the worst class of fencer: the solipsist. These are the most obnoxious athletes in any individual sport. There aren't as many in boxing or wrestling, but probably half of all fencers regard themselves as the sole determiners of every outcome. At the end of each match, they can be heard explaining to everyone present that they either "won because of my skill" or "lost because I messed up".

The delusion here is difficult to overstate. They're *so* talented that all wins and losses are entirely up to them. And not just that, but the success or failure of every attack, feint, parry, and riposte is theirs to determine. The opponent has no influence over any outcome.

Sometimes the winner and loser *both* take full accountability. I heard that in one of today's bouts. "I won because I..." and "I lost because I..." were stated simultaneously by the winner and the loser. According to both fencers, the opponent was irrelevant to the outcome.

The true masters of any sport never fall into this trap. Or true masters in anything, for that matter. "She played the better game" was the explanation given by the person who lost the championship match in regnavus on Nyros. If, instead, he said, "I lost because I made the wrong play with my berserker", it would reveal a lack of respect for his opponent. And the failure to respect one's respectable opponents promises a lifetime of losses.

Mizjak talked about something similar in Gundric's book. The value of fear and admiration. And the importance of maintaining both. Especially for the weakest opponents, who are easiest to disregard. Pompous veterans often lose to amateurs because they lack sufficient respect for them. So they don't take those bouts seriously. So they lose unexpectedly. But now the roster has been pared down to the final sixteen. At this point in the tournament, the solipsistic fencers have all been eliminated.

The performances of the winners were some of the best I've seen. The same can be said about the losers as the night went on. It wasn't just their fitness. Or their fencing form. It was their attention.

There's a type of focus I've found in the arts – visual and music – that seldom exists elsewhere. It belongs to the true geniuses. When the minstrel master finishes playing a song, you don't clap or cheer or even respond. You sit still, stunned, and think, "I didn't know music could sound like that." Similarly, when a brush belonging to Grider or some other Lonvarakan master leaves the canvas, all you can do is stare. But if you look into the painter's eyes while the brush is at work – or the singer's eyes during the song – there's a look that foretells what's coming. A depth that promises otherworldly performance.

The closest likeness I've found among us non-geniuses is when you look into the eyes of someone whose own eyes are staring into a cloudless sky. Not in fatigue, but in deep contemplation, with a meditative gaze fixed on no detail, no particular distance, and the mind behind it is open. As wide as the expanse it's peering into. As if the entirety of creation is being received without blind spots. It is that type of transcendence that can be seen in a true master's eyes during a rare moment of true mastery. And I saw it in several fencers today.

Including Bolgwin. He advanced. For a brief time, I was the youngest fencer ever to win. If Bolgwin wins tomorrow, he will be the oldest. He might be the oldest fencer ever to make the top sixteen. And if the expression he wore today – the look of artistic brilliance in action – endures, he has a chance.

In the old days, when I saw Rorrik's eyes go wide, I knew he was unbeatable. It didn't even matter if he had a weapon. Or if he had functioning limbs. There was simply no alternative to his victory.

I didn't see that look in Rorrik today, though. Instead, his eyes were adrenal. That type of focus is helpful if you want to be merely great, but greatness has blind spots. And this far into the tournament, every opponent travels almost exclusively in those spaces. So I don't expect Rorrik to earn his third pendant. But he did advance to the final day.

If Cyn and I were placing bets – on a winner and a not-a-winner, like we did in boxing – the axe handler might be the gambler's choice for the Guard. He's still in it, too. But it's a competitive group. Predicting a winner isn't an easy task. Choosing who *won't* win, however, would be simple: one of the Farhearth fencers. Two of them made it to the last day… despite themselves. Rorrik will at least beat out those Harthies. I do wonder whom he *won't* beat, though. And how upset he'll be.

After one of Rorrik's bouts in Lylir, where he won in less time than it takes me to sneeze, he asked if I could get him some lufig from the apothecary. That's how untranscendent he is at this tournament. His eyes are adrenal during the fight, but immediately after, he's thinking about drugs.

"Let me know how much it costs, and I'll pay you back", he said.

"I can't", I replied.

"If they don't have lufig, lufir will be fine. Whatever they have."

"No, it's not that. Although it probably is lufir. But I can't get it because the only place it's sold is the Pendelhall Apothecary. And I don't have access."

"Doesn't Cyn?", he asked as he gestured toward her. She was standing about fifteen feet away, close enough to hear our exchange. But I doubt she heard. She was busy. Testing the internal rotation of a fencer's shoulder at the time. But even if she wasn't occupied, it's the noisiest ring.

"I don't want to inconvenience her", I said. "If she's appointed the position, and she's granted permanent access to the apothecary, we can all go together. At some point. I'd like to pick up more solarosales seeds, too. But for now, I'd rather not hassle her."

Rorrik nodded once. A gesture that indicated his acceptance of my response. He refuses to accept my "I don't want to risk my life on an impossible quest to kill an unkillable creature" response. That, he doesn't accept. But he was immediately and completely satisfied with my reluctance to hassle Cyn. Even though it means he has no way of obtaining lufig or lufir until he returns to the West. Rorrik has spent a lot of time out here. He knows how rare each of them is, lufig especially. Although only ancestral Adonians and Lirkin can tell the difference. And Farhearth botanists. And alchemists. Everyone else regards the two collectively as "dreamveil". Or it's "the mortal mushroom" according to those who condemn its use. Beyond the borders of the West, the only place where either shroom is sure to be both authentic and correctly prepared is the Pendelhall Apothecary. Incorrectly prepared, the liver damage arrives before the dream begins.

Before I give that thought any more thought, I'll change the topic to Cyn:

At the end of the day, after she handed in her medical journal, we ate dinner. Elk and some thick, hard, salty pastries. At Elyem. With Rorrik. He still has one more day of competition, but Cyn's competitive role is over.

We sat at our table for about two hours and spent most of that time listening to Cyn describe her experience. And her descriptions helped ease my anxiety. Better than solarosales seeds could do. We discussed just about every patient. Not in a tedious, mechanical way, but philosophically. In a way that Rorrik, who has no background in medicine, could engage. Philosophy like this:

When patients arrive, a lot can be learned by how they express their injuries. There are the crude facts: this bone broke, this ligament sprained, and so on. But that's only half the story. And the patient usually knows that half already. An effective medic can interpret the other half, making sense of things the untrained are unable to see. Which almost likens them to tasseographers auguring from tealeaves. Or those old legends about Druin divining wisdom from the Western pollens. The seemingly similar sorcery of medicine is the medic's ability to read the arcane language of bodies. All those messages hidden in the patients' postures and movements. Before they even speak, there are a thousand abnormalities the highly trained can see. Subtle features of an antalgic gait or irregular sway and arm swing, for example, can indicate severity of injury and corresponding tissue disruptions. And once the patient does speak, much more can be learned from his or her tone, phrasing, and expressions.

Becoming fluent in the wordless language of medicine is mostly a matter of practice. But developing basic literacy begins in the library. The best book on the topic, and the first one Cyn read, is *Days of Sickness*. It was written by Rouska, a professor in Theology and Ethics at Farhearth. After falling ill and navigating the medical system himself, he came to understand what he called "the Pali vin Galu of medicine", referring to an old Lonvarakan play format. Literally meaning "question and answer", it's not about the questions or the answers. It's about extracting the truth from what isn't said.

Listening to Cyn at the dinner table tonight, it was clear that she has mastered medical "augury". And her audition was better than I could have ever done. Her only competition is the Incumbent.

Cyn did mention that she referred one of her patients to the Citadel Hospital for suspicion of hydrocephalus, or "dropsy of the brain" as it's often called by physicians who cling to old, vague vernacular.

I wouldn't think much of this, but I heard a different medic refer a different fencer for apoplexy. I don't know the details. And it was the Harthy-hillian who did the referring. So I can't be sure what he was evaluating. But it *could* be the same condition that Cyn saw in her patient… which would be slightly suspicious.

According to a compendium published by the Archer's Guild, there are toxins that could have this effect if ingested. It just takes a week to manifest… with a standard deviation of a few days.

"Meningimangle" is what it's called in those reports. At Farhearth, the plant is known as black risteria, but the validation experiment – poison a sample of adults to see if they develop hydrocephalus in a week – has never been tested. Because there's no way any research review board would approve that study. So, it can't be conducted in a Farhearth lab. So, we just have to trust research that comes from outside the institution.

The guild report is generally thought to be true. And if you know what you're looking for, and if you're willing to look hard to find it, black risteria can be found in the coastal mangroves in the south of the East and West, and in the northeast of the South.

It's *possible* there was an exposure. And if multiple fencers are exhibiting the same set of symptoms, which would otherwise be rare, it's *possible* there was some foul play.

The medics at the Citadel Hospital will figure it out.

As for the medics at the rings, I'm close to certain that Cyn will be appointed to the position.

We'll find out in a few days.

In the meandays, we'll watch the final sixteen fencers sort out their ranks. That happens tomorrow. And it includes Rorrik. He doesn't seem nervous. Probably because he doesn't really care. All he cares about is recruiting the right travel companion.

Then, on Lyros, nothing happens. For us, at least. It's the day of judging for the auditioning medics. We'll spend that day distracting ourselves while we wait for Cyn's ceremony. On Fyros.

But for the remaining hours of tonight, I think we can all use some rest.

Forty-Six

Aldos, Second Lufoa, Day Twenty-Five. Morning.

I woke up early. And looked at the dark sky. Made darker by an empty moon. If I believed in astrological omens, the sight might have inspired a dark mood. Instead, I dawdled over tea for half an hour, and then went to Cyn's room. She was up early, too. Earlier than I was. But instead of dawdling, she had already gone out. And bought breakfast for all three of us. And on the way, she picked up some solarosales seeds for me and lufig for Rorrik. Apparently, she heard our exchange yesterday.

I muttered some "you shouldn't have" sentences as Cyn handed me a small cloth bag. And then we ate. By ourselves. Because Rorrik hadn't yet arrived. He still hasn't. He will. On his own time. There's no rush. Today isn't like pools and the first day of DEs where it starts early and ends late. With only fifteen bouts in the whole day, the games won't begin until nearly noon, permitting yesterday's drinkers to wake up, recover, and still arrive on time. So they can buy more drinks. There's an economy behind every decision.

The final day is always fifteen matches. And it's always where the cheering is loudest, the audiences are rowdiest, and the gambling is most ludicrous… and *occasionally* lucrative.

Once upon an earlier age, the tournament served as a training ground for war. Today, most contestants would be unfit for battle. It's just an entertainment. A spectator sport. And according to the "Fourth Law of Mizjak", sports are about empathy; only war is about winning. But that's not how it's treated. For most participants, this is as close to real combat as they'll ever get. And for the spectators, in each bout, they choose a side and cheer as though their life is on the line.

Sometimes it *is* – or at least their homes and marriages are at risk – given the amount of money they've wagered. And it's not just cheering *on* one's chosen champion. It's cheering *off* the opponent. The enemy. The villain.

The vilification can get out of hand at times. I know these times firsthand. When I competed, I was no one's chosen champion. And everyone's chosen enemy. And the antagonizing didn't end with the conclusion of the games. Both Farhearth newspapers continued their campaign for weeks.

Still today, I remember every publication to the letter. Here are the opening lines of the first *Farhearth Fortnightly* article, the faculty-written periodical:

"Valiant, skilled, graceful, dignified. None of these describe the victor at this year's annual competition." It went on to say, "Too cheap to buy his victory, he battered the cashier."

The student-written periodical, *The Collegian*, printed an article the same day with a suspiciously familiar theme:

"This year's Pendelhall tournament proved a universal truism: the cheapskate always finds a way."

That's not where their similarities ended.

According to the *Farhearth Fortnightly*, "The winner of this year's games was a graceless brute; unable to thread the needle with finesse, he simply beat it in the eye, bludgeoning as crudely as a nihox clubs its prey."

According to *The Collegian*, "For the first time in the long and noble history of the contest, a hairless nihox has won the highest honor. True to its form, it swung its sword with the precision of an avalanche and grace of a rectal prolapse."

Grace (or in this case, gracelessness) is a common enough theme. But a nihox comparison? I've never seen another publication in either periodical that mentioned the animal. And they both likened me to one.

The two articles were supposedly written by different authors – a student and a faculty member – and yet they stabbed the same knife into the same flesh. Faculty often ghostwrite the student articles to build student careers while disseminating their own message into a different audience. Here, *The Collegian* was just a cruder rephrasing of the same words.

This *still* wasn't where the similarities ended.

During the Closing Ceremony, when I was interviewed, I made a couple of reverent remarks about historic fencers. Mizjak and Gundric, Rinalt, Erluk, and Olrax the First. I mentioned that I was studying their works, trying to understand them better as people. "In studying how they think and reason, there are surely insights to be gleaned about how they fence", or something like that.

Both papers – the *Fortnightly* and *Collegian* – subjected my comments to a contortionist's routine, and then published the exact same quotation, which I didn't quite say, and asserted that I was conferring myself in league with the greats after a single fortuitous victory.

"The pomposity of this young upstart!", I could hear every reader saying… justifiably if I had actually said what I was quoted as saying.

It went on from there. The crudest passage appeared in the closing lines of *The Collegian*. Too obscene to be printed in the *Fortnightly*, it was relegated to the student periodical, I suspect. Too obscene to recite here.

I was not merely thrust into the public's eye; I was forced on stage in jester garments. Because I won. And I was no one's chosen champion. Because I wasn't winning by the usual means.

Perhaps my victory cost the writer a home and a marriage in gambling debt. And he was just exorcising his frustrations. But he wasn't the only one whose criticism seemed to supersede all other life priorities. The scorn that seethed from countless other Harthies concerned my "bucking of scientific consensus and snubbing of sacred traditions."

In the intervening years, fatuous fencing traditionalism has lost few devotees. If anything, it seems to have *gained* adherents. It's worse than I remember it. During pools, practically every young fencer I saw had a "signature stance". Whenever they stood outside of striking distance, they held their sword at a weird angle, their legs were weirdly positioned, and their free arm was doing something extravagant. Attempting to appear threatening in a mystical way. As though they were channeling some sorcery, charging a "special move" they would soon deploy. Mizjak spoke of the absurdity of mythical fencing in Gundric's work. Unfortunately, those aren't works read by today's youth. So their foolishness continues. So my cringes are too hearty to contain.

While those fencers seldom make it out of pools, those who *do* advance are traditional absolutists in other ways. Most of them are either wholly ignorant of the sciences or they know a tiny fact and observe it with fierce religiosity. Having taught and published in the natural sciences, I know well the margins of any one study's finding. And they're narrow. Too narrow to dictate the strategies I used to prepare and compete. I trusted my own understanding of physiology instead. And it worked. But upon winning, the victory trailed me like an odor. As though I had stepped in a steaming pile of bykul crap and was tracking it everywhere I went.

Particularly in Farhearth. And Thevro. My reputation wasn't *as* tarnished in Pendelhall. And, if anything, it was bolstered in Estevro, where the townsfolk care little about outside news, and they're always welcoming of their own kin.

Eikir, who "authored" the article in *The Collegian*, is now a renowned writer for the *Thevro Chronicle*. To my knowledge, he's never mentioned me again. Nor has he defamed another tournament winner. Not even Holmgrin, who, not long after me, won at an even younger age. After all the contempt about my surpassing of Erluk, my own dethroning went by unnoticed. But Eikir does continue to be disparaging to Estevroans in general. Especially when it comes time for the Cookery Banquets. He calls every Estevro chef "cheap", and each instance reminds me of the article that started his career.

I did learn a valuable lesson from that experience: how viciously people cling to legacy. Erluk, the previous youngest-ever tournament victor (and still the Guard member who has served more terms as First Knight than any other), was a Harthy hero who could do no wrong. During the fifty years between his only victory and mine, his reputation was polished to a blinding sheen.

He was already celebrated in Farhearth before he competed at Pendelhall. You can still find a few engraved record slabs with the name Elgin on them. But once he joined the Guard, and changed his name, every disreputable deed was purged, every blemish cleansed, and every accomplishment was forever exaggerated.

Among those exaggerated accomplishments, his victory at twenty-one was hailed as "a feat that would never be replicated." Until it was. And I paid a steep price for my replication. Then, when Holmgrin bested us both, I heard no uproar. If there was any criticism at all, it wasn't in any of the periodicals I read. Time hadn't yet purged the smell of bykul shit from my shoes, I guess. Culture seemed almost relieved to be rid of my record.

I assume the reason was my "bucking" of tradition. Erluk was as classical a fencer as one can possibly be. And I wasn't. I was the most unclassical victor there had ever been.

A topic for future pages. Rorrik just arrived. And ate the food Cyn got him in one bite. Or at least it appeared that way. Then Cyn gave him his lufig.

And now it's time for us to head out.

Forty-Seven

Aldos, Second Lufoa, Day Twenty-Five. Afternoon.

Cyn, Rorrik, and I left for the rings shortly after Rorrik arrived.

At this point in the tournament, the bouts are staggered. One at a time, rotating through the five rings. Beginning at Arzox. Ending – after two more passes through Arzox, at Lufoa. The Moon Variation... if this were an Urzie. Everyone's favorite season, everyone's favorite movement in the Urzie, and the best of the five rings. Except, today, it won't be quiet. The two best rings – Rynoa and Lufoa – determine who goes to the finals. Who gets to fence in the black ring.

Ringside viewers typically show up early – as early as last night – to establish and defend their stations on the perimeter of Rynoa and Lufoa. Everyone else forms the outer crowd, which rotates with the matches. Cyn and I were among those revolving spectators. The elevated amphitheater steps allowed us to see clearly enough.

The crowds are too dense for the fencers to come and go, so they're stationed inside the circle of rings – in the Sanctum – where there aren't any spectators. Just like every other year, they're stuck there until they lose. Some of this morning's fencers passed the time between bouts walking laps around the black ring (but never inside of it, hardly even near it) in meditative trances. Others had different preparation strategies. But unlike the previous two days, none of the strategies were foolish. At this stage, everyone is a professional. Nobody makes it this far by the caprice of Serendipity, that scapegoat deity upon which hundreds of losses were blamed in the last forty-eight hours.

Before the first bout, the final sixteen fencers were introduced to the crowd. These introductions are nothing like those that precede the boxing matches. It's not about entertaining an audience with dazzling fibs, it's about informing them of a few pertinent facts. The fencers' names, the cities they represent, how the brackets are structured, and in which ring each contestant will have their first match. The only fiction in the speech was Rorrik's name. Olryn. And possibly the names of a couple of other contestants. Although, being the age of fame-mongering, hardly anybody conceals their identity anymore.

Rorrik's first match was the eighth of the morning. In Rynoa. The last bout in the first round.

The *first* bout in the first round – the first of the day – was in Arzox. It had that lumberman of a giant in it. His name, I learned from the introduction, is Styravesa. It sounds made up. Although I guess every name is made up, regardless of whether it's "real". He faced a Rodorite. Not an untalented one. Nor modest in stature. But Styravesa made him appear both diminutive and inept. In short time, he disarmed him by bashing down his sword. My move. In a way. Which the Eikir article said had "the precision of an avalanche". No matter how far Styravesa gets, I doubt he'll be handled as indelicately as I was – despite being more brutish – because he isn't threatening an old hero's record.

The Rodorite tried to beat him with quick feet, great leaps, and bounding. And a quick blade, great thrusts, and flurries. None of it worked. He just wore himself out. And when the weary lunge came, Styravesa bashed down the tired blade. It was a familiar move. Mine. But the next part was uniquely Styravesa's: he stomped on the sword. I could hear the ping of it snapping from where I was standing. At this point, Styravesa was facing an opponent with a dagger. The blade was now sharp and dangerous, but it was shorter than the handle. There was no way the Rodorite could close the distance against a number six. Styravesa won spectacularly. And the crowd seemed to enjoy the spectacle.

The second bout was an Eldish woman against a Pendelian man. If it weren't for Gundric's influence in the sport, this would not have been a fight we got to watch. And it was the best of the first round. Speed, wit, and endurance were equally matched. The Eldish fencer won, but it took twenty minutes. So she would be going into the second round, against Styravesa, fatigued.

The third bout was Bolgwin against a Wargee. Bolgwin won. It's hard to compete with fundamentals that sound. He has no flash, but nor does he have a flaw. Nothing to exploit. The match was so boring, it was fascinating. Like those animals that are so grotesquely hideous, they become adorable.

The fourth bout was a Kruuger against a Harthy. The Harthy did a fine job, but he was outmatched. The Kruuger won and looked like a drunkard while winning. His form was loose and unfundamental. The opposite of Bolgwin. Serious talent though.

The fifth bout was a petite but brawny woman from Ryndor against a giant even gianter than Styravesa. I don't know how I missed him before today. Fygsin of Midrodor. If he's shorter than seven feet, my eyes deceived me. His skin looked like leathery wood. An armor of hard oak laced with scars. His hair resembled a growth of nature. Like wheat streaked with saffron.

And his eyes were as green as mid-Lylir grass. If I were to close my own eyes and imagine Gaea incarnate, I couldn't picture a fitter creature than Fygsin. The Rivervalan woman did well – better than I expected – but the Rodorite was planetarily big. And remarkably skilled. He fought honorably, though. Every blow delivered was a respectful one. I guess if you're that huge and talented, you *get* to be respectful. Virtue is, sometimes, a kingly garment.

Sixth bout: Eldish and a Pendelian. Good match. Both skilled. Both tough. But the Eldish was barely tougher. So he advanced. And had to face Fygsin in the next round.

Seventh bout: a woman from Estevro and a man from Thevro. Fygsin was impressive in his enormousness, and Styravesa in her enormity. Bolgwin was remarkable for his dullness. And, of course, Rorrik is my chosen champion. But this may have been the match I cared most about. It's not just hometown patriotism. It's a rivalry as old as time. ("Rivalry" is an obvious euphemism; it's a socially sanctioned form of deep prejudice.) On my side of the rivalry, it's not enough that Estevro wins. Thevro must also lose.

This was the only gambling I did today. And I lost money.

The final bout of the first round was Rorrik's. Against a Harthy. Alnuk. Probably the weakest fencer in the top sixteen. Lucky first opponent. Rorrik had no problem advancing. And after his match, it was down to eight fencers: Styravesa, the Eldish woman, Bolgwin, the Kruuger, Fygsin, the Eldish man, my newly sworn enemy from Thevro, and, of course, Rorrik.

What's encouraging about this stage in the tournament is the total absence of argument. Those who lost blamed only themselves. Seldom does anyone in the top thirty-two voice any complaint at all, but never in the top sixteen. That's a behavior of the bruisers. Low level fencers and high-level boxers.

Which got me thinking: when has arguing ever accomplished *anything* useful? In sport, there's never been a major ruling overturned by an athlete's tantrum. But even outside of sport – in a pub, for instance – the goal of arguing is not to teach one's peers a great wisdom. The goal is victory. A ruthless attempt to make one's opponent feel the sting of loss. That's the reason we quarrel most fiercely when our facts are most flimsy. And why dignified people never participate. Nor do they participate in pub scuffles of the physical variety. These are activities reserved for the crudest class. It is their respite from the hard labor of feigning civility. Sometimes the pretense gets heavy, and they have to put it down for a bit. First, they argue. Then they ball up their fists. And after some therapeutic thumping, they resume charade of chivalry.

Arguing may be uncivil, but debate isn't. It is a sport with agreed-upon rules. The sharper the wit, the more likely it is to pierce. There is elegance to that. And the same is true for fencing. Genteel manners need not be surrendered to swing a sword at someone. The combat is practically a form of discourse. As elegant as poetry, as technical as debate, and as sophisticated as the two combined.

At least that's true for high-level fencing. And this is the highest level.

Fifteen minutes after Rorrik's bout with the Harthy, the first match of the top eight began: Styravesa versus the Eldish woman.

Styravesa won. In a pitiless way. A terrifying way.

Next: Bolgwin versus the Kruuger.

Bolgwin won. In a classical way. An honorable way. The very unclassical, drunkardly attacks by the Kruuger were difficult to read. Not just distracting, but misleading. Alas, Bolgwin was undistractable. Unmisleadable.

Next: Fygsin versus the Eldishman.

Fygsin won. Politely. But powerfully.

The last match of the top eight was Rorrik versus the Thevroan. Perhaps it's just my bias ranking the fencers, but the Thevroan appeared to be the weakest of the eight, giving Rorrik the easiest path through the final day.

He won. Quickly. And conservatively. Having spent half the time and a quarter the energy of anyone else in the final four, Rorrik was well positioned going into his next bout. Against Fygsin. But no matter how rested Rorrik was and how fatigued Fygsin was, everyone in the crowd perceived Rorrik as the pouzo of the pairing. How could they not?

Before their bout, Styravesa and Bolgwin faced off in Rynoa.

The match was surprisingly long. And difficult to watch. The lumberjacking to Bolgwin's bones would have surely felled half the Grey Woods. But he never winced. He just absorbed the blows – better than any shield could – and kept fighting. In honor of The Guard. Evidence that the sturdiest shield is not iron, but devotion. Bolgwin didn't win, but what he endured without a wince – or a subsequent limp – was perhaps the most impressive feat of the games yet.

And then it was Rorrik's turn. To face Fygsin. In Lufoa. To determine who advanced to the final bout. Against Styravesa. In the black ring.

Rorrik harbors just as much devotion as Bolgwin, but it's not to any army. Or city or religion or institution. His sole calling is killing that ruinous reaper from Thorn. He'd trade his life to see that goal fulfilled. But its fulfillment has little to do with his performance here. He came strictly for recruitment. Until an hour before pools, he wasn't even sure if he would be competing. Yet there he was in the semifinals. And then there he was, advancing to the final match.

I couldn't believe he won. The transcendent Rorrik – with the celestial stare, whom the universe deems unbeatable – didn't show up at this tournament. But the version of him that did fence was astonishing in a different way. With flashes of unrivaled brilliance – flashes of that old, wild-souled, wide-eyed wonder – he beat Fygsin. Both fought honorably. Both showed respect for the other. But it's Rorrik who will be fencing in the black ring.

He doesn't seem to be nervous. Once he passed through the thick wall of a crowd and found Cyn and me, he insisted on a trip to Elyem. "Fightin's a hungry task", he said. Most nervous fencers lose their appetites. Not Rorrik. He ate three big meals. None of them *good* meals. It's all sustenance here. Heavy chilies, dense breads. Half the foods are served in the form of pastes. Not pastries. Pastes. Which Rorrik swallowed like pills. I doubt his teeth did any work at all.

Five minutes later, he was reclining while sighing. We still have a few hours until the championship bout. Sufficient time to metabolize the excess.

After watching Rorrik beat the Harthy, the Thevroan, and especially Fygsin, I don't know what to expect in the final match. Styravesa is menacing, but it's difficult to say who the pouzo and pyloe are. Or which of the two fencers the crowd will deem their champion. But I do find it strange that *nobody* has recognized Rorrik. Everyone simply accepts the name Olryn from Laberyn, which doesn't even make sense; no one in Laberyn is named Olryn. If Rorrik enters a tavern, he is instantly recognized by at least one person. Every time. Which makes taverns a place to be avoided if he doesn't intend to perform. But here, a two-time tournament winner is completely anonymous.

I guess Rorrik is a far more renowned musician than he is an athlete. I also guess his pendants were won a long time ago. I doubt he's ever fenced any of the contestants here. Excepting Bolgwin, who probably recognized him, but he's far too formal to compromise Rorrik's confidentiality.

Most of the crowd seemed more surprised than I was by Rorrik's victory over Fygsin. Although, in retrospect, I understand what happened: both fencers fought fair. And Rorrik is difficult to beat within the bounds of "virtue" (achieving victory without undue harm). He's simply too skilled to be struck by an honorable strike. And such strikes are all that Rorrik delivers in return. In the wild, he has no qualms about inflicting harm, but during competition, he doesn't create victims. In a way, this code of conduct serves as both boon and bane. Rorrik relies on honorable opportunities presenting themselves. So if injurious attacks are the surest way to win, he hampers his success by declining them. On the contrary, he never lusts after malice, that seductress that tempts too many fencers into inferior attacks, hoping for the chance to draw a little blood. In the highest levels of fencing, malice often rebounds. Greed is too easily bested by an articulate riposte.

Reflecting on the match, I understand how Rorrik triumphed over Fygsin. But Styravesa is a dramatically different kind of fencer. The honorless kind. Cyn's most battle-battered patients were his earlier opponents. Still, I can't say which of them is the pyloe.

But it's time to return to the rings. The match won't start for a few hours, but if we want to be close enough to see anything, we have to show up now. And Rorrik is going to head inside the Sanctum for a nap. So that, when it's his turn to fight, his stomach won't be packed so full of Pendel-porridge.

Forty-Eight

Aldos, Second Lufoa, Day Twenty-Five. Night.

We watched the championship bout. There must have been five thousand people crammed around the perimeter of the rings. Our vantage was decent, but not quite as decent as I hoped it would be. Those with a better position didn't take a break for food, like we did.

The pre-championship ceremony began about half an hour before the match. An orator led us through the history of the games, honoring historic fencers. That sort of thing. Rorrik slept through it. At the end of the speech, both fencers were reintroduced. The Operating Medic had to wake Rorrik up so he would be present for that part.

Styravesa was first to be introduced. He didn't need to be awakened because he didn't bother to rest between bouts. Or speak. Or express humanity by any other means. He just stood there, granite-faced, towering over the orator, who declared no city affiliation. Sometimes this implies a lack of patriotism. Other times it's secrecy for victory's sake. If you know where your opponent comes from, you can make a reasonable guess at how they've trained. If you know how they've trained, you can make a reasonable guess at their strengths, weaknesses, strategies. And if you know these things, you have an advantage. I can't blame Styravesa for his concealment when Rorrik used a pseudonym for a similar reason.

Next up was Rorrik's reintroduction. After "Olryn, representing Laberyn" was announced, a moment of silence was requested for the lives lost on the second night of Second Lufoa. There were too many people present for a true silence to fall upon the rings. And too many of them were too drunk to silence themselves at all. But the general lull in commotion was noticeable enough to be respectful.

Most people showed further respect by bowing their heads for the duration. Not Styravesa, though; his affect held no grief or lamenting. His bloodthirsty expression seemed even more parched during those thirty seconds or so. Blood *ravenous*. Blood *insatiable*. Rorrik was exuding respect during that time, but I could tell he felt slightly patronized. He's never been a good recipient of pity. Like the rest of the Laberi, he would prefer to sing his own sorrows, rather than have an orator use up his source material.

After the introductions, the two fencers armed themselves. Rorrik selected a number three sword, Styravesa the number six, and each wore light armor. Rorrik always dresses lightly. For quickness's sake. I assume Styravesa did so out of pomposity. The only difference in thickness was their helmets. Rorrik's was a bit heavier, and it included a small gorget. Styravesa's didn't.

Then they entered the black ring.

And the fight began.

As in every bout before, Styravesa played the role of a ruthless lumberman. Adapting to his opponent, Rorrik assumed the role of a nimble tree.

If any of Styravesa's initial blows would have landed, they would have made a felling crack seem mild. But they didn't. Rorrik gauged his distances well. He wasn't striking. Not right away. The reach of his number three couldn't contend with the number six. Instead, Rorrik was playing a defensive game. Parrying, dodging, waiting for opportunities. Ways to poke him and retreat. Until an opening presented itself. And Rorrik could close the distance.

Styravesa's strikes were clearly aimed at disarming Rorrik. Figuratively, as he had done with his previous opponents. But also literally, as the felling crack detaches trunk from root and leaves behind a stump. A few of the clashes nearly shattered the swords, and a couple of them managed to clip Rorrik, but no one has ever knocked a sword from his hand. He's like a dross dog with a bone. Adon incarnate couldn't wrestle it from his grip.

The hits must have been painful, but Rorrik continued to play his distances. He continued to poke Styravesa in the knee, the arm, the hand. All the while, Styravesa was becoming visibly frustrated. His blood-insatiable expression grew more and more belligerent.

And Rorrik kept poking him. Dancing away. And poking him again.

It felt like I was watching the old Rorrik. Watching him toy with an oversized ogre whose mighty thumping was too slow and predictable. And Rorrik's distances were perfect, taunting Styravesa with seductive targets. Until finally, he overswung. And Rorrik stepped inside, where the number six sword was too unwieldy to be effective.

Styravesa switched to a half-swording position, fending off low attacks. This left the full length of his bevor-less, gorget-less neck exposed. Everyone in the crowd could see it. Surely, Rorrik could too.

But he didn't take it. Because it might have been a lethal blow. Against an opponent who had already attempted lethal blows on him.

Instead, Rorrik launched a high feint. Then, when Styravesa raised his blade, Rorrik dropped low and struck the back side of Styravesa's front knee. Hard. And nearly knocked him off his feet. His leg buckled, and he fell to a half-crouched position. But before Rorrik struck again, Styravesa lunged upward and drove the flat side of his sword into Rorrik's face. Then he stepped back, returned to his normal two-hand sword position, and took a furious swing for Rorrik's head.

Rorrik stepped away. And smiled. As though he were enjoying the challenge. But his smiling teeth looked like rows of pomegranate seeds.

And the fight resumed.

Rorrik returned to his game of distances. But slightly farther, safer distances this time. Not close enough to effectively taunt or poke Styravesa. He was moving just as nimbly, but he kept blinking. And on a couple of occasions, he wiped his eyes. They must have been watering from the hit. And he was having a hard time seeing the opportunities. So he was dragging the fight out safely while he recovered.

This lasted close to a minute. Or at least it felt that long. As Rorrik started to narrow the distance again, he landed another poke – perfectly placed – on Styravesa's hand. Quick, but hard. Beautifully executed. And I thought Rorrik was back in it. But he wiped his eyes one more time, and as he did, Styravesa bashed down his blade, then struck upward toward Rorrik's head.

It may be a brutish move, but it's hard to do. And it involves the whole body.

In my unpublished dissertation, I characterized the "spindles" embedded in the rykubs' skeletal muscles. When those structures sense rapid elongation, they generate a reflexive contraction. Human muscles contain spindles, too. They're just not as substantial or powerful. But the latency and magnitude of their stretch-flex response can be improved with training.

Accordingly, the strike-down, bash-up is not a move one learns. It's a move one develops. And Styravesa developed it. For the purpose of killing.

I trained for it, too. And I put that training to use in competition. But the only occasions I set my aim on a head were *thickly* helmeted heads. Atop opponents who would be stunned but unhurt by it.

Rorrik's helmet was not so thick. And he was knocked over. And Styravesa did not wait for Rorrik to collect himself. He launched into the most violent assault I saw from anyone. Full bodied axe hacking at Rorrik while he was down. As though he were attempting to chop a log into a cord of firewood.

Rorrik was dazed, but he was defending successfully. And he would have kept defending – he gave no indication that he intended to surrender – but the judge conceded on his behalf.

To the disappointment of both fighters, the tournament was officially over.

Cheers resounded from approximately a third of the audience. Half at most. Presumably those whose wagers proved profitable. It felt like a grotesque outcome to applaud. But wealth often inspires grotesque behavior. Just ask Bonstan.

Had Rorrik wanted to strike Styravesa in a debilitating way, he could have. There were chances. I watched him decline all of them, patiently waiting for a more valor-oriented opening. But he never got one.

After watching Rorrik's skill throughout the competition – especially how he adapted his style to Fygsin and Styravesa – I don't think he was beatable by a fencer. Not this year. Being bested by a brute is different.

After the bout, it took Rorrik a few minutes to collect himself. While he was lying down, he swam his hands through the black sand. Eventually he stood and congratulated Styravesa, who didn't return the gesture. Then Rorrik left.

I lost track of him as he cut through the crowd. But we had a plan to meet at Cyn's room after the match. So she and I just went there and waited.

Rorrik arrived an hour later. In one hand, he had a small burlap sack. In the other, a smaller cloth pouch. And on his face, he held an expression of… satisfaction? It wasn't relief. Or celebration. It was between contentment and gladness. Like he was barely pleased with the direction his life was going.

He set the burlap sack on the table, and said, "roasted eggflower seeds?"

We all ate.

While chewing my first bite, I remembered the hit Rorrik took to his face. And the bloody smile that followed.

"Do you have all your teeth?", I asked. He did. None were missing or loose. Surprisingly. He did have some bruises forming, but he wasn't that wounded. Not for a lack of Styravesa's effort. It was obvious that his intention was to maim at a minimum. Ideally kill. As though the games were a dress rehearsal for real war.

"So… are you disappointed in how it ended?" I don't know why I asked this. According to Rorrik's face, he was more than contented.

He chewed his bite a few times, and then said, "In the words of Bonstan…" He paused to chew some more, and then finished his sentence: "…defeat is just another word for delayed gratification."

Nothing seems to dampen his spirits. What would he say, I wonder, if Styravesa chopped his sword arm off? It's an opportunity to become more adept with his non-dominant hand? It would take some serious drug addling to burden Rorrik's buoyancy.

And, of course, Rorrik made one last recruitment speech. He's already put the tournament behind him. All that matters is what comes next: his hunt for the "lumbering lich", as he called it.

And, of course, I turned him down.

"I figured. That's why I already asked Fygsin. Being a Rodorite, he feels the tragedy at Laberyn intimately."

Rorrik didn't mean it as an accusation, as though my concern lacked intimacy. Many Rodorites were in Laberyn when it happened. Fygsin may have been one of them.

"You leaving in the morning?", I asked.

"Not until after the Closing Ceremony."

The ceremonial induction of Styravesa into the Champions' Guard doesn't happen until the day after tomorrow. So that means Rorrik will be here for a couple of additional nights. Technically, Rorrik will be honored in the Closing Ceremony, too. All of the reserve champions are. But Rorrik has no interest. Less than no interest: he's practically insulted by dramaturgy. The pointlessness of it. We've had this discussion before. His explanation went something like:

"If you can *act* a role, why can't you fulfill it in real life? Don't *pretend* to be a medic, *pretend* to be a soldier, *pretend* to be a contributing member of society. If you're able-bodied, you should use your body's ability."

Something like that. If you press Rorrik on his position, you'll hear hints of sexism and ageism. As in: "It's fine for a grandmother to pursue the theater, but not a tournament fighter, who is capable of contributing something real."

I didn't do any pressing tonight. Instead, I just asked, "Why bother staying?"

"Fygsin insisted."

Fygsin's insistence means Rorrik will be accompanying me to the morning ceremony – also the day after tomorrow – in which the next Pendelhall Medic is announced.

I can already feel my nerves quivering a bit. Now that everything is over, and there's nothing left to distract me. One of several reasons I'm going to sleep poorly tonight. The main reason being how loud it is outside. It's too late to leave town; even those who aren't staying through the Closing Ceremony are here for the night. And what else is there to do but join in the drinking and participate in the ruckus?

I think we'll head back out. The three of us. As ruckus spectators.

There's a new moon in the sky tonight. The first faint shaving of silver light is glowing along its edge. Perhaps that promises something?

Forty-Nine

Lyros, Second Lufoa, Day Twenty-Six. Morning.

We went back out last night. And stayed out later than I expected.

I haven't left my room yet today. We'll get breakfast in a couple of hours. The city will be overrun with people until then. Apparently, the official tally of viewers at the final bout was over *six* thousand. The largest attendance at any tournament in Pendelhall's history. I'm curious how they counted, but assuming their tallying can be trusted, there must be three thousand people ordering pre-departure breakfasts as I write this. Most would have been on the road home last night if there was enough daylight left to get anywhere. Camping two miles south of town seems foolish when a good night's sleep will get you farther the next day. By 11:00, I suspect the bulk of the crowd will be filing out of town. That's when Cyn, Rorrik, and I will start our day.

I'm sure they're still asleep, anyway. I envy their ability to adapt to bedtimes. It doesn't matter when I go to bed; my mind still crows like an advent rooster at the same early morning hour, alerting me of the coming dawn. These days, I make a habit of retiring early. So I'm not exhausted the next day. Like I am this morning. This is a feeling I remember from my old life. Back when I used to worry I would miss something – a once-in-a-lifetime experience – if I didn't join the festivities.

Had I not gone out last night, and joined those festivities, what experience would I have missed? Conversation with Rorrik and Cyn… which we could have had this morning instead. After sleeping. When it was quiet enough to hear each other without yelling.

Although I did meet Styravesa. Sort of. I didn't speak to him, but I saw him. And I saw someone *else* attempt to speak to him. Which was weird enough.

I can excuse his bizarre lack of manners on the basis that he was eating, and, since he won, he was getting a lot of attention. I know from experience how annoying that can become. "I'm trying to eat; leave me alone" is what you want to say, but you find yourself uttering pleasantries instead. At least I did. Even when people would say things like, "I can't believe you actually won." Or, "You got awfully lucky in that last bout, huh?" Instead of saying what I was thinking ("is luck how you excuse your own failures?"), I would dismiss the comment as politely as I could. "The stars just lined up for me this year."

That was a sentence I used a lot. Borrowing a boring expression – especially a silly astrological one – helped build distance between me and my accosters. It's a trick I learned from one of Rouska's books. I can't remember which. But I remember his point: if you invest yourself in a conversation, the words will follow you home. And words can be a terrible guest. How can you keep the most destructive ones from entering your house? If you have time to prepare for a difficult conversation, just put on a stage costume beforehand. A hat, a bracelet, a special pair of socks. Something you wouldn't ordinarily wear. Then pretend you're acting the part of yourself in the conversation. You're not *you*. You're playing the *role* of you. Unfortunately, preparation is a luxury we seldom have. In these instances, a polite but dismissive banality makes a fine shield. But we should keep our guard up with flatterers, too. Because pride, if you invite it inside, is an especially pernicious guest.

One rarely reaches the pinnacle of success in fencing – or anything for that matter – without heeding Rouska's warning about pride. I suspect that's why most tournament winners keep their egos dry during the waves of adulation. Instead, they attribute their victories to chance. And the most popular brand of chance is irrelevant twinklings in the sky. It was in the stars. Or the stars lined up for me. Or some such expression is uttered almost every year.

But this year's winner was different. He seemed bitter about his stars.

"Congratulations, champ", a young admirer said. Barely a teen. And clearly nervous. His first time meeting a hero. Even *firster* time speaking with one. "It's a beautiful night for a celebration", he continued, his voice quivering.

Styravesa didn't respond. He just took another bite of poultry.

The nervous kid tried again: "Prettiest night I've seen all season. Can see just about every star all lined up right." His voice was trembling even more now.

The winner swallowed his chicken, paused, stared at his huge drumstick for several seconds, looked up at the sky, and then said, "It's ruined by its scars." Not stars, but *scars*. As though the night has a complexion, and it's filled with pockmarks. Then he took another bite, refixed his gaze on his chicken leg, and released a loud, exasperated exhale as he chewed. Which clearly meant "get away from me."

Perhaps he thought the kid was accusing him of profiting from astrological luck. Even so, that's hardly a gracious way to ask that he be left alone to dine in peace... which I would understand. In the words of Rorrik, fightin's a hungry task.

Once the Closing Ceremonies arrive, this star-despising drumstick devourer will be the newest appointment to the Champions' Guard, the most selective and dignified militia across the whole of Gaea.

There are only about fifty "Champions" in it today, only one new Champion is admitted each year, and very few are former criminals. Rorrik and I both declined (me once, Rorrik twice) because lifelong fealty didn't appeal to us. *Eternal* fealty, technically. The appointment is for *all* time, not just a *life*time. According to some old-but-never-rescinded statutes in the tomes and some old-but-still-sworn oaths taken by the initiates, the Guard is predominantly populated by ghosts. Most of whom had their criminal pasts exonerated.

The ghost bit is widely known today, but not the criminal count, as people who have been charged with a class one or two crime are no longer eligible. *Formally*. But a forgiving berth is still constructed with convoluted provisos. Ages ago, however, criminality was the *only* way in. Anyone incarcerated in a Pendelhall prison could be emancipated from their sentence if they opted to fight an akira. Winners were pardoned from all former crimes and sentenced to serve in the Champions' Guard. Eventually, the Guard became so revered (every member had killed an akira in unarmed combat) that non-criminals began committing crimes for the opportunity to audition.

The incentives were meant to reduce the burden on Pendelian tax revenue. Winners became indentured laborers and losers perished, vacating their cell. Maybe this benefited the city for a few years. But at some point, Pendelhall became the crime capital of the world. Thousands of abled-bodied men who were down on their luck became burglars. There was an immediate benefit if they got away with it, and an opportunity if they got caught. The irony was the Guard – all former criminals – were tasked with policing the crime wave. In the end, the criteria for admission were changed, and within a few years, burglary all but vanished. The only way in now is to win the tournament. Or, if the winner declines, the highest-ranking contestant who is willing to swear fealty is admitted. This year, the winner is Styravesa. And after seeing how he fenced, and how he treated his admirer, I wonder: how could he not be a criminal?

That experience – watching a grown man berate a young admirer – is what I traded my sleep for. That was my once-in-a-lifetime experience. I can't say it was a good trade.

Either way, Cyn must be awake by now. Time to check in with her.

Fifty

Lyros, Second Lufoa, Day Twenty-Six. Afternoon.

We just finished eating breakfast. And then lunch. Two different eateries, one right after the other. It was nearly noon when the three of us left the inn. The crowds were too big until then. And the eateries were out of most foods by the time we arrived. So we had a light breakfast followed by a light lunch. Neither was good – all leftover scraps – but the conversation made up for it. Parts of it, anyway. At first, Rorrik was asking Cyn about her education, and I kept answering before she could respond. I should have let her dazzle him with her knowledge. But I insecurely leapt to my own defense.

"Why not Farhearth?" was his first question. To Cyn.

"You didn't stay long enough to see its downfall", I interrupted.

"I pass through at least once a year", he replied, this time to me.

"The east end of Charter County isn't the university. It's not like it was when you were there. The City and the Guildlands are more or less the same, but the university is different."

"Everything changes. That doesn't mean it's worse. A baby learning to walk doesn't ruin the kid."

"In this case, the kid reverted to crawling. And shitting all over its own legs. And screaming for an adult to wipe it up. Some changes really *are* worse."

"What specifically changed?"

"The rigor. It's gone. Passing familiarity passes the class. With no standards, there's no effort to meet them. There's no strain at all. Students aren't merely failing to learn; their abilities actually atrophy in the classroom. Just like any other bedridden tissue. In exchange for steep tuition, the academy creates brittle, osteoporotic minds that can't bear the weight of normal society."

"I think you're being too hard on them. Farhearth has to be better than the alternative: no learning structure whatsoever. It beats working the counter in their family's pawnshop until they're replaced by their own kids."

"I think you're being too hard on pawnbrokers. That environment prepares workers well for other jobs. The challenge is what matters. Like everything else in life, the shop isn't baby proofed. But the classroom is. So it doesn't equip its customers with adequate skills to cope with a jagged, difficult world. Farhearth makes all sorts of promises, but the students' hopes won't survive graduation. It's a death sentence of a kind. Commencement practically serves as their eulogy. Until then, all the faculty can do is keep them comfortable. Education has become a form of palliative care."

Something like that. I wrote it here better than I said it then. But my points were the same.

I was being defensive, as my opinions about education are a large part of the reason Cyn didn't attend Farhearth. She could have. But I discouraged her. And my discouragement surely influenced her decision. I think I was right, but I can't know for certain. Not until tomorrow, anyway, when we find out whether she will be the next Pendelhall Medic. Even if all goes well, though, it'll continue to be a sensitive subject. I've dedicated six years of my life to her training. When something that personal is being questioned, it's hard not to take it personally.

Rorrik was being defensive, too. For ostensibly different reasons, but the *real* reason is always the same: protection of self-worth. He wasn't arguing on behalf of all students. Like a champion of the people. Motivated by chivalry. Rather, he prefers to believe that today's young Harthies are just as robust as they ever were. Because he still bests their best fencers with ease. And it would subtract from his self-worth if he were beating up untalented children. And when he plays music at a tavern or theater on the perimeter of campus, and his audience weeps and cheers and swoons, he would prefer them to be bright, mature, and critical. As opposed to fools who can't tell the difference between a brilliant artist and a beginner.

Realizing the conversation wasn't going anywhere – my insecurity was simply dueling his – I changed my tack. To something I knew Rorrik would agree with:

"You have to concede there's a difference between knowledge and wisdom. The former is cheap, but the price of wisdom is high. If we want to know about pain, we must first feel its sting. Want to know about loss? Sacrifice what you hold dear. Want to know about death? That, too, has to be learned in the active. Wisdom is not passive; its pursuit is always painful, often lethal. *Life* is your curriculum. Farhearth students, though; they're raised like veal. Too soft for the world outside the cage."

Rorrik nodded in agreement, then asked about an even more sensitive topic: "What about resources? Regardless of whether students make use of them, there's no place on Gaea as furnished for learning. A lab for every science and a library that would take the fastest reader fifty lifetimes to complete."

His tone contained no criticism. Only curiosity. But I held my defenses tight. Like a Delta Reef scallop clamping down against a prying otter. "That's true", I said. "But Cyn has no use for the Geography and Horticulture labs or the Law and Governance wing of the library."

Again, Rorrik nodded, indicating his acceptance of my answer. And then he asked, "How's the learning environment in Estevro compared to campus?"

This would have been a perfect time for me to step back and let Cyn answer. But I didn't. "To me, Estevro is the intellectual capital of the world", I said. It was the most insecure sentence I've spoken this year. Objectively, I know it's false. But the most durable truths are never objective. Only subjectively held positions can fend off reality with fervor. And subjectively, I hold the institutions of Estevro – the schools, guilds, and libraries – in a sacred space. In my mind, they're completely immune to the atrophy of the veal generation.

Realizing the bias in my claim, I added a caveat: "But I look at Estevro in the way a seventy-year-old husband looks at his wife, still seeing her as beautiful. Something between devotion and delusion."

Rorrik smiled. And then he asked, "How did you set up the curriculum?" This is when the enjoyable half of our conversation began. Not immediately. Because every emotion has a momentum, and defensiveness is heavier than most. So, I *still* leapt to the response: "Early on, it was mostly liberal arts. Rouska, Kryora, Lightner, Lan, Pirazok and Pizarok, Carrin's Biodeism, Maren's Sevens—"

"All seven?", Rorrik interrupted.

"No, only Wars, Faiths, Kingdoms, and Histories."

My defensiveness began to abate. And I became more interested in my plate of "dumplings" (euphemism is too weak a word to characterize the difference between expectation and actuality here). While I attempted to carve a bite from the world's hardest doughball, Cyn finally took over the conversation. And I learned that, in her spare time, she read Cities, Guilds, *and* Societies. All three. I don't own any of them. She found them in Estevro's libraries. Again: intellectual capital of the world.

For the next twenty minutes – that's how long it took me to safely swallow one whole dumpling – I listened to Cyn describe Maren's three minor works. A topic we'd never discussed.

Before I praise Cyn's summaries and observations, let me say: when I was a student at Farhearth, and I had no budget for food, my staple was bachelor's muffins. No euphemism there. I would mix anything I deemed comestible into a pot with some flour, add sodium bicarbonate and some sort of acid – citric acid or cream of tartar; whatever was available – and bake it. It rises. And it's edible. So it suffices. What I ate today was not a bachelor's muffin. After several minutes of failed cutting, I just grabbed it from the broth with my bare hand and started gnawing on it. Even then, it would have been easier to eat a biceros hoof. I doubt a dross dog would have enough jaw strength to chew through it. A mouth that could masticate this culinary marvel into a swallowable bolus could pulverize a sword. And there were two of them. Two dumplings. I succeeded in ingesting one. I left the other behind. I was too exhausted to continue.

Anyway, back to Cyn. And Maren.

I always thought Maren ran out of ideas after her first four books. Cyn had a different perspective. Except when it came to Cities. On that, we agreed. It was her final book. Her seventh. About all seven of the Eastern cities. "For each one, she wrote a dozen pages of history, half of it questionable. Except for Charwarg: two dozen, *all* of it questionable."

That was Cyn's description. It was so accurate, I laughed. Or at least I made the noise of laughter. My mouth was too tired to smile. But I found it funny. To me, humor is an obvious truth stated in a surprising way. And Cyn did just that in her description of *The Seven Cities*.

Then she moved on to Guilds and Societies, which were perfectly factual. And global. But in those, I never thought there was a lesson worth learning. Unless you were seeking membership in one of the characterized guilds or societies. In that case, some of the facts were probably practical. But Cyn noticed several nuggets I had missed. Especially in Guilds. Listening to her describe it made me wonder why I ever thought it wise to skip. I disregarded the book – Maren's penultimate – as little more than a historical perspective of Farhearth. The uniting of seven major guildhouses. Cyn ignored that part, describing it as "a compendium of long-winded trivialities and short-winded profundities." While I chucked unsmilingly, Cyn said, "The real magic was in Maren's exploration of the *extrinsic* guilds", meaning those that didn't merge.

Cyn's description of the Poisoner's Guild – which later became the Archer's Guild, which still exists – was fascinating from an apothecarial perspective. Some fact, some fiction. Some fact that was later demonstrated to be fiction. And far more fascinating: some fiction that was later demonstrated to be fact. About ryndovyn, lufig and lufir, carrot berries, and coral from the Wren Reef. (The experiments that did the demonstrating occurred after I read the book, which is why I didn't find it fascinating until today, when Cyn brought it to my attention.)

But what interested me most was Cyn's commentary on the Gyzog Guild. When I originally read the book, I remember thinking this section could have worked as a history of Thestevro… if Maren didn't conflate fact and fable. But Cyn shined a curious light on it. First, her summary: In Old Adonian, gyzog means "grew". In Orfric, the word was borrowed, but it was assigned a different meaning, presumably owing to a translation error: radish. As in: "Gyzog Grumpkis", or, *Radish Thief*, the ancient fable shared by the East and the West (no one knows where it originated). In time, the Eastern definition of gyzog took on a different meaning: a personal food farm. And thus, the Gyzog Guild was, in practice, the Food and Farming Guild. It was stationed in Thestevro before the segregation of the cities. According to Maren, that guild was responsible for their division. Each faction created their own guild, dropping the word gyzog, which led to separate identities. Separate identities led to fierce rivalries, and those rivalries defined the residents we know today. Cooking remained central, but the core is argumentation. "Taste is secondary to debate", Cyn said, concluding her summary. I laughed a few seconds late. Once I accepted the truth in her words. Then Cyn explained the curious part. Some of Maren's passages were too fanciful for me to take seriously, but Cyn read them carefully. And her careful interpretation is that Maren anticipated several future disputes between Thevro and Estevro, which occurred years after *The Seven Guilds* was written. In the end, Cyn changed my mind on the value of the minor works – at least this one – in a liberal arts education.

Histories though. That was Maren's best. And first. She never managed to top her debut publication. Seven different perspectives on the same history. The same events presented in seven profoundly different ways. And no single set of cultural "truths" was compatible with another. In studying this, it reveals the mystery of our past. We all tell our own versions of every story. Almost like recounting a dream: we invent plots and intentions that weren't really there. We explain away the arbitrary and meaningless with meaning and purpose. *The Seven Histories* is the best work on human self-centeredness ever written. And it was the textbook we used in a course I took as a student at Farhearth called "Overcoming Solipsism". Over time, I came to regard it as the most important class in my curriculum. But it isn't offered anymore.

Rouska was the professor, and when he died, Farhearth didn't replace him. They just dropped the course. On some level, I don't understand why any department bothers to teach departmental classes anymore. The university should put math and science and linguistics on hold. And teach nothing but empathy. For one term. There's no point in learning anything if we don't begin with that. It's the foundation of humanity. And until a community is populated by human beings, narrow education doesn't seem important.

So that's where Cyn and I started. Even though she didn't need it. We used *The Seven Histories*, and I stole the academic structure of Rouska's class.

That's all I can write for now. I'm feeling too nervous to continue.

The announcement for which candidate is selected happens hours before the Closing Ceremonies. So whoever is chosen knows to attend. That means, by this time tomorrow, we'll know whether Cyn is the next Pendelhall Medic.

Breakfast and lunch weren't good meals, but they were effective distractions. The conversations took my mind off the coming decision. They helped pass a couple of tense hours. Sitting by myself, writing about those distractions, is proving less effective.

So Rorrik, Cyn, and I are heading back out now.

Fifty-One

Lyros, Second Lufoa, Day Twenty-Six. Night.

Cyn, Rorrik, and I spent the evening wandering around town. For the sake of distraction. For the sake of *my* distraction. Cyn didn't appear to be as nervous as I was. Not because of exaggerated confidence. She just accepts the present circumstance for what it is. And if Rorrik is antsy for anything, it's an eagerness to leave. Quests are urgent endeavors, and this tournament didn't put any of his questing to rest. He has a ravenous appetite sated only by adventure.

I had hoped our evening walk would be more exciting. But Pendelhall felt like a ghost town. I don't mean like Yaga-Goro. I just mean it was vacant. Even at dinner, half the eateries were either closed or out of everything but the least appetizing options.

"We're here for two more nights", I said. "Let's see if we can switch inns." I was just looking for something attentive to do.

There were rooms available at the Eldsyn Tower. Not adjacent, like they were at Pygil's. And not cheap, like they were at Pygil's. They cost twice as much and have half the heart. But we got them anyway. For the sake of distraction.

Once we had finished lugging our luggage from one inn to the other, the new environment offered no more peace. I'm just fretting in a room with a view of the Grey Delta. That's the only difference. That and I can no longer walk next door to chat with Cyn. We aren't even on the same floor anymore.

But my new room does have a nice desk where I'm writing this. And where I'm panicking about Cyn's decision in the morning. I just took caligoroot. I'll write until it takes effect. Assuming it will. *Hoping* it will.

The morning itself went by quickly enough. Because I had Cyn and Rorrik to listen to and argue with. Respectively. Really, it was me doing the arguing. I'm too defensive of my "life's work". Cyn. She's my contribution to Gaea. My effort to make the world a better place.

Now that it's nighttime, and I have no one to listen to or argue with, and I still need a distraction, I'm reflecting on Cyn's curriculum. In the spirit of Maren's Sevens, here are the seven core lessons I tried to impart:

The first lesson was to pay attention to the past. If we don't know enough about the blunders of history, we'll be condemned to repeat them. Likewise, if we're unfamiliar with our historical successes – the ingenious attempts of our ancestors to unravel yesterday's mysteries – we will have no idea how to decipher today's puzzles. Accordingly, this is where Cyn began. The first of innumerable works was *The Seven Histories*. And she never stopped surveying the past for its lessons about the future.

The second lesson was to pay attention to the present. People look at novel landscapes with wider eyes. If they've never been to the Northern snows or the Western swamps, or seen the Southern lava creeping through the clays, they look upon those scenes with keener interest. But the familiar sights are minimally observed. We only acknowledge them enough to avoid tripping on detritus. It is only when we look at familiarity with the same interest that we truly come to know it. We can start by tricking ourselves into it. "So *this* is what the West looks like" we think while journeying across a familiar East. Eventually, one learns to inspect every landscape with the same ardent eyes, read every book with interest, and engage every discussion with enthusiasm. This is a skill that Cyn quickly mastered.

The third lesson was the atrophy of complacency. The trap of feeling satisfied with what we currently know, tempted by the coziness of our bed of laurels. There are unknowns lurking everywhere. And we should greet them heartily. Especially when they feel grating to us. Often, we defend our beliefs against all contradiction. But to learn what you thought you knew is, in fact, wrong, is to become smarter. Curiosity, if it survives long enough, will beget genius. It has a mortal weakness, however: complacency. This is a poison that stifles wonder and withers the mind. But atrophy is a slow and sneaky grumpkis. It often begins its thievery at puberty. The colors of the sky inspire inquiry in the common child and the rare adult. The possibilities beyond the horizon curiositize the explorer, but not the settler. And the complicated truths that contradict comfortable beliefs are spurned by the fool and sought by the sage. In matters of unguarded wonder, I have never met Cyn's equal.

The fourth, fifth, and sixth lessons I taught Cyn, I learned from my father. Two of them intentionally, one inadvertently. And all of them are related.

On my father's side, my ancestors had two passions. Two *sacrificial* passions. One of them was transportation. The previously unmapped distances my father traveled to make *his* maps nearly killed him on more than one occasion. On more than a hundred occasions, probably. But he survived all of them. And he returned with masterpieces of cartography. The kind of artistry that can only be created by great risk.

As far back as fathers can be tracked – which turns out isn't all that far; I've done the tracking – my paternal lineage worked in transportation. That was one of their two passions. The other was fishing. And that actually did kill a number of them.

When I was young – maybe six or seven – my father took me to the Vanishing Isles. It's a long trip from Estevro, but we only stopped for horse problems, not person problems. So we made good time. And when the trip was over, I understood two of the lessons. Years later, I learned the third.

The first one didn't require any traveling. He could have just read *The Birdsong Bard* to me. At some point later in life, he did. Or perhaps it was my mother. One of them read it to me. By then, though, its moral was a reminder of the lesson I learned when my father took me to the Vanishing Isles and showed me the graves of our ancestors. *Some* of the graves of *some* of our ancestors. Those who chased Urumi, the feathered fish. Those who attempted to catch the uncatchable. Those who beckoned fame and found only their graves. The chirping bard could have been swapped with any of my great or greater grandfathers and the tale would have lost nothing of its moral. So much of my greatest grandfamily had difficulty staying alive. Because fame travels a dangerous road. And chasing it leads us off the better-beaten path. That was the first lesson I learned on that trip. When I saw how many of my ancestors fell victim to it.

The inadvertent lesson began with my realization that I lacked the character to join those graves. Not because I was destined to live an un-bard-ly life, but because I couldn't catch a fish. Or ride in a boat. By the time we reunited with the mainland, I had vomited much more sustenance than I had caught. My stomach was as empty as my hook. "I just can't catch a fish", I said to my father when I had finished vomiting. "I didn't expect you to", he said… without acknowledging my seasickness. "If the gillies aren't diggin' any bugs, the fish aren't bitin' any bait", he finished.

At the time, I didn't know what gillies were. I later learned they're a species of bird. Their formal name is rynkos, but everyone knows them as gilly birds. And they're practically fish. They just can't swim. The gills are decorative. Probably vestigial. Excepting those who call them rynkos, people believe them to be descendants of Urumi. The only evidence of Urumi's existence is her offspring. Those scantily feathered birds with a fear of water are the closest creatures to those that dwell within it. And nature's rhythms seem preserved across species. If one herd is hungry, its counterpart is probably feeding, too. Thus, if the gillies aren't diggin'…

Upon learning this, years later, my inadvertent lesson matured into wisdom that I could pass on to Cyn: a fisherman's success, like every other pursuit, has little to do with luck. There was a time when I thought regnavus was a game of skill, fencing a sport of aptitude, and fishing a vocation of chance. But then I came to appreciate that only birth is a matter of luck. The life that follows is not. With the severing of the umbilical cord, we're separated from the bulk of our fates. Very little in life owes fealty to the seasickening waves of luck. Not even luck itself arises entirely by chance; it's a matter of position. We can posture ourselves to receive chance's fortunes and evade its hazards.

Once I learned that, I applied it in every pursuit, including my profession. When I became a professor, instead of a transporter or a fisherman, my father demonstrated a kind of pride that implied he would have been disappointed had I become anything else. Because my paternal legacy was not about fishing or transportation. It was about committing to one's calling. When he first expressed this pride, I came to appreciate that we don't need to abide by the expectations of others. That was the sixth lesson I taught Cyn. Her journey, like mine, has veered from its ancestral path. But as long as it doesn't veer in the direction of fame and celebration, and it stays true to her own passions, she's making the right choices.

Then came our final lesson. The seventh. The science and practice of the profession itself. This is where everyone else begins. They go to Farhearth and start memorizing facts about their field, eager to enter the workforce. But this is the last thing any of us should be taught. Specialization absent a foundation results in dangerous practitioners. Today's aspiring apothecarists insist on learning prescription independent of alchemy, botany, and biology. And the same is true for each other branch of medicine. It's equivalent to teaching astronomy without math. In separating them, you'll fail to calculate anything of value in the cosmos. Good luck predicting the next eclipse, or even the coming nightfall, let alone making any substantial contribution to our body of knowledge. Similarly, separating medicine from statistics, and a dozen other foundational disciplines, creates practitioners who comprehend nothing of illness or its remedies. Once learning on this final lesson begins, it should last a lifetime. For Cyn, I know it will. Soon, history will not know her equal. And she will reshape medicine across all of Gaea. She has already demonstrated a degree of mastery in her Pendelhall audition. And I've never been prouder of anything. Nor have I ever been more optimistic of a future. I have nothing left to teach.

As for tonight, it is past my bedtime. The caligoroot is working well enough that I'm going to attempt some sleep. *Attempt.* In the morning, we find out if she is appointed as the next Pendelhall Medic.

Fifty-Two

Fyros, Second Lufoa, Day Twenty-Seven. Morning.

Last night's attempt at sleep was unsuccessful. Later this morning, the next Pendelhall Medic will be revealed.

This is what we've been working toward since we began. When the last sun sets on Second Elyem, it will have been a Thevro dozen years. A quarter of an Estevro dozen. (Or an ordinary half dozen.) And soon, the decision will be revealed. Despite the caligoroot, I couldn't put it out of my mind. I just rolled around, trying to find a position in which my heart didn't feel like a shrieking infant being held captive in a cradle of ribs, its cries for attention resonating throughout my chest.

I never found the position I was rolling for. So I'm too tired to write anything of value. So I'm writing about divisions of dozens instead. Trying to distract myself from the ruckus of my still-shrieking heart thumping in its cage.

I wonder if Cyn slept. If she's as nervous as I am. Or if she's still sleeping.

I'm going to head to her room and find out.

When we were staying at Pygil's, we were neighbors. The walls were so lean, I could have probably pressed my ear against the one that divided us to hear if she was up. But it was just as convenient – and perhaps less intrusive – to walk next door and look. Here, we're on different floors. Which makes it a rather large errand to see if she's awake.

I'll pick up breakfast first. That'll give me something to do. It'll occupy the better part of an hour, letting Cyn rest a little longer. Assuming she managed to make better use of the night than I did.

Some of the eateries must have restocked their pantries by now.

Then, after breakfast, we'll head to the Archives for the announcement.

It doesn't start for several hours, but we'll show up early. Unnecessarily early.

Fifty-Three

Fyros, Second Lufoa, Day Twenty-Seven. Afternoon.

Cyn and I went to the Archives, where the decision of who would be the next Pendelhall Medic was revealed. Rorrik met us there. The appointment will be *ceremonially* honored in the Closing Ceremonies, but it was revealed here. Not without ritual, but not as formal or extravagant as it will be this evening. It began with a brief introduction of all five candidates. Then the Operating Medic made the announcement. Not by stating the chosen candidate's name aloud, but by silently fastening the official pin of the Pendelhall Medic onto the winner's coat.

There was the day I won the Pendelhall tournament. There was the day that I graduated Farhearth. My *first* graduation. The Degree of Lower Licentiate. There were the days that I finished my next two degrees: Higher Licentiate and Magister's Degree. And there was the day that I was hired as a professor. Each of those was fulfilling in its own way, but today leaves them all behind. Today is the most rewarding day of my life. When I watched Cyn receive the pin of the Pendelhall Medic, I wept. More than I expected to. Silent streams of tears flowed down my cheeks like Eastern rivulets winding toward the sea.

During the introductions of the candidates, we were informed that everyone except Cyn had a Magister's Degree from Farhearth, was a valedictorian in their Lower Licentiate, and they were all decorated with academic awards. Plus, all of them had the Bonstan Medical Certification and one of them was the Incumbent. Cyn was the last to be introduced, and her introduction was awkwardly terse. And still she was selected over all of them.

As I watched the hole get poked into her coat – ruining it a little but honoring the body that wore it – I felt more accomplished than I ever have. It was like watching a formerly twinkling star ignite into a nova, super-ing itself across the sky. This is the single most sought-after and prestigious medical position anywhere on Gaea. And Cyn is only twenty-four years old. She might be the youngest appointment ever. I'm not sure. But I *am* sure that she has already accomplished more than I have. And she's just getting started. This means, after she presents her work at the Farhearth Faire, I can retire. At least from my role as a teacher. Which pleases Rorrik, as he interprets this life change as a newfound freedom to accompany him on his adventures. As I once did. But that's not my intention. My short-term intentions are to rest on the bed of laurels that I spent the last six years making.

Not forever. Just long enough to figure out what to do with myself as I enter the final act of my life. Then, once I decide, I'll get started on whatever that decision is. I suspect it will involve my garden. And whenever Lonvarakan notes can be heard ringing on the distant wind, I'll go watch Melindroth play. Abendroth would be as proud of her as I am of Cyn.

As I write this, I'm realizing why I wept. As dehydratingly as I did. It's that my life's responsibility feels complete. I reside between Abendroth and Cyn, my mentor and my mentee. If I ever had a destiny, I was meant to be the link between them. And today, upon the puncturing of Cyn's coat, that role has been fulfilled.

Cyn's role – her "destiny" if we're to be whimsical about it – still lies ahead. Especially in the coming year. There's no better place to balance academics and clinical practice than at Pendelhall. Which is to say: there's no better place to learn, as participation in both gets us further in each. Teaching keeps us current in our knowledge. If we don't advance at the same pace as science, we fall behind in our instruction. And that constant amassing of knowledge arms us with skills for the clinic. Conversely, there is a type of insight one only gleans from practicing the trade. To set aside one's books and do doctoring in the active is to understand the practice on a deeper level, which makes one a better academic. And beginning with the first sunup of Arzox (Arzox Syofa literally means "first sun"), Cyn will be combining academics and clinical practice better than any medic who has ever come before.

Ten minutes after the pinning of Cyn, I needed a nap. I had been so tense for so many days. And last night, I might have slept an hour. Standing at the entrance to the Archives, anxiety was all that was keeping me upright. The moment she won, it felt as though a hundred miles of emotional levees holding all that anxiety inside broke. And a thousand emotions flooded free. And all I wanted to do was collapse and sleep. Cyn and Rorrik could see it on my face. And in my posture. And, while accompanying me back to the Tower, they could see it in my gait. It took all the energy I had just to walk. So Rorrik did the talking. More of a congratulation speech than chatting. "According to some very old fables", he began. This is a common beginning for him. No matter the setting, no matter the topic, he has a line from an old fable that's perfect for the occasion. He continued: "There are continents across the sea. They lie at the precise antipode of our own. And it is from those lands that our ancestors emigrated."

"Pilgrim's Day", Cyn said, referring to the day of rejuvenation and blossoms on the last day of First Lylir. It's one of six holidays celebrated by all Geans. In the East, celebration means nobody works and everybody eats.

"Correct", Rorrik said. "In years long past, we celebrated the landing of our ancestors on our shores. In years shorter past, afraid of appearing foolish, we discarded our history, but kept the holiday, replacing it with sunshine and flowers and bunnies. Which says something about what's really traditional in our traditions."

"We celebrate Pilgrim's Day in the South, too", Cyn said. "Not as the arrival of our ancestry, but as vernal equinox. We don't work any less, but we eat twice as much."

"We celebrate with food in the West, too. A feast for the day our ancestors landed. Because they would have been famished when they finally arrived. According to those fables, traveling from the Dark Isles to our lands…." Rorrik paused, and then asked, "Is there a biological word for relocation?"

"Assuming you don't mean migration – the whole body doing the traveling – if a protein or vesicle goes to some other location, we call that *trans*location", Cyn said.

"Since you're the Pendelhall Medic now, we'll put it in your parlance", Rorrik said, and then he gave his speech… in a way that sounded nothing like Cyn, excepting the two words she loaned him: "It supposedly took half a year to translocate that vesicle of pilgs, delivering them from one world to the next. Six dreadful months of the same sights, the same company, the same food. Cramped sleeping quarters. Endless swaying. The rum bottles gone empty. Six months without a break. Until *land ho* finally delivered them to a better, brighter world. And it was suddenly worth every moment of their suffering. By comparison, you have been on your present journey for almost six years, and I know the waters were rough at times. In every quest of self-betterment, the path from novice to master is a trying one. There are struggles worse than seasickness plaguing those pursuits. But today, you've nearly arrived. Tomorrow, you'll be even closer. There are only a few more months until this year ends and you set foot in your new world. So make the most of the time you have left in this one. For memory's sake. Everyone thinks they'll go back, relations will remain, and life will always be the same. And all of them are wrong. All we keep is our memories. And our lessons. Six years' worth in your case. Of memories and lessons stowed in your heart and mind. So as you *land ho* upon the shore of your next world, remember to always keep your compassion close. To always be fair and generous to those who remain stuck in the world to which they were born. Those who haven't had the same opportunities. Go win – take the moon from the sky if you can – but do your winning both graciously and gracefully."

It went something like that. I don't know that the end of Rorrik's speech was Cyn-oriented. She's the humblest creature ever orbited by the moon (regardless of whether she takes it from the sky). But the rest of the speech was good. And the delight exuded by Cyn was even better. She deserved it. And deserves what comes next: conquering the world. Not in the way of Northern tyranny, obviously, but by purging Gaea of all that ails us.

On the subject of the memories we take with us, this is a day I will forever hold dear. And one I would like to be reminded of every time I look out of my bedroom window. So, as we were walking back to the Tower, I wearily crouched and plucked a stone from the ground. More of a rock than a stone. Brown and plain. There are millions just like it. But it doesn't need to be unique to serve as an idol of my experience. Physical objects, no matter how plain or special, mark a time and place. They're relics I can look upon to better conjure those memories in my mind. Some sorrowful, others joyous. I have one from Pendelhall, the day I won the tournament, unaware it would come to be remembered as a rather upsetting day. I have one from each of my Farhearth graduations. A bunch from my young travels with my father. Including one from our trip to the Vanishing Isles. And the rock I took today will perhaps be the fondest on my sill. I'll place it there when we get home. Before we immediately leave again. To Farhearth. To submit Cyn's research. I'll take a stone from there, too. Representing the last day of my mentorship, and the first day of her independent journey.

And now it's time to go to the Closing Ceremonies.

That hour came quickly as I spent the bulk of the afternoon napping.

Rorrik spent those hours with Fygsin. Planning their escapade.

Cyn and I will meet him there.

Time to go.

Fifty-Four

Fyros, Second Lufoa, Day Twenty-Seven. Night.

Cyn and I went to the Closing Ceremonies together. We met Rorrik there. And then she and Rorrik had to go to the roped-off region behind the stage, since they were both being honored. Among the three of us, I was the only audience member.

It began with a speech by the mayor. He confirmed that it was, in fact, the most highly attended tournament in recorded history. This was followed by some cursory "thank you for attending" remarks. And then he introduced the current Pendelhall Medic. She spoke briefly about the importance of the position, its scrupulous selectivity, and its long legacy. Then she introduced her successor: Cyn of Cinderheim.

I wept. Again. But I did a better job containing it this time. I wrestled my quivering until it submitted to stillness. I subdued my breathing into silence. And I angled the brimming wells in my eyes toward the breeze so evaporation would help manage any spillover. The smaller ceremony this morning also provided some emotional sandbagging, which helped prepare me for tonight. The two events were almost identical. As though this morning served as a dress rehearsal. The current Operating Medic even reapplied the same pin, poking a second hole in Cyn's coat.

Then it was time to announce the winners of the sport and regnavus contests. Cyn and the Operating Medic took seats at the back of the stage, and Bonstan stepped forward. And stood beside the mayor. "Of course Bonstan is here", I thought. And may have said out loud. In a tone of exasperation.

At this point, the mayor announced the reserve champions and the winners, and Bonstan shook their hands (reserve champions) and placed the pendants around their necks (winners). The traditional regnavus pendant is silver, wrestling is given gold, and the fencing pendant is amber encased in wood. Boxers are honored differently. Bonstan coronated the champion with the traditional wreath.

Cyn was the only victor that Bonstan didn't congratulate in some capacity. He seemed to ignore her completely. I wondered if it was because she didn't have his certification. She wasn't part of *the family*. And so he snubbed her. Or maybe it was just a coincidence; that's how the ceremony was planned.

The contests were celebrated in the same order they occurred: wrestling first, then boxing, then regnavus, and finally, fencing. For each one, the mayor began with a brief speech honoring the contest's history. Then he introduced "this year's additions to the roster of historical contestants!" He exclaimed that exact quotation for all four events. In a feigned dramatic tone that would induce a powerful cringe in any Lonvarakan.

Tauro, the reserve champion in wrestling, was the first "addition to the roster of historical contestants" to be announced. The mayor gave a few words about his city and legacy while Bonstan shook his hand. And then Rugyn, the winner, was announced. As Bonstan placed the medal around his neck, I cheered loudly. Embarrassingly. It was an undignified holler of hometown patriotism. But I don't regret it. Rugyn then had the opportunity to speak. "Thank you" is all he said. Then he bowed, indicating his speech was over. He left the stage and hugged a Rodorite.

Next up: boxing. The mayor announced Tyfir, the reserve champion, and Bonstan shook his hand. Then Lanko, the winner. While Bonstan placed the wreath upon his head, some people cheered. I was not one of them. Lanko started his speech before he was offered the stage. Before the cheers had died. Before Bonstan had even let go of the wreath. It went on for at least five minutes. And the entire time, Tyfir wore an expression of irritation. Like he wanted an immediate rematch. Each minute that passed, his glare at Lanko grew more rancorous. After a couple of minutes, I finally remembered where I knew him from: Lum. He almost attacked Lum about ten years ago. He wasn't as big then, but his silent fuming was no less noxious. A story for another time.

When Lanko was finally done talking, the mayor introduced the regnavus reserve champion: Hembolt, a Western woman whose hair was the orangest thing in the world. Oranges themselves must envy its hue. Bonstan shook her hand. Then it was Lydria's turn. Bonstan had already provided a prize, but this time, he placed the medal, and she, too, was given the stage to speak. If Lanko was narcissism incarnate, Lydria seemed wholly possessed by some god of bitterness. Just as unlikable a champion.

Lastly, fencing was honored. Bonstan didn't give this award, but he shook Rorrik's hand. And I could tell this was the last place Rorrik wanted to be. The person who *officially* bestowed the honors in fencing was the First Knight. Limited leader of the Champions' Guard. It's a single-year appointment, and once elected, they are no longer eligible to compete in the Pendelhall games. Because losing would break the mystique. After Bonstan let go of Rorrik's hand, the First Knight extended his own in Rorrik's direction.

It was Erluk. I wonder how many times he's been elected. It's as though the Guard is compensating for his first fallen record by establishing one that *really* cannot be surpassed. He must have served fifty terms by now.

In the old days, the Morning Sword was tantamount to king. Today's version, First Knight, wields far more honor than power. But tradition still regards the post as the best living knight. Whose sword is sworn to protect all from injustice.

By my math, Erluk is eighty-seven years old. But standing tall and proud in his regal suit of armor, he still looked young and adept. Although I doubt his skill and mettle will ever be tested in combat again.

Erluk gave a short speech, outlining the history of the Champions' Guard. I've heard some iteration of that history every time I've been here. He then announced that Styravesa would not be appointed to the Guard. The word "disqualification" was used. Which could technically be true, as winners who fail to attend the Ceremony forfeit their right to join. And he wasn't there. But I assume there's more to it than that.

Having had a brief encounter with Styravesa, he didn't seem fit to a life of civic duty. So I wonder if he rejected the Guard, and Erluk was saving face. Or if there is some information known by the Guard that's unknown to the rest of us. Either way, the announcement clearly came as news to Rorrik, who wasn't expecting the invitation.

Rorrik can hardly stay put for a week. Let alone a *life* of sworn put-staying. He opted out. Obviously. But graciously, too. With reverent showmanship. He took a knee and bowed his head to Erluk as he declined, implying he is unworthy of the invitation at this time. It's the same gesture he made in both of his previous offers. Three rejections now. Given that Mizjak was never given the choice to reject – he was bestowed with an honorary appointment upon his first victory, which did not restrict him to Pendelhall – I wonder if this makes Rorrik the refusingest candidate in history.

But this created a complication Rorrik didn't plan for: since he and Styravesa both refused – in Styravesa's case, Pendelhall may have done the rejecting – the offer was extended to the third-place candidate. And that was Fygsin, who was present. And who was supposed to be Rorrik's quest companion. And he accepted. His swearing in took ten minutes. Ten *very* formal minutes. During which, I watched everyone on the stage. As I said earlier this month – before we left on this journey – one can learn a great deal about someone based on what they assign attention to.

Cyn was focused on the ceremony. In her face, I could tell she was learning. Fully present. Fully focused. Developing an understanding of the customs of the city in which she would soon be living.

Bonstan was standing beside Cyn. He was focused on his smile, his posture, his presence, trying to represent himself as one of us.

The wrestlers and boxers were bored to death.

The regnavus players were deep in their heads; their bodies may have been on stage, but their minds had already left the venue.

Fygsin was elated in a quiet, dignified way.

And Rorrik was scanning the audience intently. Searching for a substitute.

When it finally ended, Rorrik found me in the crowd. Ten minutes before Cyn did. "I got you something", he said. And he handed me that cloth bag he's been carrying for the last couple of days.

I opened it up. And instantly knew what it was.

"For your windowsill", Rorrik said.

I stared at it, caught in a state between surprise and shock. Noticing I had been disarmed by disbelief, Rorrik renewed his recruitment efforts.

"What are your plans now?", he asked. "Cyn is moving to Pendelhall soon. What will you do then?"

I was still staring into the bag. Too distracted to answer.

"Tell me you aren't just going to sit at home by yourself", he said.

I looked up and mumbled something about getting my life in order.

"Order is a trap for the apathetic. Productivity makes a mess. Organize your closet all you want; you'll ruin it when you get dressed. You can't eat and keep your kitchen tidy or read and leave your bookshelf pristine."

"I don't mean *order* like I'm going to organize my library and never read again. I just mean I need some time to reflect, and figure who I am without my role in Cyn's life. And, of course, I would love your company while I do it."

"Are you inviting me to be cooped like a hen?"

I looked back in the cloth bag while Rorrik said that. So I didn't respond. He continued: "Your life has so much value… if you do something with it. But you keep it in a box like a jewel. You'll take it out on special occasions, like a trip to Pendelhall, but then it goes right back in its box, locked away for fear of losing it."

I kept looking in the bag. But I nodded in agreement. Rorrik wasn't wrong. Not much happens in my life these days. I used to be able to tolerate more. My allostatic armor was thick. But I no longer cope as well with excesses of demands. I can write better than I ever could, teach better than I ever could, and probably fence at least as well. But the *amounts* of those activities… that's where I can't compete with my younger self.

I was thinking about this at the time, staring blankly into the cloth bag, when Rorrik said, "Come on, let's find Cyn and celebrate."

We did.

I had one drink. Cyn had two. Rorrik had at least three.

That was our first round. It's hard to keep up with Rorrik. His moderation masquerades as an indulgence of excess. Somehow, he's always managed to extract more life from his liquor than it extracts from him.

Cyn saw me clutching Rorrik's cloth bag, guarding it as though a pickpocket were lurking nearby. "What's in it?", she asked. Rather than explain, I opened the bag a tiny bit and showed her. She looked inside. Then she looked up and met my eyes, and smiled, communicating her understanding that it was Baguzu-level contraband.

Then we ordered another round. Cyn and I each had one. And Rorrik had another three. If this were Moonkruug, I might join Rorrik in his pursuit of inebriation, but Pendelmeads and Pendelales are hardly worth the hangover.

After round two, we went to another tavern. And then another. I stopped drinking after the second, but the merriment grew brighter and louder with each new destination. And I had no reservation for *that* gluttony.

As the night went on, Cyn and I both developed headaches. I knew I would, but it was unexpected for her. And Rorrik was fine. Every passing hour, he seemed even younger, every drink revitalizing his spirits a little more.

The only reason I was able to keep up with him socially is that I napped for so long earlier today. I rarely sleep between morning and night. (As opposed to *barely* sleeping between night and morning.)

Ordinarily, if I fall asleep at some point during the day, I'll be up all night. I'm hoping that won't be the case tonight. If so, tomorrow will be difficult. I can hardly move my hand to write another sentence. I need some real sleep. Bed has been calling me for the last hour. It's time to heed its call.

Cyn and I will meet in the morning, eat one last bad Pendelhall breakfast, and then we'll start our trip to Farhearth to submit her research. With a brief stop at Estevro.

Rorrik said he'll join us for breakfast. After that, who knows where he'll be. At some point, he'll have to pick up Gyfur. So I'll see him again.

Fifty-Five

Nyros, Second Lufoa, Day Twenty-Eight. Late Morning.

We stayed out *late*. When I went to sleep, the sunrise wasn't too far away. And I was hoping I wouldn't rise before it. I almost always do. If I stay up an hour later, I get an hour less sleep. Two hours later? Two hours less sleep. My morning mind refuses to adjust for the previous night's bedtime. Just as tomorrow's me won't accommodate tonight's.

I was prepared for this morning to be glum and groggy. Maybe two hours of sleep at the most. Hoping for more. But expecting less. When I awoke, though, it was light out. *Bright* out. Just a few seconds after closing my eyes. Or at least that's how it felt. Midday is almost here, and I just got out of bed.

And I feel... good. Surprisingly. Only Westerners are granted access to those forbidden slumbering acres, but last night, I feel like I trespassed a tiny bit. Just on the perimeter. For the first time in my adult years, I slept deeply. And I emerged from bed a different person. I sound the same; the timbre of my voice hasn't changed. I look the same; my hair is no longer or shorter. The world sees me the same. But I see it differently. And hear it differently. That's what changes. The world. Not me. Except for my ability to *perceive* those differences. The ability to see things and understand their meanings. That's what yesterday's me couldn't do. That's what yesterday's me would envy if he knew what he was missing. And tomorrow's me will surely mourn the passing of today's. Although I wonder if this is what it feels like to be Rorrik. And I wonder if my waking self would begin to resemble him more if my sleeping self were capable of consistent imitation.

I don't think the quality of my sleep had anything to do with the room itself. The luxurious amenities, the softness of the bed. I didn't even sleep under the blankets last night. Or take off my shoes. I just collapsed, fully dressed, face down, diagonally across the top of the bed. And I felt years of anxiety suddenly unshackled. My spirit had been lugging a hundred pounds of stress everywhere it went. Leading up to this moment. And suddenly it was gone. After six years of relentless effort, the accomplishment of Cyn's appointment washed over me. More than a mere washing, it swept me out to sea. I could barely keep my mind afloat. So I just sank into that sea of Western dreams.

I hope Cyn slept as well as I did. I know Rorrik did. Because he has never failed to do so. But Cyn deserves a Western night more than either of us.

It's time to meet Cyn. She and I will be leaving Pendelhall later than expected. I assumed we'd be a few miles south of town by now. But I'm glad we're not. Even if it means a late start, we should enjoy our final day here together. Not the food. We won't enjoy that part. But the city itself. Soon, it will be hers. And I will occasionally visit. As an old friend.

I hope Rorrik is still here. And that he'll join us for our noontime breakfast. Even if it means I'll spend half the meal fending off his recruitment speech. And the other half trying to persuade him to put his own adventuring aside. At the end of every dispute, he thinks his arguments were more persuasive, and I think mine were. Neither of us ever changes. But one last friendly tiff before we depart wouldn't dampen my mood.

I should hide his gift before I head out. In case the Eldsyn Tower employees assume I've vacated my room, and they come in to clean it for the next guest. The last thing I need is for someone to find a sack of black granules from the center ring. Taking a handful of that sacred sand is surely the most illegal act committed at Pendelhall during the games. The most illegal act committed at Pendelhall this year. So I'm going to hide the bag now. And then it's off to Cyn's.

Fifty-Six

Eldos, Second Lufoa, Day Twenty-Nine. Night.

I haven't written lately.

We're on our way to Farhearth. Rorrik is here. We just stopped for the night.

I took some mayor's journal. I don't know how. I don't remember doing it. I have no idea if I did it on purpose. And if I did take it on purpose, why? Did I think it was mine? There are two different sets of handwriting in it and neither one looks familiar. I don't know why I have this. But I do.

I also don't remember checking out of the inn.

I asked Rorrik if he knew whether we did. He said he took care of it.

And he packed our belongings.

I'm too distracted to think. I thought writing would help but I'm finding it hard to write anything. I'm just going to lie down.

Fifty-Seven

Seros, Second Lufoa, Day Thirty. Morning.

My eyes are burning. I didn't sleep. And I still can't.

I'm sitting inside the wagon with Cyn. Rorrik is driving us to Farhearth.

I can't diagnose anything. My mother was a Pendelhall Medic, so I grew up with medicine. And I taught medicine and physiology for years. But I can't even identify a swollen finger from an uninjured one.

We spent a whole day at the Citadel Hospital.

For combat injuries and detriments related to overexertion, it has no equal, but the medics were untrained for this.

That was the day before yesterday, I think. I can't keep track of time.

All I have with me is a rock, a sack of sand, a mayor's journal, my own journal, and the clothes I'm wearing. And a lingering nausea. I can't cope, let alone think, let alone write. I don't know what we have for food. I haven't eaten since Pendelhall. It looks like we're a few miles north of Estevro. We'll stop and pick up some resources but won't stay.

Fifty-Eight

Seros, Second Lufoa, Day Thirty. Probably early afternoon.

I don't know what time it is. We got to Estevro. I got out of the wagon and looked at the house, but I couldn't bring myself to go inside. I intended to. But I just stood there. I don't know why. Maybe I was worried it would feel like closure in a way. Home is where I was supposed to go when this trip was over. And I could sit at my kitchen table, drink my tea, and fill the room with my contentment. I didn't want to go inside like this. And fill the house with these feelings. That's probably the reason. But that's not what I said to Rorrik. "I would just slow you down", I told him. And I thought it was true at the time.

Rorrik didn't mind. He unpacked everything we had with us, and repacked everything he thought we'd need. A couple of boxes of food, some water, oats for the horses. His and mine both. I don't know what else. He made several trips carrying luggage back and forth. And he checked on Abbie and Gyfur. Said they were fine. After twenty minutes, half an hour at the most, we were back on the road. Couldn't have been later than 10:00. Rorrik is still driving, and I'm still riding in the back with Cyn. And it feels like I'm wearing the heaviest suit armor in the world… which protects me from nothing. I can barely move and yet everything pierces it. Everything hurts.

A few years ago, there was a windstorm. I remember walking home during the worst part. When I turned onto my street, I was squinting my eyes against the gusts, trying to look ahead. To see if my house and Abbie and Wylmot and the wagon were all okay. But it was too uncomfortable. I had to turn my head and look somewhere else. Today, it feels like I'm squinting my thoughts and attention against something far worse than a fierce and relentless wind. And I can't do anything at all. I feel helpless. And numb.

In these situations, I try to split the difference between realism and optimism. And I fail, deciding there is no solace for death's random malice. I just need a sign to convince me that life is fairer than it seems, justice more just than it appears to be. And I don't expect to encounter one. Sometimes I wonder if life costs more than it's worth.

Fifty-Nine

Seros, Second Lufoa, Day Thirty. Night.

It's nighttime now. I'm not sure where we are. Somewhere along the North Grass Road. Rorrik is constantly updating me on travel progress and plans. Where we'll camp, when we'll arrive. He's using my father's maps, so his plans are precise. But I haven't been paying attention. I don't even respond when he tells me the updates. I'm grateful, but all I can do is nod or make a noise of acknowledgement. Not a word. Just a vowel sound, barely more than a breath. Still, he keeps me apprised. Keeps reassuring me that we're making good time. I think that's his way of trying to minimize my worries.

It's about sixty-six miles to Farhearth from my porch. Over low, rolling hills and around lazy bends. This stretch of road is beautiful if you take it slow, and it's hard on horses if you take it fast. I couldn't be bothered with scenery, and Rorrik pushed the horses as hard as he could. Since we left Pendelhall, Wylmot's age has been tested by the pace. And Rorrik's horse has proved to be a true solyre: it doesn't have the temperament of a wagon puller. So this hasn't been an easy job for Rorrik. But there's no point in me taking a shift. Because a solyre that pure won't obey an Easterner either.

Rorrik has been stopping regularly so the horses can drink and eat some oats. And each time we stop, he assures me we'll be there the day after tomorrow. Before nightfall. That's his effort to ease my worrying.

What would ease my worrying more is if I could stop myself from dwelling on what caused it. If I'm to blame. Maybe I pushed Cyn too hard. I've never taught anyone as capable, nor have I enjoyed teaching anyone as much. She seemed able to handle twice what I put on her, and I've never pushed anyone half as hard. In my time at Farhearth, there were some promising students, but I've only ever met one Cyn. Never an equal. Not even close. That's why I pushed. And I'm worried I pushed too hard.

I just gave her some water. She's able to swallow fluids in small amounts. But no whole foods. So I've been squeezing fruit into her water. Her breath is still soft. But her heart is beating strong.

I can't write anymore today. I doubt I can sleep either. But I'll try.

Sixty

Aldos, Third Lufoa, Day One. Morning.

I still don't have an appetite. I'm sure some food would do me well. But I don't think I could keep anything down.

I joined Rorrik for breakfast anyway. Not for the food. Which he had clearly gone to some trouble to make. I got out of the wagon and sat beside him as an attempt to be companionable. An attempt to be emotionally present for the first time since last Fyros night.

Failing that, I managed to be *socially* present. I wasn't coherent enough to say anything of interest, but I tried. It took way more effort than it should have to come up with some boring sentences about the horses. How they seem cooperative with our pacing. And about the weather. How we seem to be having fortunate skies. And about our luck with wildlife. How it's surprising we haven't had any encounters.

Rorrik responded politely to the first two. But he didn't say anything about the third. Which said enough. In the politest possible way. There *were* some encounters. Rorrik just dealt with them and didn't mention it.

He was checking in so often – updating me on the distance we had covered, how the horses were holding up, how much farther he thought we could push them before setting up camp, where he expected to camp, and so on – I assumed he was mentioning everything.

"What was it?", I asked.

"A trapjaw basking in the road. It was a good time to feed the horses anyway, so I stopped. Far enough away. And I dispatched it while the horses ate."

"Is that all?"

"A couple of lumpy-milk wombats. They were easy to deal with. No reason to mention it."

It's hard to find gratitude for anything, but I'm grateful Rorrik is here. This would be a lot harder on my own. I don't know if I could cope without him.

Cyn's condition doesn't seem to be improving. She can breathe on her own, but her breaths are shallow. Her swallowing reflex is intact, but she can't eat solid food. She has somewhat of a cough response. It doesn't sound like a sick person hacking, but it's not merely a reflex arc. And her eyes are open, and she's able to track moving objects, so I know there's conscious activity. But her face is disengaged from any emotion. There's no expression at all. It's just blank.

I never realized how much of our personalities are held in place by our facial muscles. Those small, static contractions communicate more than surprise and focus and anger and gladness. They reveal who we are. As clearly as any written language can express. Our ambition, our generosity, insecurities, every formative experience. All of it is written across our faces. Erased by paralysis, Cyn looks like a different person. Similar enough to be her sibling, but not herself.

I keep staring at her, waiting for something to change. Searching for a sign of a familiar face.

Loss is always difficult. But old loss is easier to bear. With each passing year, one expects it a little more. Time is our innate prophylactic; we accumulate our acceptance gradually. A ninety-year-old's funeral is emotional, but not tragic. A twenty-four-year-old's is both. And it's the tragedy that really stings. Because it strikes without warning. If you know you're about to be slugged in the stomach, you can brace yourself. Hold your breath, take a wide stance, clench your muscles, and prepare to absorb it. You can't do that with an unexpected gut punch. It's the same impact, but the difference in expectation makes all the difference.

Sixty-One

Aldos, Third Lufoa, Day One. Afternoon.

We continue to make good time. Or good distance in a given time, I guess. Rorrik is still pushing the horses as fast and far as they'll go. We're loping along the milder stretches of road, but around the sharper corners, I can feel the wagon careening a bit. And I know the horses are straining over some of the steeper hills. But I continue to pay very little attention. And Rorrik continues to update me anyway. Every twenty minutes or so, he hollers some trip commentary over his shoulder. I can tell he doesn't expect a response. And I have yet to give one. I have been talking to Cyn, though. I don't know if she can hear me. Whether her brain can make sense of incoming sounds or if it's just basal functions. Even if it is the latter, I would still talk to her. Because I wouldn't know what else to do.

When I taught at Farhearth, there were so many students whom I spoke to daily, knowing there was every chance they would hear me and no chance they would listen. Yet I kept trying to instruct them anyway. Knowing it would accomplish nothing. It was just a matter of course.

Cyn is the only person I've ever met who has actively listened to everything she's ever heard. And I believe she's listening now. Attentively. So I keep talking. Mostly, I've been telling her how proud of her I am. The extent is not possible for me to explain, but still I try.

She has been so much more important to my life than I have been to hers. For nearly six years, I have had the honor of playing the role of Abendroth for Cyn. That is the most rewarding accomplishment of my career. Perhaps of my life. Short of reviving Abendroth herself, it's the single greatest gift anyone could have given me.

Sixty-Two

Aldos, Third Lufoa, Day One. Night.

We're camping. We have a little over twenty miles to go according to Rorrik. Which is, by extension, according to my father. And I know those are reliable estimations. So, by this time tomorrow, we should be in Farhearth.

I've been thinking about our medical strategy when we arrive. Where to go first. Whom to see, what to ask, how to answer the questions I'm asked... but my thoughts have been jumbled. I'm too disoriented to plan effectively.

For years, I have served as an intermediate. Between mentor and mentee. My purpose was to take Abendroth's legacy across the bridge to Cyn. Now it feels like that bridge has suddenly collapsed beneath me. I fell into the water, and I can't see land on either side. Anywhere. I have no idea where to swim.

The last time I felt this adrift and directionless is when Abendroth died. She shepherded me through all three degrees. Then, right before I graduated with my Magister's, she passed. So young. So unexpectedly. With heartbreaking surprise, I lost my guide.

That day, my ability to take pleasure in functionless entertainments vanished. The charm in my childhood joys – novels, songs, and other arts – seemed to pass with Abendroth. For years, I lacked the ability to insert meaning into the meaningless. I saw things only for their utility. Even food tasted bland. I had no idea how to move forward, how to navigate on my own. So I went through a period of struggling and blind exploration.

While I taught at Farhearth, especially in the early years, it felt like I was living someone else's life. Until I finally found my path again. I discovered a young woman whose eyes were so huge and curious, whose hands understood real work, and whose mind was sharper than anyone I knew.

I found my purpose. All the effort Abendroth put into me – all those lessons she imparted – were ultimately for Cyn. I wasn't smart or talented enough to actualize her teachings. All I could do was carry them for a while, be a good steward. Until Cyn arrived. Then I would become the bridge between. But now it feels like that bridge has collapsed. And I'm lost at sea. If Rorrik weren't with me, breathing the water would be preferable to treading it.

Sixty-Three

Lyros, Third Lufoa, Day Two. Morning.

It's late in the morning. We're on the road again. Our last day on this road.

I couldn't sleep last night. Maybe two hours total if you sum the fragments. The rest of the time was spent staring up at the waxing half-moon, bright in the cloudless sky. I was wide awake for at least an hour before the sun hinted at rising. And while I lay there, motionless, waiting for the morning to arrive, my appetite returned. Just barely. But I decided it would be wise to act on it. So once the horizon began to glow, I got up and started looking for food.

I hadn't even bothered to look *at* the boxes Rorrik packed, let alone inspect their contents. The first one I opened had non-essentials. Including ink and paper for me. A lot of each. More than I could use if we were making a round trip to Laberyn or Cinderheim.

Behind that box was one I didn't expect to see. All my old journals. I had wrapped them up before we left and was planning to give the package to Cyn when we returned. My congratulation gift. Rorrik brought it with.

I opened it and started looking through the pages. The light was dim, but I wasn't really reading. I was just holding a relic from an earlier time. Looking at something that belonged to an earlier me. Remembering that it was real. And imagining myself there again. I flipped through the pages until I found the entry I wrote on the day I met Cyn. Life was far more complicated then, but it felt like a simpler time. Definitely a brighter time. Before all this.

I was still going through my journals when Rorrik woke up. I forgot I had been looking for food. "I thought you might want that", Rorrik whispered when he saw what I was holding.

I nodded. In a way that meant: *I did, thank you for packing it.*

"I'll make breakfast", he whispered next. Along with a gesture that added: *you just keep reading*. Then he reached past me and opened a box I had yet to check. And half an hour later, I was being summoned to eat.

Eggs. Not the omelet I've been wanting for weeks. But he scrambled some. With chunks of meat that seemed fresh. I didn't ask what he killed.

Rorrik is a terrible hunter. He's a marvel at killing what is trying to kill him. But sneaking up on unsuspecting animals and puncturing holes in them so they bleed out, collapse, and become food? Rorrik is terrible at that.

No matter what species of animal it once was, what we ate was "porch pork". That's what Lum calls it. Eating whatever meat greets you at your door. Or, in this case, whatever unfortunate creature got in the way of the wagon. I can only assume it was recently dangerous. If not to us, at least to our horses. But it made a fine breakfast. Breaking a several-day fast. Once I swallowed my first bite, my body realized how hungry it was. And I finished my plate before Rorrik had even started his.

He took one bite, then said, "We should get moving." And he emptied his plate onto mine.

I gave him a look that meant: *are you sure?*

"I'm not hungry anyway", he said. Then he stood up, stretched, and started packing for departure. Getting ready for the last leg of our trip.

After I finished eating, I climbed into the wagon and sat beside Cyn. And my mood began to change. My despair hasn't faded, but my thoughts are clearer. And I'm overcome with appreciation for what Rorrik is doing. He's currently driving. As I sit with Cyn and write this.

Until Cyn's accident, Rorrik's Thorn-mongering was relentless. His singular priority was to enlist me as a companion on his quest. But that's just Rorrik following his heart. And it's not a tyrant's heart. Because now he's here. With me. Without question. Without hesitation. I'm sure his recruitment will resume someday. But not today.

Sixty-Four

Lyros, Third Lufoa, Day Two. Afternoon.

The gates of Farhearth are about five miles away. We just stopped at a creek so the horses could drink. And Rorrik gave them some oats. But we didn't stay long. Rorrik is pushing the horses as hard as he can today. Hard enough that it would compromise their ability to pull us tomorrow. Which is fine because we don't need them tomorrow. They can spend the day stabled, recovering.

After breakfast this morning, I went through some more of my old journals. And read many of the entries aloud to Cyn. Much of it was poorly written, an obvious effort to sound smarter than I was. And many of the observations I thought profound then seem pedestrian today. And the science I considered advanced is now obsolete. But there were occasional passages – raw, honest paragraphs I wrote without any reader in mind – that were surprisingly deep.

I told Cyn this collection of old musings was for her. And someday soon, she'll be able to read them herself. That's not the most inspiring incentive for recovery, but it's all I have. Perhaps I'll leave her with *these* journals, too. Today's musings. Which I began writing on the tenth day of Second Lufoa, chronicling the end of our six years together. Despite the dearth of scientific and medical information, it may be a more meaningful gift. But if I'm leaving these journals with her, I should write something worth reading. To do that, I need to be present. I haven't been these last few days. I've been dwelling on tragedy. Which isn't helpful. Ruminating on suffering seems only to worsen the pain of loss. And stifle the promise of hope.

After tragedy, people often spend the rest of their lives in a perpetual eulogy. And I don't know if that honors the loved ones who were lost or harmed. Or if focusing on the loss and harm prevents us from remembering them as brilliant and vibrant. So, rather than slogging through some sorrowful mire of my own making, I'll try to be more positive and present. Starting now.

Not by forcing merriment into somber circumstances. I don't trust people who have high spirits in low places. The medic whose patient is screaming, the miller whose mill is burning, the kedger whose boat is sinking. If I see a smile beaming on their faces, I'm going to think they pose a threat to their communities. In a healthy mind, emotions track with reality.

And depression and anxiety are reasonable emotions to feel. We all know the fate that's coming. Everyone will die, the sun will burn out, and our Gaea will become frozen darkness. One by one, every twinkling star will snuff. The Starless Crossing will stretch and stretch until it eventually engulfs the farthest reaches of existence. And all that will remain is a vast, lightless, lifeless nothingness. There's nothing we can do to change that and nothing we can do to survive it. Happiness!

Fixating on inevitable endings does not enrich our lives. But sheer bliss amid present catastrophe is the countenance of a scary person. In between those extremes lie acceptance and inner peace. Much more complicated emotions. When I say I will try to be more positive and present, that's what I mean.

Even in the darkest, coldest day of Arzox, if I experience a warm moment, I'm reminded that there is warmth in the world. And in difficult times, the search for warmth can nourish our hope.

Sixty-Five

Lyros, Third Lufoa, Day Two. Night.

We arrived at Farhearth. Earlier than I expected. The horses may be haggard, but they can rest tomorrow. If Rorrik had showed them a bit more mercy in his pacing, we wouldn't have gotten Cyn into a hospital bed tonight.

When we reached the gates, we headed straight for the Commons Hospital. Not the Common*wealth* Hospital. That's not affiliated with the university. You're better off getting treated by a barber. The Commons Hospital is the only place I can think of that might have an answer. And with an answer, there might be a treatment. And with a treatment, I maintain hope.

So, we went straight to that hospital.

It wasn't there. The university has done some rearranging since I left.

I began asking people for directions. Which would not have taken more than a minute or two if I were asking flatties. But I was asking Harthies. And they can be uncooperative for no reason at all. Or at least no *reasonable* reason.

The first people I asked were civil servants, assuming they would be obliged to provide this civil service. Not pleased, but obliged. At Farhearth, the tax and tuition collectors double as general enforcers, and they go by a more commanding name: Justiciars. Always capitalized, even as a common noun. Out of self-importance. Not even "mayor" is capitalized unless it is properly preceding a specific mayor's name.

In addition to untalented boy-giant fencers, the Justiciary Office is populated by former rowanoki players whose truest passion was pushing people around, vigorously exerting their dominance. But after graduation, they discovered the wanton aggression they thrived on to be punishable by every city's law. So they found a solution: become a Justiciar. That way, they would get *paid* to push people around.

It's best to avoid them. But this wasn't the best of times. I needed their help. So I asked for it. From the first pair of officers I saw. In their fancy hats, cudgels at the ready.

"Excuse me, will you direct me to the Commons Hospital?"

"State your business."

I stated my business. Not every detail. That's none of *their* business. But my statement was sufficient. And it was followed by a rather strict interrogation. As though I were a criminal plotting my crime.

We were clearly arriving from out of town, towed by some knackered horses, we didn't know where a major facility was, and my solicitation for directions had a tense tone. But none of that should have been perceived as threatening. None of that should have resulted in my sick companion being perceived as a ruse. This response wasn't merely hurtful, it was delusional. Whatever they imagined we were rusing, I'm having difficulty imagining myself. Were we feigning a health crisis to…… I can't even think of how this would fit into a criminal plot.

When I insisted that all we needed was directions to the Commons Hospital, my insistence was met with more resistance.

Realizing further interaction would only serve as escalation, and escalation would only waste more time, I sincerely apologized for the hassle, insincerely thanked them for keeping the city safe, and then excused myself from the conversation.

As soon as we were out of sight of the Justiciars, I asked a group of students.

They cowered, mumbled incoherently, and scurried off like feral cats.

I looked at Rorrik with an expression of, "You see how pathetic they are? Being asked a direct question by a disheveled elder is enough to instill panic. This is who you're beating up in the fencing rings." I didn't actually *say* that. It was just a look.

The smile Rorrik returned told me he interpreted my look correctly.

Then I began scanning the crowd for someone with more confident posture. Assertive young men tend to exert themselves in helpful ways if there is an audience to see them do it. Like insisting on helping a middle-aged woman load her luggage onto a carriage when she didn't need the help. Or want it. But behold!, your savior resolves your luggage crisis!

I found one: a boy of maybe twenty who stood two inches taller than he was. And wore jewelry. Excesses of it. Every young man whose wrist gleams and jingles with an array of bracelets will come to regret it if he lives long enough.

Or at least that's what I tell myself about jewelry of this kind. Wealth flags. Those gem-studded bracelets of gold and silver that reveal far more insecurity than they conceal. The kind of decorations that promise endless retaliation should one mutter the slightest of slights in his direction.

That was the student I chose to ask.

"Excuse me, sir", I said, loud enough that nearby strangers would overhear. And participate as audience members. "Might you direct me to the location of the Commons Hospital?", I finished, bowing my head a little. I was sure this would result in detailed instructions. For the cheap and quickly payable price of dignifying his authority. I was wrong. Very wrong. My ability to read people used to be so finely tuned. I guess I'm out of practice.

It wasn't his words exactly. Or even how he said them. It's what he looked like while saying them. It's difficult to explain, but his brow framed his expression in a way that made trust an impossible interpretation. His eyes might be soft or sympathetic, but his brow hardened and devious'd them. When someone has bags under their eyes, it makes them look overworked. Loyal, maybe. Busy, at least. This wasn't that. It was like bags *over* his eyes. It made him look underworked. And disloyal. Anyone can put on a mask and communicate something their words do not. And that's what this was. His brow was overt, unmistakable. So I didn't trust his words.

The conversation did go on for a minute or so. I responded, he responded, me again, him again. While I can't recreate the exact words, my memory of how he said them is clear. Like a Thevroan elite, he began most sentences with "actually", meaning, "let me correct you." There's no more pompous a first word in any utterance. But the pomposity only got worse from there. Between every breath, he managed to brag about his station in life. Which had nothing to do with my question.

The one thing I *was* right about: he was in this for the audience. His gestures – waving around his well-braceleted arms – were too theatrical for a private conversation. They were clearly meant to capture attention from a distance. But his voice was even worse. It wasn't just his amateur thespian enunciation. Or the barker's volume, booming from his imaginary stage. It was the *sound* of it. Not timbre, exactly. That was obnoxious, but not creepy. The creepy part was the noises he made that *wouldn't* carry to the balconies. Every word was emitted from an audibly wet mouth. "Moist" does not capture the extent of its ickiness. As though every sentence attempted seduction of its hearer, but only accomplished revulsion.

"I appreciate your time", I lied. Loudly. Then I complimented his bracelets. Just as loudly, but less convincingly. I shouldn't have. I should have resisted the urge to insult. But when I encounter arrogance of Thevroan proportions, the temptation is often too great.

That interaction was more irritating than my encounter with His Excellency, the Justiciary Officer (does that confer enough respect to escape oppression?).

After two failed solicitations for directions, I started looking for a third person to ask. Ten years ago, everyone would have been willing to help. But today, I have to be more careful in my selection process.

So, I began scanning the crowd with a bit more scrutiny.

Then I saw a type of student I knew I was reading correctly: the Farhearth damsel. Those delicate maidens who concoct their own tormentors. And endure – nay, *survive!* – such imaginative persecution.

It's not avaricious, fire-breathing dragons or jealous, cackling witches or anything else so… tangible. Her plight is far more fictional: the very way of the world, as though Gaea itself has selected this poor young woman to endure a life of targeted suffering. A life in need of rescue. How does this sweet, tender inamorata reveal her plight? By making herself uncomfortable. Deliberately. To inconvenience her partner. She is often found standing dejectedly in the rain, an inch or two shorter than she is, to see if her partner will acknowledge her situation and make a sacrifice toward its resolution. Surrender his hooded rain cloak, if he has one, for the unnecessary reason that his companion has decided to stand beyond the awning. Day after day, greater and greater sacrifices are demanded as sustenance for her insecurity. And he dutifully pays. Until one day, when he is on the brink of utter defeat, unable to bear the weight of one more bloodletting of his soul, he brings light to the realities of the relationship. And again, as ever before, she positions herself as a victim. Except now, instead of insisting he rescue her from the make-believe wrath of nature, *he* has become the source of her oppression. I know this damsel well. And I saw a few, and I knew it wise to avoid them. But I also saw the queen of this class. There's always a queen.

I've decided to call today's Violet. Because of the color of her dress. I know nothing about fashion, but I can tell the difference between home-stitched fabrics bought from a common market mercer and regal attire acquired from a patrician's couturier. Violet's was the latter. And when I saw her, she was pretending to be victimized by a faculty member. Maltreatment so egregious she will never recover!

The professor was clearly apologizing. I couldn't hear anything he was saying, but I could see his expression. He was nearly in tears. His whole face was furrowed into a mix of panic and remorse. And he kept touching his chest and bowing and clasping his hands together. All the histrionics of a cowering adult. It was sad to watch. But I still watched. For probably half a minute. And then Violet excused her tormentor. He bowed one last time, and then shuffled away.

That's when Violet revealed her queenly malice. The expression of anguish vanished from her face. And it was replaced with a cruel smile as she began whispering in her fawners' ears. I couldn't hear what she was saying any more than I could hear the professor's apology, but she was clearly mocking him. Every whisper was followed by subservient laughter. Not genuine laughter, but groveling trying to pass as giggling.

I did not approach any of them to ask for directions. Or watch their display any longer. Instead, I resumed my search for a better-natured member of the crowd. It took another minute, but I finally identified one. A young woman who appeared to live here, but not belong. I could tell she was a student, but she was few years older than her peers. And she stood at her *exact* height, which was short enough to make her look younger than her age. And, most importantly, she was completely indifferent to the theater of the walkways.

"Excuse me", I said. And she jumped. But once she was done being startled, she politely aimed all her attention at me. Her face was gentle and speckled with light constellations of freckles. Not the tenants of our own night – the serpent, the albatross, and the firefly – but new constellations. Her cheeks looked like an unmapped sky of distant twinkling stars. Faintly visible.

"Can you direct me to the Commons Hospital?", I asked.

She didn't respond immediately. She just held an empty expression, as if she had no idea what I was asking. But after a few seconds, her soft, star-fretted face lit up, and she said, "Oh, you mean the Fentin Infirmary."

Apparently, it's not called the Commons Hospital anymore.

Despite the initial confusion, she turned out to be the right person to ask. She didn't merely provide directions… with a bunch of haphazard pointing and a list of ambiguous landmarks to guide our reckoning. She escorted us.

It was in the opposite direction that she had been walking. And it was not a short trip.

Along the way, I got to know her a little bit. Although everything I said felt awkward while I was saying it. Which made me self-conscious. Which made everything I said feel *more* awkward. Which flustered me enough that I forgot to ask for her name. So I never learned it. Even so, this interaction was the highlight of the evening. But its light didn't linger long. When we arrived at the hospital, any brightness I briefly held was dimmed.

Tomorrow will be a new day. But here's tonight's experience:

Rorrik parked the wagon at the entrance and helped me carry Cyn inside. After we placed her on a portable bed, he put his hand on my shoulder and said, "I don't want to get in the way, so I'm going to find us a nearby inn and stables."

I nodded. Then my effort to obtain a diagnosis and treatment for Cyn began.

Most physicians had already left by the time we got there. But the few that remained were easy to see: they all wear white. And no one else is allowed to. Even the patients are draped in alternative garments if they show up in white. They're forgiven if they arrive unconscious, but for everyone else, it's less uncouth to attend a wedding wearing a gown more elegant than the bride's. Or at least that's how it was when I lived here. And it doesn't seem to have changed in the intervening years. Nor has the job title changed. Outside of Farhearth, there are doctors and healers and medics and a dozen other names the practitioners go by. Here, they're all "physicians". And failing to address them by that title is as unpardonable as wearing their colors.

I approached a man in the lobby who was flagrantly unoccupied (leaning against a wall, inspecting his fingernails), and whose snow-white coat gleamed as brightly as a bride-to-be standing at the altar under a full Lufoa sun.

"Excuse me, Physician Alneg", I said. That might not have been his name. It could have been Aldul or Alkar. I just remember his nametag having one of those Al names common among Harthies. "May I have an appointment?", I asked.

"You'll have to go through proper scheduling", he said while pointing in the direction of the scheduling counter, operated by people in dark brown attire.

I pushed Cyn's bed to that counter. And I explained that she was the patient, but since she is unable to speak, I'll be accompanying her to the appointment. And may I please schedule one?

Less than a minute later, Physician Alcon or Almyr or whatever his name was approached the counter and greeted me. "I'll take it from here", he told the reception staff. Then he led me to a diagnostic room. "Please sit", he said. I did. Cyn wasn't with us yet. The staff would be transporting her shortly.

"Now... where does it hurt?", he asked me. This is a terrible question on so many levels. First, did he not notice the woman I had been pushing in the portable bed? The woman whose bed was right next to me at the counter? The woman who was obviously the patient? But even if I *were* the patient, diagnosis should never begin with such a leading question.

As I began explaining that Cyn was the patient, not me, a member of the staff, who was wearing a red uniform, pushed Cyn's bed into the room. Back when this was the Commons Hospital, only physicians and interns had designated colors. Today, it seems the entire hierarchy is color coded. And for some reason, they've chosen to dress the auxiliary staff in the hue of spilled blood.

"Is there anything else I can bring you, Physician Al-whatever?", the woman who appeared to be wearing a blood-soaked uniform asked.

"Nothing, thank you. I'll take the patient's history now. You're dismissed."

Take was the word he used. He'll *take* her history. Not collect it or receive it or discuss it. But *take* it.

The staff member bowed slightly in his direction and left the room.

Then the physician attempted to pilfer Cyn's medical history. By asking some even-more-leading questions. I answered them, but I also provided details I thought would be more relevant. Such as Cyn's age, her recent stressors and possible environmental exposures, and the timing and setting in which her present condition developed. "She and I both experienced headaches on the night of the Closing Ceremony", I said. "But the next morning, mine was gone and hers was worse. She was briefly alert and able to articulate what she was feeling, but then she lost consciousness."

"In the days when hounds tracked criminals..." the physician began without looking at me. Then he stopped talking and struck some of Cyn's tendons with his tiny hammer to check reflexes. Half a minute later, he finished his sentence: "There's a story about one clever criminal evading the dogs using the odor of smoked fish. The smell of it misdirected the sniffing dogs and he got away. What you need to understand about medicine is that it's full of misleading clues, and we call them..."

"I know what a red herring is", I interrupted. "I'm just trying to provide the relevant details, trying to give you the context."

"I can see the context for myself, thanks", he blurted in a sharp tone.

I didn't respond. I wanted to insult him, but I didn't want to incense him. Because that would *certainly* distract his diagnosis. Wrath is a crimson herring. And I needed him to stay calm, compassionate, focused on Cyn's condition. What he doesn't seem to understand, though, is that herrings come in more colors than there are uniforms at Fentin Infirmary.

Society has agreed that red is a distraction. Let's say blue hints at the truth, but it's an ordinary and obvious truth. While silver is just as factual a color, but it's inconspicuous and counterintuitive. A hidden clue to a secret truth. Unless physicians pay close attention to silver herrings, they'll fail to uncover anything of meaning. In my experience, most physicians only take notice of red and blue. They arrogantly condemn the former while using the latter to justify a diagnosis with more pomp than precision.

That's what happened this evening. "Your friend is afflicted with idiopathic neuralgic syncope", he said. As he handed me the bill. In which I appear to be paying by the syllable. I don't know what's more absurd, his diagnosis or his fee. If a condition begins with "idiopathic", I don't care what it ends with. In five covert syllables, the physician is passing the onus of understanding onto civilization. An honest answer to "what caused this illness?" would be "I don't know. Someone might have an answer, but it isn't me." That's not what they say though. With great self-assurance they report, "it's idiopathic", which is a fancy way of calling it an idiot's pathology. Which isn't as insulting as it seems. Idiot bears its original meaning: one's own. This is *your* condition. And no one else's. As such, civilization cannot possibly know a cause or cure for what ails you.

All I could do was sigh. Because he's the idiot if he can't admit ignorance or inferiority. In the place of honesty, he concocted the mother of all herrings: "idiopathic neuralgic syncope". Hospitals continue to be one of few natural habitats in which the golden herring still thrives. Its scent is used to distract patients from the realization that they aren't getting what they paid for: truth.

After receiving the unexpectedly expensive bill, it was time to leave.

I'm not despondent though. Because that was just one physician. There are at least sixty others who work here. And we'll see another tomorrow.

For tonight, Cyn is staying in the hospital. We're renting a bed. Not a room, but a bed. In a shared room. With three other patients. I'll come back in the morning. I'm hopeful this will be the only night we have to do this.

Once Cyn was settled in her bed, I left. To find Rorrik. Who had already found an inn. The Commons Tavern. It's a new inn owned by an old family. In honor of the old hospital, a short walk from the new one.

"I thought this the most fitting residence on the street", Rorrik said, and then added, "Just tell the boniface you're with Olryn. I already paid."

"Olryn still?"

"I'd rather pay for the room than play for it. And I'd also rather avoid the conversation in which I have to explain that."

I should have known that already. I don't know why Rorrik had to explain it to me.

"Where are you going now?", I asked, assuming he had some errand to run before joining me.

"I'm sleeping in the wagon tonight. Don't want to leave it unattended."

Then we parted ways. I went to the Commons Tavern, and he headed toward the stables.

I continue to be grateful for Rorrik's help.

"What brings you to town?", I was asked by the boniface when I walked in... with no luggage of any kind.

I told him I was with Olryn.

"And what brings you to town?", he reiterated his question, in a polite tone, as he began riffling through a small chest, looking for the key to my room.

I stumbled through an answer, providing a few cursory details of a medical emergency interspersed with some general cursing of Adon and His peers. (Or *Her* peers, depending on whom you ask.)

Recognizing this was a difficult subject for me, the boni was polite enough to avoid further probing.

Instead, he placed his hand on my shoulder, donned the most sympathetic expression I've ever seen on a face, and said, "Tell me, where are you from?"

The tension that was knotted into my posture loosened a bit. "I've lived in a few cities", I said. "Here for a number of years. But I was a flatty at birth, and I'm a flatty at heart."

Without losing any of his sympathy, he said, "I'd prefer if we used a more respectful term than flatty."

"But... I'm describing *myself*."

"Still, it's more proper to say Estevroan."

"Have you ever been to Estevro?", I asked.

The answer was no, but it took him a while to get there. Actually, he never got there. But I managed to deduce.

He was still holding my shoulder. And how he spoke was so tender, it would have been impossible to take offense.

"I got used to *Estevroan* while I was living abroad, but I've been back home for several years now", I said. "And you just rarely hear that word from the mouth of a... an Estevroan."

"I prefer to keep the dialog proper here, so why don't we address each other on more formal terms", he said with a tone of compassionate finality. The tone of an old member of an old family who conflates tradition and respect. And insists language is how we preserve the former and express the latter.

I understand that "flatty" harbors a splinter of deprecation. But who has ever protested *self*-deprecation? Still, I honored his request for antique civility. Because I could tell it came from a gentle place.

Before referring to myself as a flatty, I muttered a few lordly names in vain, and that didn't bother him. I suspect because his family's wealth isn't a source of personal pride like it is for every hillian (sorry, I mean Thevroan).

The boni sees Estevroans not as inferior, but as victims of random poverty. With little hope of climbing the lordly ladder. And it's mean spirited to mock the hopeless. So, "I prefer to keep the dialog proper here."

But the penniless prodding the prosperous? That's satire. And what is the most prosperous creature in the world? God. So those expressions are okay. Any lord worth his estate can tolerate a peasant's sarcasm with grace. Surely, God can too.

What about "Lirkers" and "hillians" I wonder.

I've never addressed those wealthiest Westerners as anything but Lirkin – my city and theirs are not locked in eternal rivalry – but it does seem to be the same thing. A *very slightly* derogatory collective noun… for a citizenry defined by prosperity. Would that, coming from a flatty – a member of the struggling class – be excused as satire?

I don't know. But I should try to get some sleep. I managed to hold myself together today, but tomorrow will be just as difficult. And it'll surely be worse if I'm up all night writing.

Sixty-Six

Fyros, Third Lufoa, Day Three. Nearly morning.

I didn't sleep at all last night. It's still last night. Another hour until morning. At least. But I've given up the effort to sleep.

Visceral stress is an understatement for what I've been feeling. I have been ulcerally stressed. But I've been distracted by duty. People to interact with, tasks to perform, a purpose to pursue. All of that was diverting my attention from panic and depression. My wits were held together by responsibility.

But when I climbed into bed, every distraction departed. I was left alone in an empty room with nothing but my thoughts. And anxiety is a nocturnal animal. As I closed my eyes, fears and regrets began lurking in the darkness. When it became unbearable, I got out of bed, got dressed, and went outside. Farhearth never quite rests. And walking among the bustle for a few minutes put my fretting at ease. So I returned to bed. And shut my eyes. And, again, attempted to sleep. And, again, those anxious thoughts crept into my mind. So, again, I opened my eyes and let the bustling world in. And, again, those skulking emotions scattered like roaches in a suddenly lit room.

Back and forth. Again and again. Under the blankets and out on the street. That was the pattern for the whole night. The silence inside felt louder than the crowds, and the stillness was far more restless. And I just couldn't cope. While we were on the road, headed here, we were doing *something*. Rorrik was busy driving, and I was watching over Cyn, providing whatever care I could. Now, I'm alone. With nothing to do. And I'm finding it difficult to bear.

There was a professor who taught at Farhearth when I was a student – she'd retired by the time I taught – named Unaga. She spent her whole tenure blind. She could see; she just preferred not to.

"Open eyed, the world rushes in", she said when I asked why she lectured with her eyes closed. "And all commotion is distraction", she explained… without opening her eyes.

At the time, I just thought she was weird. Now, I can appreciate the power of a rushing world. I guess she wrote in an even more distraction-free environment. Eliminated every sensation she could. Sounds and smells. And tastes. Long bouts of fasting were a normal part of her routine.

"The mind abhors silence, so it fills the space with its own noise", she wrote in one of her books. I don't remember which. I read a few. The same few I had Cyn read. It was probably the last one, but Unaga wrote dozens more. She's among the most prolific faculty members ever employed at Farhearth. And I remember that line specifically because it has since been counterfeited by countless imitators. The mind abhors a void or a vacuum, and it fills the empty space with thought or imagination. And so on. Whatever version of the quotation, no one has ever had a quieter, tidier, more fertile mind than Unaga, and she filled every inch of that vast and vacuous space with words. On the topics of theology, ethics, and "Passing into the Darkness" (that was the title of her final book). In the small amount Cyn and I read, there were countless premises no one else would have thought of had Unaga never lived. Whether one agrees with them, or perceives them wise, is a different matter. But I think I now understand the wisdom of *this* premise. Instead of basking in the blissful spaces of my own void, however, I just hear anxiety skittering around like rats in the shadows.

When I finally quit trying to sleep, I sat at my window and watched the sky. Sometime during the night, a lightning storm was born. It was a humble birth. It didn't announce its arrival with a bunch of clatter. One flash after another, all of them modest, none of them applauded by thunder.

I watched in a meditative trance for probably half an hour. And felt at peace. But then the storm drew closer. And closer. And closer. And I could tell the heavy footfalls of thunder would soon come crashing down. It was like watching a frantic infant preparing to cry, breathlessly gathering up despair. The longer that silent frenzy lasts, the fiercer the subsequent wailing will be. Not unlike a lichfruit accumulating heat. If the pressure isn't released early, the explosion will ignite the forest.

During this moment of stillness, I had a thought that was at once worrisome and sobering: what if this time with Cyn isn't the peak of the storm, but the gathering? That thought was interrupted with the first crack of thunder. Shortly after the flash. A minute later, the flashing and thunder synched and seemed to amplify the whole. Another minute later, the lightning focused its attack on the Language and Literature campus. I guess the arms race is still holding true to its truce.

The university comprises nine colleges, and a flagpole stands *proudly* in the campus of each one. Those poles used to be made of wood. A single beam of pine, fir, or cedar. So they could only rise as tall as the tree grew. But they built them as tall as possible because it attracted students for some reason. I've never understood why. But I know nothing about marketing.

What I *do* know is that it was the most overlooked, least notable colleges that built the highest poles. Because they needed to. They were the least enrolled. And how else could they *possibly* recruit more students? Again: I will never understand marketing.

At some point, the poles in front of the humblest colleges began to exceed the limits of ordinary logs. At first, they were inserted into elevated bases. But that only raised them a few feet. The height could be doubled if multiple logs were fastened end to end. But those poles swayed and groaned in the wind, and occasionally collapsed. Which *wasn't* good for recruitment. Again: for reasons I cannot begin to comprehend… except for one instance in which the top half of a shattered pole fell on a student. And the student was permanently disabled by it. That's why there's a Halrond Building in the College of Music and the Arts. Becoming an eponym at Farhearth requires either a fortune or a tragedy.

Halrond's tragedy did not slow the arms race, though. The poles continued to grow. Year by year, inch by inch, year after year, inch after inch.

In the nearby Grey Woods, every tree is locked in eternal competition with its neighbors. If the tree beside you is taller, it will be gilded in sunlight while you're dressed in the garments of its shade. Less dignity, reduced sustenance, destined for humility. One must grow tall to continue growing at all. Taking this lesson from the forests, the flagpoles grew. As did the flags themselves. They became larger and more elaborate, too. More symbolic but also cruder. Larger crests made room for the addition of esoteric glyphs. And larger fields made room for artless slogans. The only flag that stayed simple was that of the College of Language and Literature. Solid green but for a stark white ring.

But it was *that* college – the least enrolled with the plainest flag – that ended up building the tallest pole. The first one not made of wood. It resembled a giant sword blade with an angular silver shaft that reached up to the sky and seemed to stab the clouds. They didn't build it themselves. Or commission an Easterner to build it on their behalf. It was made by Cinderheim smithies. After which, the Harthies went to literally great lengths hauling it all the way back to campus. Then, in front of Farhearth's smallest, humblest building, they sheathed it deep into the scabbard of Gaea. Ten feet down and still it towered twenty feet above every other pole.

That happened when I was a student, and even then, I thought it was absurd. The College of Language and Literature was founded by flatties. Still today, most faculty and students hail from Estevro. But in went the pole. Into the flattest, most unfitting stretch of Farhearth's landscape.

And that's when the lightning took notice.

It's almost as though that magnificent Eldsyn storm – eternally imprisoned in its bay – finally escaped. Instead of striking elegantly and indiscriminately over the breadth of the seas, it chose an enemy. Carefully. And made a long, silent journey to Farhearth. And directed the full force of its assault upon… the College of Language and Literature.

Good for the poets, I guess. But the clichés that came from it are unbearable. "Alit by pride" and "lightning strikes the prideful" and "sneaking beneath the thunder ceiling" and on and on. And on. And on.

The storm I watched in the night struck no other college. Which means no other college has dared to raise its flag higher.

About fifteen minutes ago, the storm finally ceased. With one last spectacular strike. Then, as if the pole fought back, it was suddenly over. Suddenly silent. No creature stirred. Even the wind stopped breathing. For a few minutes, at least. Then the advent roosters started crowing.

According to some old fables, those fire-colored fowl summoned the first sun to touch Gaea's soils. Now, thousands of lifetimes later, they still sing their summoning song. A moment before the horizon glows. Well before the hospital opens. The "infirmary", I mean. Either way, it's time to put my writing aside. I'll check in on Rorrik, try to eat something, and then wait for the red-uniformed staff to unlock the entrance doors.

Sixty-Seven

Fyros, Third Lufoa, Day Three. Afternoon.

The storm never returned. The entire city felt calm when I left my room and checked on Rorrik. It would have been a perfect day for a peaceful stroll through the nine campuses. Instead, I spent the whole morning inside. Dealing with physicians. And the student workforce. And those were not peaceful settings. And I was not calm.

When I got to the hospital, the only employees present were the brown coats, red coats, and grey coats. Grey is the color of student interns. There must be sixty physicians employed, and not one of them was there when it opened. I asked a brown coat how long it would be until a white coat arrived.

"An hour... at the earliest."

After about half a minute of waiting, I grew impatient, so I tried to work with a grey coat, and I was punished for my impatience. The experience reminded me of Aetheldorf's line, "The acorn, thinking itself mighty, sees no reason to sprout."

It was the last sentence in *Aphorisms*. Which was the last complete book that Cyn and I went through together. I had no idea then that its messages would be so applicable in such short time. The students today remain cloistered in their nutshells. But they imagine themselves to be mighty oaks towering over their communities. Way too confident in their conduct. One should always retain a degree of insecurity. Lest all self-betterment be arrested. Mistakenly believing arrival to have already occurred only ensures it will never come. Or, as Cyn put it, the macramog vine that blooms its pride in darkness will never find enlightenment. Something like that. I don't remember her exact words.

Cyn wasn't from Farhearth. She wasn't planted against a lattice and promised a life of easy climbing. Today's interns, though. They arrive on campus with the pomposity of a pebble lion. Far too proud for guidance. No berry ever blooms, but they think they're feeding the nation.

"I don't think we're going to keep her admitted; she probably just choked on some food."

That's what the first intern told me.

Without calling him foolish or unqualified or worse, I explained how that wasn't the case. How it couldn't be the case. Refuting his claim with what must surely be the single most cogent minute of medical reasoning he has yet encountered. Inside, I was fuming. But I didn't show it. My casual posture was a perfect counterfeit of a careless bystander. I spoke clearly and slowly. My gestures were calm. Perhaps my pupils didn't participate in my theatrics, but otherwise, it was a Lonvarakan performance. And since he couldn't argue against it, he dismissed it as "a rant!" Then he marched away, audibly huffing. Even his gait was huffing.

A concise and articulate argument delivered in a dispassionate tone in defense of a defensible position is not what "rant" means. Today's youth don't seem to realize that.

After he huffed away from the exchange, I met with two more grey coats. Neither dismissed my explanation as a rant. Because they didn't let me finish. They simply talked over me. About science or medicine or hospital resources or anything else that might be helpful? No. Instead, they gushed descriptions of their brilliance, then regaled me with tales of their medical heroism, then assured me that everything they had to say was infallible, life-saving wisdom.

If you actually were heroic and brilliant, there would be no need to declare it. The truth doesn't need champions. Only lies need advertising of that kind. There's no way Orfric went around telling everyone "I'm skilled at language!" or Mizjak bragged about his fencing skills or Bonstan boasts of his prosperity. In my experience, marketing is loudest where the truth is furthest. So when I'm assured of someone's infallible medical brilliance, that tells me they make a lot of mistakes. And the worst place for a mistake to be made is a hospital. Because the clinician is sorry, and the patient is dead. Only the coat wearer has the luxury of getting over it. And if they think of themselves as infallible, they're not learning from their errors. And if they aren't learning from them, they'll inflict the same harm on the next patient.

Recklessness, mindlessness, selfishness... whatever the reason for your error, you should never have chosen this career. You should not be allowed to work with anything that lives.

Unfortunately, yesterday's grass grads are tomorrow's physicians. So this is a problem that will only worsen.

Whatever optimism I preserved yesterday had already turned rancid by the time the white coats finally arrived. But Cyn and I were able to see one almost immediately.

I told him about our experience last night. And what the diagnosis was.

"Sounds like spittle from the pig to me."

That's what he said. Not the two-word iteration we all know today, but the full, unabridged expression. Had I not been looking at him while he said it – if our correspondence was in writing – I would have known his generation. Today, time has excised the six expendable words, but this physician comes from a culture before Orfric was subjected to the scalpel. I'm sure he also addresses misbehaving children by their full name. "Gylot Oro, son of Krark, you are in trouble!"

This was a physician I could trust to be comprehensive.

He asked me to provide details about Cyn, her medical history, the setting in which her condition occurred, recent exposures, and so on. I did. For several minutes, I described every faintly pertinent detail about her.

He sat across from me on his stool, listening attentively. Leaning toward me, nodding on occasion, only breaking eye contact to look at a notepad on which he would write a brief note. Then he would resume focus on my narrative.

When I got to the part about Cyn's headache, he tilted his head and leaned in a little closer. Like a dog would if it were trying to decipher your commands.

As I kept talking, he stopped taking notes. He didn't stop paying attention, but he leaned back, and his nodding grew more exaggerated. He had clearly decided on his diagnosis.

He politely waited for me to finish. Then he said, "The matter at hand is a treatable one. It's a matter I've seen before. Not uncommonly. Shall we proceed to the treatment?"

I was overcome with relief. My heart felt suddenly light, emptied of the grief it had been carrying so gravely.

I barely had the strength to mutter, "Yes, what's wrong with her?"

And then I was told the diagnosis: acute pancreatic insufficiency.

My respite was a brief one.

My heart was suddenly stricken again with the crushing weight of grief.

I taught Clinical Physiology while I was at Farhearth. And how the pancreas influences metabolism was a central concept in that course. I've read most of the research on this topic, and I've even contributed to it myself.

This was not an accurate diagnosis. Had the physician reflected on the state of evidence, he might have realized that. But physicians aren't taught to think. They're taught facts. And in healthcare, facts only last a few years. Then they start to decay.

Physiological truths are more durable. If the experiments are done correctly, they're invincible. But those truths are tiny. And they lack clinical application. Deriving broad diagnostic and therapeutic utility from a narrow laboratory discovery is an abstract process that involves a considerable margin of error. Sometimes, new scientific findings build upon preexisting principles; other times, they overturn what used to be conventional. But Farhearth physicians were trained by rote memorization rather than deep consideration. So, they hold all conventions as eternal. They don't believe in "science"; they believe in *themselves*. "Does my belief contradict the evidence that has emerged since my graduation? That means the evidence is wrong!" Some say that out loud; others simply imply it.

To challenge a physician's diagnosis, however, is to be dismissed. No matter how ludicrous it is. Further challenge elicits anger. And still further challenge prompts a *new* diagnosis: the questioner is exhibiting signs of acute delusion, and should be medicated accordingly, or at least monitored until it passes.

I know this. And yet I questioned. Because the diagnosis he gave was clearly incorrect. And I tried to explain that. As humbly and reverentially as I could. Hoping it would be received as an invitation for further discussion.

It didn't work. Instead of discussing, he scribbled something in Cyn's chart. And I knew it was about me. Adon forbid someone who reads, teaches, and publishes on the subject be permitted to inquire on it.

I didn't press him further. Drawing additional attention to his mistake would not correct it. All it would do is increase the bill.

So I thanked him for his time and effort – tried to make it sound sincere – and accepted the bill as it was written.

Then I returned to the scheduling counter and spoke with a brown-coated member of the staff. And found a new physician who was willing to see Cyn. It was a woman who had the appearance of a sympathetic listener.

Walking into her office, my hope was restored.

And then it was re-squashed.

Her posture and expression both gushed compassion, but it was a deception.

She subscribed to that business-first belief that whatever the patient reports suffering from is not a real condition unless it is treatable with medication. If a product cannot be peddled during the appointment – a pill, a poultice, a tincture – the physician is either in error, or the patient is crazy.

Although "crazy" is characterized in heavier syllabled vernacular. Words like supratentorial or psychosomatic are used. And dismissive diagnoses such as Eldug's disorder are assigned. Which means, "You're making all of this up; dishonesty is the pathology." Other patients have Ucretia's disease written in their charts. That one means, "You genuinely believe these symptoms to be real, but you're mistaken." Scrawled in other charts is Cedyl's syndrome: "There *is* something real here, but you're doing it to yourself for attention; by not giving you the attention you seek, I'm curing you."

In every case, the patient is blamed, and the physician remains unchallenged.

In *this* case, Cyn's diagnosis was Cedyl's syndrome. Cyn did this to herself. Drugs of some sort.

That's not even close to true. Not even close to close. And I argued as much. Or at least I tried. Before she even said the word "Cedyl". I could tell that diagnosis was coming, so I tried to thwart its deployment. Unsuccessfully.

At least the visit was brief, which left enough time to see one more physician: a well-bearded man who lacked the appearance of an attentive listener, but his appearance was deceptive, too.

He sat and listened quietly as I explained the details of Cyn's condition for the fourth time.

He didn't interrupt me or write anything. As I talked, his squinting eyes just stared ahead. At nothing. While he slowly stroked his beard.

Then I got to the Pendelhall tournament. I explained how Cyn dehydrated herself – very slightly – to avoid the need to urinate. And how we both drank ale and experienced headaches after the Closing Ceremony.

Finally, the physician asked a question: "How much coffee, tea, milk, and ale does she ordinarily drink?"

Before I had finished answering, he said, "I know the cause." And then he explained that dehydration was the culprit. "For months leading up to the tournament, her consumption of water in the form of water was insufficient. Coffees and teas, milk and ale: these do not hydrate us. They're all diuretics to varying degrees, causing us to excrete more than we take in. The amount may be small, but over time, these incremental reductions in blood volume will cause our blood pressure to decline. Uncorrected, it will keep declining. Until it ultimately crosses a symptomatic threshold in which it can no longer overcome gravity, so we must lie down to adequately perfuse our brains."

As he handed me the bill, he winked and said, "Restoration is a matter of rehydration."

As I took the bill, I explained – as respectfully as I could – that a century ago, these beliefs about diuresis were thought to be true. But that was the last time they were believed.

"I'm familiar with the work by Unsoth and Gamel", I began.

That's the everything-but-water-is-a-diuretic study... which was published a century ago. I doubt the physician knew the reference, so I provided context: "Their report on hydration and diuresis really got the conversation started."

At this point, the physician resumed his beard stroking. As though he had reverted to a diagnostic mindset. Except, instead of deciphering the clues of an illness, he was trying to figure out where the conversation was going.

I continued: "But there was a recent study in *Farhearth Frontiers* that compared urine retention after consumption of water, milk, coffee, and ale." As I began my explanation of the methods and results, I was interrupted.

"I know what *science* says!" He did not wink as he barked that.

"I don't think you do", I wanted to say. But didn't. If this physician really did understand the science, he wouldn't continue to report such unfounded claims. Perhaps he's heard rumors of scientific conclusions that contradict his beliefs, but that would be the extent of his knowledge. The mechanisms certainly elude him. Otherwise, he would be embarrassed by his diagnosis. It's akin to saying *germ theory is a hoax! I know what science says, but it's a hoax!*

Still, I didn't argue. That wouldn't accomplish anything. It would only ruin our ability to see anyone else. So I just nodded deferentially in his direction, put his bill in my pocket (along with the three other bills containing incorrect diagnoses), and left.

Except for emergency patients, the hospital closes for a midday meal break, leaving me with nothing to do for an hour and a half. So, I'm currently sitting at the eateries.

This morning, when I stopped by the wagon, Rorrik said he'd try to meet me here for lunch. "If I'm not there by the last song, don't wait for me", he said, referring to the bell tower songs that play all morning.

From six o'clock to noon, every hour chimes a half-minute version of the Hail Farhearth Hymn. After that, the bell tolls once for each of the next twelve hours. On the hour. One toll at one o'clock, two tolls at two, three at three, and eventually, it tolls twelve times for midnight. Then silence. Until six o'clock the next morning. Those are the "idle hours". Or, as they're referred to in the storybooks, the "untolled hours" or "atolling hours".

Rorrik didn't show up. So, instead of complaining to *him* about my morning, I've been chronicling those complaints on the page. For six pages. But now it's time to return to the hospital. I hope I have better luck in the second half of the day.

Sixty-Eight

Fyros, Third Lufoa, Day Three. Night.

When I was a child, my mother said she was making chicken and dumplings for dinner. It's soup with a tiny bit of chicken and a couple of biscuits in it. I protested. I'm not sure why. I'd never had it before. So I wasn't speaking from prior revulsion. And "dumpling" is a very edible name. It might have been how she answered the question, "What are dumplings?"

"They're like gooey pancake balls."

"No, not those!", I shrieked. "Anything but those!"

She did not heed my plea. A few hours later, I was being served dumplings. I ate the chicken, drank most of the soup, and then grudgingly bit one of the gooey pancake balls. And found myself chewing the most delicious lump of finely ground wheat I had ever tasted. But I couldn't reveal that. Because I had already established a position – in the form of a tantrum – against the dumplings. And I had pride to maintain. So I held firm. Dumplings were a dinner to be detested. To demonstrate this, I left one dumpling in the bowl. Untouched. As my mother cleared my bowl from the table, I felt the sting of my sacrifice. But at the time, I thought my behavior preserved my honor.

In bed that night, I dreamed of dumplings. And I mourned their wastage. Never before nor since has my pillow absorbed so much saliva. And never again have I put pride before gluttony… or anything else.

I was seven.

Cyn and I saw three physicians this afternoon. They were all older than I am. And they continue to berate dumplings. By which I mean: they prioritize pride above patient care. They stick to their initially established positions no matter how ludicrous they're later revealed to be.

Everything they've ever said out loud – to me one minute ago or to a different patient last year – is a claim to be repeated. A claim they must fortify against all future evidence to the contrary. The less defensible it becomes, the more strident their endorsement. If they once admitted a distaste for dumplings, they must champion that statement until the end of their days, at which point, it might as well serve as their epitaph.

In patient care, pride is the most debilitating handicap there is. With general physicians – meaning those without specialty – it can be difficult to predict the manifestation of their debility. But with specialists, it's easy to anticipate where their bias will lead. And that describes my experience this afternoon. All three specialized in different branches of medicine, each had a different diagnosis, and each was *sure* of it. As sure as I was about gooey pancake balls.

The first physician said it was Cyn's heart. This was followed by a reasonable explanation of how a stroke or aneurism would result in this presentation.

The second physician said it was Cyn's liver. This was followed by neither reason nor explanation. "This is a classic case of lufir stalk toxicity", he said. Then, after a well-rehearsed pause, he added, "Dreamveil poisoning, as it's often called by users and poisoners alike." He was making two assumptions. First: I wouldn't know what lufir was. Second: I needed someone to blame, and this diagnosis would satisfy that need.

The final physician said it was Cyn's kidneys. This was followed by a detailed lesson on renal function, which concluded with an explanation of how uremia developed and led to every symptom we see today. The least believable of the three. The latter two came with medications. All three came with a bill.

When I presented counterarguments to each physician, they disparaged me, asserting that I'm "too caught up in the papers!" Then they "educated" me on how *actual* medicine *actually* works. Apparently, "the laboratory" has no place in patient care. A system that puts blind faith in beakers and formulas is a system that needs to be bucked. A system these physicians *are* bucking. Because they know better than those white-coat novices who lack instinct and compensate for that shortcoming with obedience to the latest "science". They hissed that word like a snake. They weren't merely scoffing at research; they were *bragging* about scoffing at it. It sounded like a seven-year-old boy boasting of his ignorance after a poor performance on a mathematics exam. That's how the boy signals a rebellious sensibility to his more popular peers, and in doing so, garners social esteem without having to accomplish anything. The same is true for the physicians. It's just sadder. Because they aren't seven.

I was polite, but I didn't accept divination as justification for their diagnoses. I wanted evidence. So I asked for it:

"What tests are you running?"

"None."

"Well, what evidence do you have to support your diagnosis?"

"I just *know*."

"Okay, that's a start. But I would *also* like to know. And one's instinct only convinces oneself. So, for me to join your conviction, I would need a more objective justification."

This incited the tirades on "science" and the bragging about its bucking. All three specialists clearly perceived themselves to be mavericks, unique in their approach to patient care.

Physicians don't often diagnose each other. And if they do provide counsel to a colleague, I suspect they conduct themselves very differently. So they have no idea that every other physician is incanting the exact same cliché. Only the patients are aware that this august "infirmary" is packed full of indistinguishable mavericks. I've been here for a little over a day and I'm already tired of the repetition. I doubt I'm unique in my feeling.

More physicians to see tomorrow.

In the meantime, Rorrik met me at the hospital as it was closing. He insisted we get dinner somewhere away from here. So we went to the Square.

If there's a Lir in the East, this is it. A cobbled circle surrounds a park that's filled with the flowers of every season. Tonight, Lufoa was blushing its finale. In the center of that park stand two ancient ash trees. Ancient enough to predate the university. For ages, their branches reached out to each other, but never touched. "Generations pass patiently by awaiting a perfect union." That's the famous last line of *The Longing Trees*, a fable that either took its tale from those perennial paramours or it lent its name *to* them. No one knows. Tonight, however, when Rorrik and I walked by, we saw that the patience of generations was put at ease. The trees' reaching branches now intertwine in matrimony. The lonely unrhyming line has finally seen its couplet complete.

Somehow, the sight seemed both joyful and sad. Like a great love was found, but a poetry just as great had to be sacrificed to find it. No happy ending is ever purely sweet, I guess.

I'm sure the curmudgeons of the campuses are eagerly awaiting their divorce. But I'm even surer that the roots are far more entwined than their branches. But what I am *most* sure of is that Rorrik and I were the only two people in the Square who were thinking about the trees.

The circle-shaped Square is where a lot of the student communities do their communing. So it's often crowded. But not always. The throngs arrive and depart like tides. Although their presence has nothing to do with the moon's orbital period. So there's no need to consult a scientist whose name begins with Ol to predict the entry and ebbing of traffic. You just have to check Farhearth's course schedule. The Square will be sparsely populated during heavy curricular times and teeming when the classrooms are empty. Tonight, it was teeming. With lunacy. Of a non-lunar variety.

On the way there, we saw several signs telling us what to think and instructing us what decisions to make. Mostly about voting. It's a mayoral election year. And we're made to think that our votes count. They do for lots of measures. But for mayor? I doubt it. Still, there were posters telling us whom to elect, which judicial revisions to support, and which ones we must disapprove of. And if that's not enough, there were lobbyists beside each poster expounding on their messages, every one of them on the university's payroll. Every one of them also holds a degree from Farhearth. That's why they're campaigning. Once upon a time, students who graduated in the lowest quintile were called "grass grads" because they graduated into the workforce as groundskeepers. Today, the grounds are overstaffed. So these alumni lobby on behalf of the institution instead. Vote no on this, yes on that. Protest this, donate to that. Dense hordes of lowly-lettered dunces pay off their tuition debt by telling the masses how to behave.

As a faculty member, I'd make all my decisions contrary to their instructions. Not for the pleasure of being a contrarian. Nor the satisfaction of rejecting authority. It just seemed like a shortcut to morality. The point of lobbying is to persuade people to behave in a way that is inconsistent with their nature. Why would anyone pay employees to convince people of what they already believe? Lobbyists are only useful if the desired outcome contravenes the people's integrity, their values, their sensibilities. Thus, I assume anything they tell me to do is the opposite of how I would act if I were being true to myself. And I vote accordingly. What I learned tonight is that I'd support the ballot measures for institutional proceeds reporting and coastal wetland protection. I'd oppose the measures for literacy reformation and expanding the authority of the Justiciary Office. And Ceryd and Alvos are not mayors I would vote for. Alas, I'm not a voting citizen.

I did see a *Wanted* poster though. "The Singing Sisters". There was a reward. A big one. Offered by Atrok-Ilrum, which is an old club of old, rich families. The sisters aren't wanted by the *law*. Just by the club. But rich people tend to be more threatening than law officers.

In the Square, we were free from campaigning. Instead, we were enswarmed by the out-of-class students. Some were coming, others going, but most were loitering. Either socializing or attempting to attract the socializers' attention.

There was one who was worse than the others. Perhaps I'm biased because I encountered him yesterday. The one with the bracelets whom I asked for directions. I pointed him out to Rorrik, and we both watched. And listened.

He had a sword that he barely knew how to handle. And he was explaining to his immediate coterie – in a voice far louder than necessary – that it was a great legendary weapon. "It is imbued with the spirit of its previous owner", he said... loud enough to address everyone in the Square. Then he named that owner. While staring smugly at the blade. Then he paused, looked up, and repeated the name: "*THE* Dember Unspell!" He practically shouted it. This was followed by an uncoordinated flurry of attacks in the air. It startled a student who was passing by at the time. She let out a brief scream as she dropped a stack of loose papers. The braceleted boy didn't help her. Instead, he laughed and said, "en garde."

She didn't say anything. Or even glare. She just scooped up her papers and hustled away, looking both embarrassed and afraid.

"I tell you what", the boy said to his small group of goons, "Dember Unspell can be unruly if I don't keep her under control. She's only just come to me, so she's still learning to obey her master." They made a sycophantic noise that could be confused with laughter. Then the boy returned to his boasting: "Dominating this blade will be like taming a wild stallion, and I've broken a thousand in my day. Give me one good ride, and by the time I'm through, all the life will have drained from its eyes."

What a fool. He's clearly trying to impersonate some sort of masculine hero, but the only impression he's creating is that of a boy who thrives on creating impressions. And "Dember Unspell"? Nowhere in any fable or history tome does that name appear. And even if it did, only self-important buffoons insist on being addressed by two names.

While this boy was certainly king of his class, he wasn't the only showoff in the crowd. Rorrik and I didn't listen to anyone else's conversations, but the flamboyance was visible from a distance.

When a teenage boy styles his hair to resemble a snake stripe or flail spikes, hoping it will make him look mean and dangerous, it only ever accomplishes the opposite.

Rorrik and I tried to think of a single powerful person throughout history who took an interest in fashion. A northern warlord, some militant mayor, a winner of the fencing tournament, or even a revered Southern blacksmith. We couldn't think of a single person who carefully tailored his wardrobe and styled his hair to appear imposing. I doubt there has never been a tyrant who groomed himself into the image of tyranny. And yet there is no shortage of Farhearth boys who play dress-up in the Square.

The other feature of the boys trying too hard to exhibit manliness is beards. Later in life, when they become old men, they'll groom their faces so smooth it's as if they're attempting to counterfeit prepubescence.

Between these two phases of reputation curation is where Rorrik and I reside. Neither of us has any interest in our appearance. And the same seemed to be true for everyone else near the nydel of their lives. All of us were in a mild state of dishevel.

Eventually, Rorrik and I sat down to eat. At an outdoor table. And as we ate, we continued to observe the crowd. And discuss them. Our conversation was lighthearted until we saw a professor we both recognized. One we both had as students. One we both detested. I met her my first day on campus. She was already old then. She must be in her eighties now. But there's one compliment I can't deny: she still in phenomenal physical health. If she were a horse, I would bet on her to win the Salt and Stone.

I doubt we would have recognized her if it weren't for her twirling arms. It's a gesture she does while thinking. Her elbows are stationed in front of her, forearms angled straight up like pillars, fingers extended, palms aimed toward her face. And then her hands begin to perform little pirouettes. Like they're orbiting a tiny, invisible planet. Six-inch circles. Over and over. I watched her make at least fifty tiny orbits before she finally extinguished her silence with another sentence. And returned her arms to rest.

There are really only two classes of Farhearth faculty. There are those who grow humble through the accumulation of knowledge and experience. Those who learn their modest place in a mighty world. And then there are those whose despotism is nourished by knowledge and experience. Those academic warlords who squash everyone they perceive as a threat. Picadillo is from the latter class. I've always blamed her for Rorrik's decision to leave Farhearth without a degree. He was always the brightest one. And that's what made him a target. She focused all her insecurity on him. That's what permitted the rest of us to "sneak beneath the thunder ceiling".

All right, it's time to put my journal away and get into bed.

Rorrik is sleeping in the wagon again. And I'm back in the Commons Tavern. I suggested we trade places. Take turns. But he insisted. "You're the one working tirelessly. You need a more restful place to sleep."

Then he told me some Farhearth students did try to steal the wagon last night.

When I asked for details, he said, "Initiation into a fraternity, I assume. They left with urine in their shoes."

Sixty-Nine

Nyros, Third Lufoa, Day Four. Morning.

When I was a child, "go find an adult" was how I solved every problem.

The worst part about being a grown-up is that, when I encounter a problem, I have to solve it myself. *I'm* the adult. Especially here, at the infirmary, where I seem to be the *only* adult.

Another day of medicine ahead. Six physicians yesterday, one the day before, and I don't know if I'm going to get an answer. Or if I've already gotten it. But I have to keep seeking. Because the mystery is often what hurts the most.

In sickness, there are knowns and unknowns. And even if there's nothing you can do about the knowns, they feel more controllable. It's the unknowns that feel completely out of our control. Because we don't know their extent. And if all we have is our imaginations to contemplate our conditions with, the pain is a hundred times sharper. Knowing the cause and cure, the extent and duration, the biological mechanisms: this takes away some of the sting. In uncloaking it, it loses some of its power to wound.

Or at least that's true for me. Like swimming in the ocean, it's a fear of the unknown that holds our attention. If I can't see what threatens me, it could be anything. The imagination is the scariest thing there is. And the hardest thing to ignore. Until my imagination can be replaced with facts, it's going to keep churning. And churning. And the butter that comes from it is pungent.

I suspect most people would have already accepted one of the diagnoses, but I'm not most people. At least in this sense. No one has ever accused me of being *under*-analytical. I just wish someone would do the analyzing *for* me. That's the whole purpose of coming to the most advanced hospital on Gaea. I wish one of the physicians here, who are being paid to diagnose, would take it seriously. But they don't. The only thing they take seriously is the bill.

People who go into medicine for the money or esteem or, in the case of most physicians, both, will never be skilled. They'll be *wealthy*, but never respected. Because they're bad at their job. Consider music. People who go into music for fame and finances are bad musicians. Nobody wants to hear their songs. Because they lack passion. Maybe they're passionate about other things, but not art. So their art is bad. They care about the trappings, not the product.

Many of today's physicians, just like today's students, are stunted vines that will never bear edible fruit.

Instead, they just believe in themselves. I don't mean "hold oneself to a high standard"; I mean *believe* in oneself, standards be damned. That's the kind of religiosity one defends vigorously.

Too many physicians erect thick walls around their fragile egos. So pristine and brittle, those egos will shatter with the tiniest penetration of opposition. So they erect protective ramparts. Thicker and thicker. Higher and higher. And they populate the battlements with guards. Criticism can neither pass nor climb those fortifications.

What those walls *really* keep out, though, is information. Sustenance for a growing mind. When denied that nutrition, the mind will decay a little more every day. Just like anything else that's freed from challenge, the slow poison of atrophy takes hold. The deadliest nemesis of progress is always arrogance. If you fill an ego with air, it'll never contain merit. And that's why pride is a particularly perilous threat to public health.

There are old fireside stories about changelings. In a common cottage in a common city on a common day like today, a mother puts her infant in a crib. A *common* crib. Then she averts her eyes. To iron her gown or brush her hair or polish the dinnerware. And her infant is suddenly snatched from the crib, replaced with a lookalike. That humanoid beast now wriggles and cries where the child once did. And that's where the stories usually end. If they go on, the mother's life only gets worse. As the days go by, the creature festering in the crib grows uglier and uglier. As the years go by, the creature she's rearing grows more and more corrupt. And *then* it ends. Or, if it goes on from *there*, the mother dies of dejection. And that's the final ending. It's never happy.

I didn't understand the moral message of those stories until now:

If we aren't vigilant custodians of our souls, they risk being snatched from our cradle of ribs. And replaced by a pile of nobles and crowns. And that will corrupt us from the inside out.

Or maybe the stories really were meant to be pointless horror. But the souls of the physicians we've seen so far were swapped for coins long ago. And that never ends happily. For anyone.

When patients come to them, they're vulnerable. They're broken, defeated, helpless. They're usually desperate, almost always too exhausted to go on.

So, the physician, recognizing their position of power, takes a perch. From on high, they look down on those in need. Over time, they grow comfortable with their perch, and begin to look down on *everyone*. Soon, the whole world is beneath them. But they never learn much up there. They aren't that smart. Or talented. Or even useful. What they are is *superior*.

There's so much deference given to them. They're the ones who underwent medical education, not you. Therefore, you must accept anything they say as the clinical equivalent of Druinian prophesy.

And if you politely challenge them, it might as well be a declaration of war.

"I have a different view" says the student. The professor wants to hear it. Because we don't want to hold an inaccurate or incomplete belief any longer than we must.

"I have a different view" says the patient. The physician does not want to hear it, and they'll come up with the most absurd ways of silencing the asker.

This is the exact problem Cyn has been training to fix. For six years.

There's nothing she couldn't do. If the world had a bigger crisis, she would be preparing to confront that instead. Until that day comes, medicine is what needs fixing. But before Cyn can take it on, the broken medical system has to fix her first. That's the tragedy of it all.

When I was a child who relied entirely on grown-ups for my problem solving, I thought becoming an adult would be empowering. But it's not. It's just frustrating. Because many of life's problems remain unsolvable without help. And the help I need can't be found. Because I need an ethical grown-up with medical training. And I'm having trouble finding that here.

I'm already getting upset and I haven't even left for the hospital yet.

But I'm hoping for a better outcome today.

The eighth attempt is generally a *charm*, is it not?

Seventy

Nyros, Third Lufoa, Day Four. Afternoon.

Arrived at the hospital early again. But I had no interest in interacting with the grey coats, so I sat and watched them. What did they do for a full hour? Pretend to work. Pretend to "be busy" by shuffling papers and saying sentences like, "I'm really busy."

To squander so many hours posturing without succumbing to depression, one must believe life is eternal. If your hours are infinite, there's no urgent reason to make use of the one you're in. Contrarily, if you're made aware of an approaching terminus, you ask yourself if each hour was wisely spent. Could you have done more? Are you making the most of your life?

These are not questions the grey coats burden themselves with. Their primary concern is appearance: how productive they *appear* to be. Why even show up if you have no interest in productivity, though?

I guess I know the answer: to climb the rungs of the hierarchy. Without the support of your colleagues, it's an unscalable ladder. And those colleagues won't support you if they never see you. Rank favors the present. But history remembers the absent: those ghostly curmudgeons whose utter avoidance of society enabled them to contribute to it without distraction.

If the entire world were populated by grey coats, whose collective life goal is to be *perceived* as productive, we would be living in dank caves and flimsy huts, and the most advanced technology would be sharp rocks bound to sticks.

One needn't be productive *every* waking minute. No one is. Me least of all. I think distractions are fine in moderation. Like many nutrients, a little bit is required for human health. As part of a balanced diet. But an excess is detrimental. And the grey coats don't seem very balanced in their behavior.

But I did learn one thing from their morning prattle: there is a documented case of shepherd's fever. In the hospital. A patient was admitted last night wearing the pale wreath. So far, it's just one case, but if it spreads, it could present a much larger problem. In part, it will reduce the availability of beds and personnel. But also, I can't risk Cyn getting it in her present condition. And I would prefer to avoid it, too. I know people who have been infected and recovered from it. But I know *more* people who got it and *didn't* recover.

Those who survived spent several weeks alternating between cold sweats and hot sweats, cold shivers and hot shivers. The headaches and frozen bones are the first symptoms to resolve. The cough might linger for a few months. But one symptom always lasts: "I used to be so active", every survivor says... a year after recovering from everything *but* the fatigue. "My health, which used to be typhoon-proof, can now barely withstand the breeze", is how one of my old friends described it. Risha. She contracted shepherds' fever the last time it came through Farhearth. I wonder if she's still there. She worked in the library. The library *complex*. The equipment part. Not the book part. Although I would wager that environment is more bookish than the hospital. These days, anyway. It used to be that physicians had Magister's Degrees. Now, they get two-thirds of a Higher Licentiate, then dawn their grey coat, beginning an apprenticeship for which they are paid little and deserve less. Depending on their field of study, they won't have their white coat ceremony for one to five years. And at no point do the greys have any incentive to read. They gradually grow obstinate in their knowledge, and soon become obsolete. Then they spend their careers misdiagnosing patients. And how do they react to their errors? Blame, berate, and bill. Then yell, "Next!"

If a blacksmith bungles the blade, they don't charge you for it. If a mason or cobbler or cook makes a mistake, and they don't correct it, a disparaging story will appear in the next issue of the local paper. With a physician, however, if you visit them a second time to correct the error of the first appointment, they'll just bill you twice. "Next!"

I was already frustrated when I arrived this morning. And it only got worse. Each physician Cyn and I saw had a document with all previous diagnoses, and probably some comments about me. At the very least, they know I don't trust any of the previous diagnoses. Perhaps that motivates them to come up with something new. But it also puts them on guard when I walk in.

Upon meeting the first physician, I began my well-rehearsed explanation of Cyn's condition. And he stopped me. Immediately. "I don't need the story; I have it all here", he said without looking up from his chart. In a tone that indicated he thought of me as mentally unwell. He must have been reading something about me.

Then he sat there, unsociably, reading the document for half a minute more. If I could read lips, I would know exactly what it said. Because the physician's mouth was silently reading along. In the way that children's lips move when they try to read quietly. Finally, he spoke, agreeing with one of yesterday's physicians: "It's a pancreatic disorder."

No, it isn't. Obviously, it isn't. But I didn't say that. Instead, I tried to ease into a respectful conversation on the topic: "I appreciate your expertise here. I'd like to discuss this diagnosis further. I've published a bit on the pancreas, mostly how its function differs in sedentary and—"

"Who's the physician in this room?", he interrupted. His voice was angry.

I didn't respond. We just held eye contact for a few seconds. My look must have conveyed confusion. His was clearly meant to intimidate.

Then he looked down and began scribbling frantically in his chart. His lips were moving just as frantically, sounding out the words as he wrote them. Again, like a child. Except he wasn't doing it silently. He was whispering the words aloud. It was hard to make out much of it. Only the words that sizzled with rage: "authority" and "delusion" were among them.

He wrote that I'm delusional, knowing it to be false. He was just retaliating for the crime of questioning his authority. One can easily tell which patients are delusional by looking at their faces. It's a matter of attire. The faces of the deluded are inappropriately dressed. They can be seen wearing surprise, disgust, fear, elation, anger... when the situation calls for different apparel. It looks like swimwear in the middle of Arzox. Or fur in the heat of Lufoa. An inability to clothe one's face in the appropriate expression reveals a lack of circumstantial understanding. And he saw nothing of the sort on my face. I understand the weather and I'm dressed for the occasion. Yet he scribbled (and whispered) about me bitterly. Then he handed me bill number eight. Eleven if you count the three grey coats. But those bills are cheap. And still overpriced for what you get.

I didn't even look at this bill. I just put it in my pocket. Then I scheduled another appointment. With another physician. At that point, I *was* on the brink of delusion, having been pushed to that brink by this ludicrous series of encounters. So my expression probably did look like the clothing of an incoherent mind.

When I met with the next physician, she seemed to think that's what needed diagnosis. "Why don't you recount your experiences for me", she said.

I did, assuming she wanted to hear the details of our Pendelhall trip herself. Perhaps she was looking for something more than was written in the chart. When I got to the part where I found Cyn, the morning after the ceremony, she interrupted me to say, "I'm so sorry you've had to go through this."

"Thanks", I said. Then I started describing other details about Cyn that I thought might be relevant. And she periodically interrupted to patronize me with more "I'm so sorry"s, each phonier than the last. She wasn't listening to what I was saying. Or taking the situation seriously. She thought I was there to be consoled. So that's what she was doing. But I *detest* fake sympathy. And I resent being billed for it, as though it were a treatment. If I wanted someone to *act* caring, I'd go to Lonvaraka, not Farhearth. That would be cheaper and more compelling. This was just insulting. In retrospect, I wish I had said, "I accept your apology" or "I forgive you" or maybe "I *don't* accept your apology" or "I'm not ready to forgive you." Or "I appreciate you taking accountability for your actions." But I said none of those things. I didn't respond to her syrupy interruptions at all. I just imitated a woodstove and fumed from within. Until finally, she put her hand on my shoulder and said, "Time always repairs our pains. Sometimes it doesn't seem that way because it doesn't do its mending at our pace. We just need to be patient."

That put another log in the belly of the stove. Exalting "Time" as the great healer of all wounds is a terrible pretext for inaction. It should never excuse physicians from doing their job. Innumerable wounds are irreparable to the mending powers of Time. Even minor injuries are seldom repaired in full. Time may scab over the gash and ultimately restore *most* function. But that's not the "healing" that's being implied. Most wounds leave behind clumps of collagen. Lumpy, inflamed scars that you feel with the turning of the weather. And emotional scaring is imprinted even deeper. Time does not regenerate those structures to their pre-wound condition.

I might have maintained my equanimity if this were the first physician I had seen. But it wasn't.

South of Death's Meridian, the horizon always promises an oasis. And those oases always reveal themselves to be mirages. So one learns never to indulge a thirst. Otherwise, you dry up faster. Like how the sound of running water makes urination feel urgent if you have a half-full bladder. Today, I realized it is similarly wise to evacuate hope before embarking on a medical journey. Otherwise, if it goes unrequited in appointment after appointment – all you experience is *dis*appointment after *dis*appointment – the frustration can be too much to bear. For me, it was. I snapped at her. "I'm not the patient!", I nearly yelled.

"I know", she lied. Calmly. "I just wanted to make sure you felt heard, too. Now, tell me more about the night of the ceremony. I'm especially interested in what she ate and drank."

I explained everything I could remember. Including the details I knew were irrelevant. When I was done, she said, "I have good news and bad news."

I sat quietly, waiting for her to explain.

She also sat quietly, waiting for a response. But I wasn't asked a question. One should never pause after making that statement.

After about five unnecessary seconds of silence, I said, "Okay?"

"It's her liver", she said. I've heard this already. Last night. Except this time, it wasn't lufir poisoning. It was a different cause, but otherwise the same. That was the bad news. Which wasn't true.

Then came the good news, which was based on the false bad news… so it didn't matter.

"The good news is that she's likely to recover. The liver is the noble organ. Just as the struck dog reliably returns to its owner, so too will the liver be restored if you simply treat it well and give it time."

Then, with one last "I'm so sorry you've had to go through this", she handed me the bill. I put it in my pocket, left the hospital, and returned to the Square. To the same place where Rorrik and I ate last night. That's where I am now. Where I've been writing ever since. Where I continue to nurture frustration.

But the hospital will be reopening soon. So, it's time I head back.

In the interest of my own emotional health, I will resist the mirage of hope that's tempting me.

Seventy-One

Nyros, Third Lufoa, Day Four. Night.

The rest of the day's appointments were not uplifting. There were only two. Three if you count the grey coat, but I don't. I have a difficult time treating the greys – those early-twenties kids with scant academic training – as experts. That's not the same thing as treating them with respect. I can respect infants as precious lifeforms despite regarding them as experts in nothing. And that's how I see the greys.

I don't blame them for their ignorance. Not entirely. The system is probably more culpable; it seems designed to foster confidence in the absence of merit. All those "coat" ceremonies they do between matriculation and graduation. There must be a dozen events of celebration and congratulation before they even accomplish anything.

At first, the exceptionalization of every student seemed innocuous. "You're extraordinary!" doesn't cost the institution anything, and it keeps the students paying tuition. But if you compliment the incompetent, they'll believe you. If parents praise everything their child says – "you're so smart and funny!" – the child will believe them. *Everything I say is clever and entertaining,* they think. When this child grows up a little, leaves home, and expects everyone else in the world to continue applauding their ordinariness, they'll be struck with a painful truth: *I'm surrounded by idiots who can't appreciate my brilliance!* That's not the *actual* truth, but it's what they glean from the experience. If enough people kneel before us, no matter how humble we used to be, we come to believe the kneelings are deserved. And at Farhearth, when "exceptional" stopped being a comparative term – when it became a right of every student – their attitudes changed. They morphed into something both helpless and harmful. The student body today is a vast and briny sea of mediocrity, but every drop believes itself to be a diamond in the deluge.

I'm pretty sure that was a strategic mistake in our effort to train the next generation for the workforce. But we didn't stop there. We didn't stop when the feeble believed themselves to be powerful. We actually gave them power. Each semester I taught at Farhearth, more and more clout was siphoned away from the faculty and funneled to the students. By the time I quit, the students wielded far more authority than the faculty did. And empowering anybody too early will cripple their intellectual development.

But the worst people to empower are those who perceive themselves to be exceptional. Because how many young pouzos indulging that delusion would refrain from abusing their power? At Farhearth, the answer turned out to be a slender minority. And it didn't take long for the faculty to grow fearful of the majority.

Early on, it was frustration, not fear, that vexed the faculty. Students in the lowest quintile became infected with a pathological apathy when they learned they could force any professor to advance them through the curriculum – no matter how poorly they performed – provided their tuition was paid. There is idleness in safety of that kind. And idle minds are strenuous to instruct. So the classroom gained a few hassles. Nothing immediately menacing, but unresolved hassles have a way of growing. And idleness wasn't an exception. For a couple of years, it was endemic to the lowest quintile, but it eventually began to spread like shepherds' fever. Until it reached pandemic proportions and Lower Licentiate education became an exercise in heaving lectures at unresponsive students.

The power discrepancy did not stop widening at this point. Soon, students towered over their faculty members. Once they realized it, the tyranny began. At that point, if a professor said anything that a student preferred not to hear, or imposed a challenge that a student would rather not face, that professor risked termination.

Aetheldorf wrote about this phenomenon decades before the second person observed it. In both *Aphorisms* and his *Treatise on Progeny*. And he was also the first victim of termination on the grounds of disagreeable publication. Decades before the second. He was uniquely abrasive, though. And much of his abrading was against the delicate reputations of Gaea's most affluent. And one must expect retaliation after slighting a hillian. But the termination of a Ranked Professor apparently came as a surprise to everyone in that post. When Thevro exerted its wealth, and it worked, it was a strike of dominance. Today, considerably smaller fortunes exert a similar amount of dominance: a single semester's tuition is sufficient to enforce servility among the faculty. I guess coppers spend as crowns these days.

During my last couple of years, I saw faculty being reprimanded for the most absurd reasons. And that changed their profession. The goal was no longer education, but preservation. How do I keep my job? Student satisfaction. How do I accomplish that? Do not disturb the students. And how do I accomplish *that*? Do not challenge them, do not overwhelm them with ideas, and most of all, do not encourage their betterment, because that would imply they are not already exceptional.

That's what it was like when I left. I'm told it's only gotten worse since then. Which brings us back to this afternoon:

Every exceptional grey-coated dunce has the ability to discharge Cyn, which would prevent us from further consultation. So I played nice. Even after his supratentorial diagnosis. Which he didn't come up with himself. He saw it in the chart. Then plagiarized it with the pomposity of an overlord.

I shook his hand and thanked him for his time. And began seeking someone with more humility. Humility – far more than power – is earned. It is a status that can only be achievable by actual accomplishment. I don't know what color it wears, but it's not grey. At least not here. So I waited and waited. Until I was able to meet with an old white coat. It was a woman with a tender expression. And in my experience, women take more notice of a patient's narrative than men do. They enter life with more empathy, and that makes them better listeners. Or so my bias has me believe. So I was at first relieved. But then I saw her amulet, and I hold a different bias about amulet wearers.

"Tell me about your experience here so far", she said, after noticing that she will be the tenth physician.

I did. And she listened.

After I had finished explaining all the reasons I was unhappy with the first nine physicians, she said, "I have a more holistic approach than those you've seen so far."

I have what I would describe as a holistic approach to holism, but I listened. Sincerely. Until her explanation of what ails Cyn took a turn for the magical. Or something close to magic. She was basically a sorceress. And her therapy involved crystals.

"Will you help me understand how you came to your diagnosis?", I asked.

"You're just going to have to trust my methods", she said. "What you don't realize is that diagnosis is every bit as much art as it is science."

Way too many physicians say this. None should. Because they clearly know less about art than they do about science. So they would do well to focus on the science part of their practice. Unfortunately, they don't learn real science at any point in their education either. They *think* they do. But training to be a surgeon or memorizing apothecarial applications doesn't teach you the scientific method any more than it makes you a credible astronomer.

I was polite. I smiled the whole time. But only with my mouth. And I held that expression as I took the bill and asked if Cyn could stay one more night.

The physician arranged for occupancy.

I thanked her, turned, and left.

My mouth stopped smiling as soon as I turned my back. I even shut my eyes as I released a sigh. But before I had finished exhaling, I ran into another physician. Physically. Because I was walking with my eyes closed.

I was still apologizing to him when the medical enchantress I had just seen left the room and walked past us.

"Was that the physician you just saw?", he asked.

"It was", I said, happy to stop apologizing.

"Did the treatment have something to do with rocks?"

"It did."

"Do you want me to take a look?"

"I do."

He did.

He didn't ask me any questions. But he did take a look. And then he declared his diagnosis. And wrote his prescription.

It may as well have been magic rocks.

I opened my mouth and took a long, deep breath in, exhibiting the universal gesture of, "I'm about to speak." But the physician interrupted before I could make use of my breath: "Diagnosis is like a game of regnavus", he said while putting his hand on my shoulder. "It's much more complex than you think."

Condescension aside, how is diagnosis anything like regnavus? One would never say "diagnosis is like a game of rowanoki", but that's the same thing. They even have the same number of pieces, the two games. The goal of both is seizure: you advance your commander to seize an opponent's home turf. What part of that resembles medical practice?

While these thoughts were quietly roiling inside of me, he gave me the bill. Number eleven. And I'm no closer to an answer than I was before the first.

I haven't heard of any of these physicians. None of them publish. None of them teach. No one I've seen has any esteem in the scientific community.

Where is everyone? Many of the best physicians in the world should be here. Why haven't I encountered any of them? Even in passing.

Maybe tomorrow. Although if tomorrow is anything like today and yesterday and every other day lately, it will be long and frustrating.

So I should try to get some sleep.

Seventy-Two

Eldos, Third Lufoa, Day Five. Morning.

I couldn't sleep last night. I was too frustrated. Most of the physicians won't listen to anything I say. But even if they did, they don't seem knowledgeable enough to be of any use. They have impressive vocabularies, but they don't know what they're saying.

By way of comparison, if you can recite the title of every book on Farhearth's shelves, and you've memorized a one-sentence summary for a thousand of them, but you've never read a page from any of them, you're not a scholar. You're a braggart. That seems to describe most physicians here.

In school, they had to memorize every organ's vessels, lobes, and chambers, every muscle, every protuberance on every bone. Hundreds of illnesses and corresponding medications. They learn the whole lexicon of a new language. And they memorize a thousand phrases. But they never learn any grammar. Because grammar isn't taught in the clinic. It's learned in the lab. And if you aren't in the lab, and you aren't reading the publications that come from it, you'll have no idea how to create an original sentence. Until these physicians know how bodies work, they can't diagnose anything that wasn't memorized in school.

Years after I admitted a fondness for dumplings, I published my first paper. And in conducting research, I had to read all the previous work in my area. With some of these diagnoses Cyn is receiving, I've read a hundred pages of study results, but I've never had a conversation about it. Because I've never practiced medicine (because neither of my Pendelhall auditions resulted in an appointment). The physicians seem to have the opposite set of experiences: they've never read a page, but they've had a hundred conversations. And they play to that strength. When I begin to question a diagnosis, I'm interrupted. "Actually, it's pronounced…", they interject about some word I just said… before I finish the sentence it was in. Apparently, my vowels were wrong. I've only seen the word in writing, so I'll trust their authority on the matter. But why does pronunciation matter at all? Why is it imperative that our mouth noises be exactly the same? Why are we prioritizing that over an understanding of physiology and chemistry and truth?

"Wouldn't a patient with Cedyl's syndrome typically have—"

"Actually, it's pronounced SEE-dill, not seh-dull."

How is that helpful? Its pronunciation has nothing to do with the patient. It's not a magical spell from a children's tale where the witch must incant it perfectly or it transforms the patient into a newt. It's an arbitrary word. Had I pronounced it kid-DILE, it would be just as irrelevant to Cyn's condition.

This is like astronomers who can only tell you the names of the constellations. They can't explain gravity or star formation or the properties of light. But they vaunt their knowledge of pointless names assigned to bundles of stars. As though it's important.

Interruptions of this kind – *actually, it's pronounced SEE-dill* – are assertions of dominance. Nothing more. And asserting oneself seems to be what these physicians do for a living. They prioritize reverence over patient outcomes. Which is why they refuse to be challenged.

It's not always corrections of pronunciation. Other common phrases include, "Why don't you let me be the physician?" and "Who has the medical degree?" Sometimes their dominance isn't masquerading as a question. "I'm the one with the medical degree", they assert. "You'll just have to trust my knowledge on this."

That's not how knowledge works, though. It can't be awarded in degree form. It must be learned. I don't care if the physician has two brains, each bigger than mine. If at least one of those brains didn't read the published reports on this subject, there's no way this subject could be known. Yet somehow, they know *everything*. Because they own a diploma. And that's what a diploma means: infinite knowledge forever.

I'll admit: one of the eleven physicians we've seen may have been correct. But no more than one. Because no two diagnoses are entirely compatible. Despite this, every physician is *certain*. And what happens when evidence contradicts their certainties? Do they reexamine their beliefs? Of course not. They just state them louder. To their credit, when the volume of their voices reaches a bitter barking, they continue to pronounce their fallacies flawlessly! And that's what *really* matters. Who cares about biology or healing or truth. Reverence is the profession. The physicians we've seen so far are just idols in a sanctuary. You may bow to them, but they're not to be disturbed.

Those who believe themselves too smart to read anything new have always endangered the devout. Just ask the corpses who were killed by filthy hands. Germ theory is widely accepted now. But what group was first to accept it?

Researchers. The last group? Physicians. Just a decade or so after fishermen. The facts convinced everyone but the physicians. In every other profession, the workers accepted the importance of clean hands when handling wounds and foods. Only physicians knew better. They were *certain* of it. That's why they wore the previous patients' blood proudly while operating on the next. What evidence finally came to light that convinced them to wash their hands? None. The physicians of that age never changed their minds. Those minds simply expired at death. They entered the grave still ridiculing the belief that infections were spread by "invisible monsters". The succeeding generation was taught different facts. That's how the final group of people came to accept germ theory. It's a phenomenon scientists refer to as "the funeral march of progress".

And today, much of what physicians continue to assert (with certainty) still collides head on with scientific facts.

That's been my experience so far. But the facts as they relate to Cyn remain a mystery to me. And this hospital is the only place where I have any chance at solving that mystery.

So I'm going to keep trying.

Seventy-Three

Eldos, Third Lufoa, Day Five. Afternoon.

I spent the entire morning trying to get an appointment. It's not a matter of money or availability. They just won't see me anymore. They see her chart and decline to meet. After several hours of pleading – occasionally begging, one instance of bribing – a white coat finally agreed to see Cyn.

He glanced at her quickly, and then declared conclusively, "it's head trauma."

"There was no trauma, though", I replied.

"So you *did* see her each second of every hour and minutes of each day!"

The phrasing was more bizarre than it was hostile. But it was a lot of both. And I didn't know how to reply to the hostility *or* the general weirdness. So, in the place of a verbal response, my face started assembling an expression of confusion.

He let the silence float in the air for several seconds, and then he popped it: "*Exactly*! It's head trauma."

Then he handed me the bill. Which was ludicrously expensive… for an encounter that couldn't have been more than a minute.

It took me three hours to get that appointment. And afterward, no amount of begging or bribing could persuade another physician to see Cyn. Until ten minutes before the hospital closed.

I was standing in the lobby. I may have been staring dejectedly into an abyss.

"Are you being helped?", a white coat asked.

"Not now."

"Do you need to be seen?"

"I'm not the patient. But the person I'm here with needs to be seen again."

"I'm available now. Why don't we have a look?"

The physician and I walked to Cyn's room. When we got there, she waved at a woman in a red coat, who hustled over. "Will you bring me the chart for this patient?", the physician asked.

As the red coat hustled away, the physician gave me a sympathetic look and said, "Why don't you tell me why she's here."

I started telling the story. But I had told it so many times in the last few days, the narrative had leaned out and taken on something of a five-act structure, typical of Eastern tales. The whole thing sounded rehearsed. Because it was. Twelve white coats worth of rehearsal beforehand. Not counting the greys. Still, it didn't sound authentic.

Her expression was difficult to interpret, but I'm pretty sure I could see doubt in her eyes.

It reminded me of a passage in Rouska's *Days of Sickness*. It goes something like this: Nearly all patients who have been sick for an extended period have learned to control their delivery in a manipulative way. Through repetition, they learn of the emotional floor one must rise above to get the attention of the practitioner. If they aren't tense and emotional enough, they're dismissed. So, they heighten the tension of their delivery. In the next encounter, they're more panicked. The situation is more urgent. When that proves insufficient, they increase the panic and urgency again. And again. In small increments. Until they finally get the attention of the practitioner. Unfortunately, in rising above the basement, they've crossed the ceiling, above which all patients are dismissed as having a fit of hysteria. Excepting those with enormous wealth, the ceiling is always lower than the floor.

While I was reflecting on this, the physician received Cyn's chart.

It was thick.

As she flipped through it, her mouth and brow joined her expression, which made it much easier to interpret: "You tricked me into seeing this patient." She refrained from voicing that accusation, but her face enunciated it clearly enough. I guess trickery is more effective than begging and bribing, but any deception was unintentional.

I tried to explain that: "There have been a lot of diagnoses… as you can see. But there doesn't seem to be any consensus… as you can *also* see. It makes me think there's still more to this case. More than what appears in her chart. That's why I'm so grateful you're willing to help."

She didn't respond. Not right away. Her face just reverted to its former shape of vague skepticism as she continued to skim Cyn's chart.

When she reached the last page, she stared at it for longer than it would take to read. The silence lingered. At first, it felt contemplative. Then it became awkward. Then it became tense.

I was about to speak again. I took an audible breath to do so. But before I had finished inhaling, the physician took an even deeper, louder breath. So, I bated mine. And waited.

And continued to wait.

Finally, she released her breath in the form of a long sigh, dropped the chart, looked up, held my eyes in a patronizing gaze, and said, "I think I can provide the consensus you're looking for."

She then explained her agreement with the previous diagnosis, but she added a seizure disorder. "That's what *caused* the head trauma", she concluded.

Although the addition of a cause may sound more plausible, it's less probable. Because it requires the previous diagnosis to be true (head trauma) in *addition* to a second diagnosis (seizure disorder). And two is not more likely than one.

A series of expressions began kneading themselves into my face. It started with a blank stare of passive denial. Then active denial. Then frustration. Then disappointment. Then sadness.

At no point did I respond.

I wasn't flustered by the improbability of the diagnosis, although it's close to impossible. What rattled my emotions was the association. That's exactly how Abendroth died. So when I was told the diagnosis, I was struck by an unexpected shock.

That's when I was handed the bill. My thirteenth. Without an answer.

I walked out of the room with an empty spirit. And no idea what to do next. So I gathered up all the prescriptions I'd been given, went to the apothecary, and purchased several of them. Some were for specific diagnoses that Cyn obviously doesn't have. So I ignored those. But anything that had a general application, I bought. Medications that mitigate *general* inflammation or ease *general* pain or help with tissue regeneration... *in general*. I bought those.

Then I left the hospital and went wandering. Past the College of Language and Literature. And the great storm pole towering amid its old, stately bricks. Past the College of Law and Governance. And the Farhearth High Court that resides beside it. Past the library. And the quiet cemetery sprawling behind it. Across all six of Farhearth's boroughs, the percentage of cemetery real estate allocated to medical malpractice is stunning. If physicians don't start learning science soon, we're going to run out of graveyard acreage in my lifetime.

If we don't understand the methods of science – the theory, research design, and mathematics of analysis – we cannot comprehend the medical literature that advances it. If we fail to advance along with it, our beliefs and abilities will lay dormant. After a decade of dormancy, we become obsolete, and an obsolete physician is a threat to the public's health... as I have experienced firsthand.

Those were my thoughts on my walk around campus. Which eventually led to the Square, where I sat on the stone ledge and stared into the crowd with a kind of hollow-hearted apathy that's only accessible to the newly hopeless.

The fragile positivity I had been protecting so dearly these past few days finally shattered.

I didn't blink. Or sniff. Or make any sound at all. Tears just appeared on my face. As though a levee flooded over without breaking, spilling silently down the slope.

Some tears were for Cyn, some were for Abendroth, and others were for me, forever stuck between my two losses.

I don't know how long I sat there. But I know the sun was in a different spot in the sky when I was interrupted. By Herrin. Whom I hadn't seen in years.

I didn't recognize him at first. Or acknowledge him when he sat beside me. I just assumed he was a stranger trespassing into my personal space. So, I ignored him. Until he spoke. In that unmistakable Herrinian tone that gently explores your chest until it finds the calmest chambers to resonate in.

And I was instantly pulled out of my daze. In a very soothing way. Although I was surprised that he recognized me. We don't usually recognize people outside of the contexts in which we expect to encounter them. And there's no way Herrin expected to see me sitting on the wall, plumbing the deepest, darkest places of my daze. But I'm so glad he did.

I spent the next hour explaining why I was here, sitting alone in the Square. And he spent that hour listening attentively. In a way that only Herrin can. It's a kind of attention that doesn't patronize or sympathize. It just joins you wherever you are. And treats you as the most important thing in all of Gaea. For as long as you remain in his company.

Once I had finished recounting my entire story, he told me he would do what he can to help. He still has some authority on campus. Some favors that can be called in. And he would do that calling. "But you should get some rest for now", he said. Then we agreed to meet for breakfast tomorrow morning. Here. In the Square. "I'll let you know then if I've managed to arrange any help", he said.

So now I'm back in my room at the inn. With a little bit of my hope restored.

Seventy-Four

Eldos, Third Lufoa, Day Five. Night.

I had planned to rest for the evening. But I was too restless. I tried pacing, walking circles around my room. But it didn't accelerate the passage of time. So I aimed my pacing abroad, wandering around campus, looking at familiar sites. That worked for a while. Then, as the novelty wore off, it worked less. So now I'm writing. Which is working so far.

While I was out, I realized the hospital isn't the only building that has a new name. My old academic building is now called Reder Hall. It used to be the "Life Sciences Building". Those utterly uncreative and plainly explicit letters were etched into the stone edifice above the front doors. Faded by time, they were difficult to read. But the building wore its name like stately grey hair. Now, the once-dignified edifice wears a cheap wig. It's been bricked over. And chiseled boldly into those cheap bricks are the words: Reder Hall.

I have no idea who Reder is, but I dislike him already. It seems reasonable to assume it's a him. A rich and unaccomplished him. Because what else but insecurity could motivate anyone to carve their name so deeply into anything? And who else would be so driven by insecurity but a contemptable elder son whose only accomplishment is inheritance?

Maybe I'm being too hard on this fellow. Perhaps the eponym honors some old, dead professor whose scientific contributions merit his immortalization. Although I doubt it. Because I can name every notable professor in my field. And there's no "Reder" on that roster.

Granted, I'm less familiar with the lists of legends outside of the apothecarial and natural sciences. I'm sure there are hundreds of influential historians and humanitarians I've never heard of. And people from every other discipline, from geology to theology and everything in between. So maybe Reder was a great litigator who spent every penny he had defending the disadvantaged. Or maybe he was a great liturgical scholar who united some warring faiths. Or maybe he's a contemporary astronomer being hailed as the next Elsiel. "The first cartographer of the sky!" or some such designation.

Although I doubt all of those. Because why would a life sciences building be named after a notable figure in a totally different field? That's why I suspect Reder is an insecure inheritor of a substantial family fortune.

When I was a student, half of Farhearth's buildings had plain, perfect names. Alchemical Laboratory. Conservatory of Music. Historical Studies Building. Statistics House. And so on. The other half had names that made no sense unless you knew the history. Some were references to old, natural landmarks. Birchwood Block was built out of sapstone where the birch woods once grew. And Sapstone Hall was built out of birch wood atop the old Sapstone Hill... after excavating all the stones. I was given similar explanations when I asked why Woodbridge was made of stone and Stonebridge was made of wood. The remaining buildings were named after obsolete cartographical locations. Thirty-Seven North. Thirty-Two East. And so on. While these names were confusing, they had character. Relics of a rich history.

"Reder Hall" has no such character. This is just a rich person *erasing* history. Or, in the case of "Life Sciences Building", erasing clarity.

The sale of building names is a relatively new form of fundraising. The first one sold was the Archive of the Regnalects and the Contralects on the Law and Governance campus. A small but historic facility. With an unimaginative but intuitive name. In exchange for an undisclosed sum of money, it was plastered over and replaced with "Bowan Gallery".

I was a faculty member at the time. Lots of my colleagues protested. I didn't, but I *was* opposed. On an emotional basis. Nothing so serious as nostalgia, as I had never entered that building. But there's a sanctity of memory that can sometimes be conflated with sentimentality. And that was the basis of my opposition. I just didn't want history to change. I don't mind the future undergoing great transformation, but I want my past to remain the same. And I still feel that way today. Which is why I refused to enter "Reder Hall".

Instead, I visited the library, one of few remaining landmarks that has yet to be sullied by vanity. It is still called, simply, "The Library".

It does have another name – Grogador – but that name predates "Farhearth". It's a vestige from the guild days. And it's worn like an elegant gown: rarely. On very special occasions, the banners might be hung, honoring its history, but every other day, it's just The Library.

I went in through the P.O.C. entrance. That's the wing of the building where scholastic equipment can be rented. It's basically a giant, staffed closet with one door to the outside and one door to the inside. As if to say: "we prefer you to come and go through the service quarters since you're not *really* part of the library... but in case of an emergency, here's a backdoor to Grogador."

I didn't recognize the person working. It seemed to be a student employee. But when I looked at the staff board, I saw Risha's name on it.

"When does Risha get in?", I asked.

The student worker didn't respond. She just pointed to a smaller board, which had everyone's schedules listed. Three days until Risha's next shift.

I suspect we'll be gone by then. But I wrote the schedule down anyway.

Then I left the library and wandered around campus for a while, observing the behavior of the crowds. The people here are similar to those at Pendelhall in that they can be divided into the same three classes: residents, tourists, and sentimentalists. But those in that last group were failing to find familiarity in the radically changed landscape. "It used to be right here" or "I could have sworn it was over there", they would say to their companions. The memories they cherish are of a vanished world. At Farhearth, maps mark a point in time every bit as much as they mark a point in space. One can never really return. But everyone still tries. They graduate, embark on a long hike, far from home, and never stop looking back, over their shoulders, at where they came from. Making sure they don't get lost along the way. And just like every other hike, they ultimately return to where they came from. Except here, they find their world changed.

When I got tired of watching the sentimentalists, I started reading the posters. There were a lot of them. More than I'd ever seen. Some were advertising the upcoming faire. I saw a second *Wanted* poster for the "Singing Sisters". And there were election posters everywhere. Most belonged to the current mayor… whom everyone should vote against. As a demonstration that the public's ballot doesn't matter. These elections are pointless pageantry.

It would save a lot of time and paper if the office were simply given to the richest candidate. Bonstan, would you like to be mayor of every city in the world simultaneously? Just say the word!

To date, Bonstan has never said that word. Probably because he can exert greater influence by *not* serving.

But if I *were* a voter looking at these posters, I would have no idea what I'm voting on. Mayors and measures alike. The posters provide no information. They tell me exactly what my vote should be and then fill the rest of the space with vague words such as *change!* and *progress!*, neither of which means "good".

After reading a dozen posters, and listening to the lobbying of the grass grads, the only thing I learned is that political campaigning has become a particularly pernicious form of romantic courting. Seductive promises are freely given, seedy flaws are carefully hidden... until the knot is tied. Then you're stuck. And prenuptial flattery does not promise a thriving marriage any more than successful campaigning ensures a thriving economy.

The Science Faire posters weren't much more informative. They were only advertising the Inventor's Faire half of it. Nothing about the dissemination of recent experimental evidence. While that's what has always interested me, I realize the average passersby would be more enticed by illustrations of air and submarine travel. That's what the posters were of. Which doesn't mean either mode of travel will be there. They've been aspiring to debut both since I was born. Since my parents were born, actually. I wouldn't be surprised if their parents came to the faire expecting to see underwater and overair ships. Despite the decades of elaborate art, no such ships exist. Most inventions are just a bunch of shiny garbage. Yet somehow, people continue to get excited.

While standing at one of the posters, I listened to a student talk about how gold is going to be worthless now. "Because the alchemists can convert pretty much anything into it." This was met by an argument that alchemists figured that out a long time ago. "That's where Bonstan got all of *his* gold!"

Conspiracies of this kind reveal a lack of understanding of what alchemy is. For some reason, people still think it's a secret assembly of robed warlocks with long beards who incant spells over nuggets of copper and iron. It's not.

Half of them are Laberi for some reason, but all of them are scientists with Magister's Degrees in Apothecarial and Natural Sciences performing tedious biochemical work. They use completely normal biological means to induce chemical changes. For food. For medicine. And once upon a time, for war.

It was alchemists who made Farhearth's archers the most feared on Gaea. They used puffers to generate a potent toxin to coat the tips of their arrows. It wasn't even those quasi-mystical puffers that wash up on the Eldsyn shore once a decade with the bladder that's forty feet across. They were using the common one-footers that inhabit the strait. If their diet is right, a chemical reaction will occur in the gut, which synthesizes the poison. Kept in a clean aquarium, they won't produce it. But alchemists were able to artificially manipulate the captive environment to maximize synthesis of the toxin. And harvest it. And paint thousands of arrowheads with it. Today, this is illegal. Just like the iron berserker... which was devised by alchemists in Midrodor.

The point is: whether for war or medicine or food, alchemy is not magic. Nor is it about gold. Or any other metallurgy. It's much more about feces.

Those Magisterian Laberi scientists oversee the conversion of one substance (often an ingested substrate) into another (the excreted product).

Our excrement may not be good for much, but yeast's sure is. And the same is true for lots of other critters.

"I heard the serious alchemists quit doing metallic conversions a while ago", one of the poster-side students said. "What they're all chasing today is the *apotheosis* of alchemy. Transmuting sin into sanctity!"

At that point, I sighed and returned to the inn.

Now it's time for bed.

Seventy-Five

Seros, Third Lufoa, Day Six. Morning.

It's Departure Day. The hospital is open, but most businesses are closed.

I'm going to meet Herrin at the hospital soon. I don't know what to expect. All I can do is hope for something different. I've seen thirteen white coats and received nothing but disappointment. And bills. Lots of bills.

If anyone can make a difference, it's Herrin. There are few faculty as capable, and none more compassionate. He's half the reason I quit Farhearth.

In the early days – both as a student and as a young faculty member – Arzox tested my patience. I just wanted Lylir to come. Not for the usual reasons: Arzox skies are grey, and its branches are barren, while Lylir brings Gaea her blues and yellows and greens. That's nice. But what I really looked forward to was Lylir's *semester*. So I could resume my academic routine. There are no classes during Arzox. The whole school – at least the academy part of it – shuts its doors and shutters, boards up for the long night.

In the middle days of my faculty role, I stopped looking forward to the return. At least not in an eager way. We can all see the future ahead, but I no longer awaited Lylir's routine with excitement. Arzox and Lamenting were enjoyed.

In the later days, I looked forward to breaks and dreaded their ending. But I wouldn't have quit over that. I still had hope that conditions would change. The students, the resources, the environment. I retained hope that it would all be restored.

Even back then, Herrin was the most caring and capable faculty member in any of the nine colleges. And the most loyal to the institution. If anyone was going to renovate Farheath's crumbling integrity, it was him.

He used to walk to campus. He didn't live particularly close, but he walked. On the way, he would pass the place where I was staying. Just before sunrise, I would see him. Then, just after dusk, I'd see him again on his way home. Every day, he toiled more hours than the sun did. And he was delighted to do it. That delight was visible in his gait and posture. On his way to work, he stood taller than his biological height, and no amount of candy has ever made a child step as briskly.

When the bell tower tolls the end of the day, Estevro children race from their schoolhouses with more vitality than a hooked fish fleeing against the line. Yet compared to Herrin's headed-to-work enthusiasm, those boys and girls appear listless.

Then, hours after Herrin's last class, as the night was shading the landscape, he would begin his walk home. His pace had slowed – the carriages could now keep up with him – but his spine was still propped up with satisfaction, contented by his day's contribution.

Since the founding of Farhearth, there has never been a purer professor.

That was in my early days. And in my middle days. But at some point during my later days, his pace and posture changed. There came a semester where pure glee stopped passing my window just before sunrise.

If Herrin were a stranger to me, it would have looked like an ordinary walk to campus. Just like everyone else. An ordinary height. An ordinary stride. At an ordinary hour. But he wasn't a stranger. And that ordinary walk was hard to watch.

The semester after that, his campus commute was an after-breakfast amble. And during his still-light-out walk home, he stood taller. As though his spine had just been unburdened.

It's hard to imagine how much disrespect it took to deflate the enthusiasm of someone that committed. But Farhearth administrators accomplished it. And they were my employer too. And Adon knows I had no ability to reverse the hurtling downfall. If anyone could set the university right, it was Herrin. But when I saw the changing of his gait, I knew hope was a fool's dream. And when our heroes lose their hope, that's a reasonable time for us common folk to quit. So, I did. But Herrin didn't. He's still showing up. Still trying. Not for hope's sake, but because no true Ryndor captain would ever abandon a sinking boat.

That's Herrin's relationship with Farhearth. It's the most honorable one I've ever known. Someday, I'm sure he'll finally retire. And return to Midrodor. That's where he was born. The land of soft-spoken heroes. The spirit of that city lives in his bones.

But for now, while he's still here, I'm off to meet him for breakfast. I'll find out if he still has enough power to make a difference in Cyn's medical care.

Seventy-Six

Seros, Third Lufoa, Day Six. Afternoon.

I met with Herrin. We planned to have breakfast. But everywhere was closed. When Departure Day falls on a Seros, it's difficult to find an open business. Fortunately, hospitals seldom abide by holiday standards. Although it was only half staffed.

On the way there, Herrin said, "I have an appointment set up, but it's not for another hour." We spent that hour in the cafeteria.

Then I met the physicians who would be working with Cyn. Two of them: Cliwen and Kara. It's a married couple. They work as a team. Always have. And they're two of the most renowned physicians at Farhearth. There are countless conditions and treatments named after them. Half the discoveries in the last two decades wear one of their eponyms in the medical dictionaries.

I'd heard of them both – having read much of their work – but I'd never met either of them. When I was at Farhearth, they rarely taught, and they took on few patients. They were primarily researchers. These days, they apparently *never* teach or treat patients. Unless the need is great. Or the favor is greater. But everyone seems to owe Herrin a favor. Even the great Cliwen and Kara.

They came to the cafeteria to meet us and discuss a plan for Cyn's diagnosis. On its own, this revealed humility. Most physicians wouldn't discuss *anything* outside of their diagnostic throne room. And they certainly wouldn't discuss scheduling. Being asked to do the work of a brown coated scullion would be an insult to a white coated sovereign.

Cliwen and Kara weren't wearing coats of any color. They were dressed in normal human clothes. And at no point did they declare themselves to be different from the rest of the physicians, which tells me they actually *are* different. Half the physicians we've seen so far have referred to themselves as "against the grain" during our appointments. But what they really are is against the facts. Because the facts are unknown to them. They boast of their honed skepticism, but they only distrust information they have yet to learn. And accordingly, they refuse to learn it. Their behemoth egos are confined to such tiny parochial cages. Learning and self-betterment are difficult in that kind of captivity.

If you really want to be against the grain in medicine, learn science. And then behave like a scientist: devise a theory, then attempt to prove yourself wrong. By comparison, Farhearth physicians try to prove themselves right to justify their decisions, straining their ingenuity to concoct believable support for the unsupportable.

Their diagnoses and explanations *are* believable, though. In the way that all fiction tends to be. Freed from the constraints of fact, it can be presented in simple, understandable terms. Whenever a physician tells a perfectly clear and tidy tale, it's safe to assume it's false. Because real biology is complicated. Fiction is easier to believe. So that's the medium of medicine. It's decisive. It's authoritative. And it's populated by people who are unafraid of mistakes. As long as they're never obliged to admit one. And they never have to apologize to a patient or suffer the grief of a job poorly done.

From what I knew about Cliwen and Kara, this was not a problem I'd have. And after meeting them, I'm even *more* encouraged. They're taking the case seriously. And taking my concern and input seriously as well. When I met the previous physicians, it was obvious they had been told "what I'm like", and that colored our interactions. Not Cliwen and Kara. They were more interested in my account than anything in Cyn's chart. All they needed to know about the other physicians is whether any of their treatments had been administered.

They were relieved to hear the answer was no.

"Did you want to read the chart anyway?", I asked. "In case there's a useful test result or something in there?"

"We'll be doing our own tests. All the chart would do is bias our thinking", Kara replied. "Now, walk me through the trip from Estevro to Pendelhall. Step by step. Tell me everything you remember."

I did. And then I explained the tournament, the ceremony afterward, and every day since. Cliwen and Kara each took their own set of notes that was at least double the length of Cyn's entire chart.

When I had run out of things to say, they put down their pens and explained how they would move forward with the case. They would be approaching it in two parts. First, they would each gather as much evidence as they could. Independently. They would not consult the other until they had each settled on a diagnosis. Then they would come together. To discuss.

If their diagnoses perfectly concurred, they would accept the answer. But if they came to different conclusions – even about the tiniest detail – they would undertake a comprehensive, systematic debate. The way they described it resembled how the legal system works at Farhearth. After "Publications", where each team gathers evidence, the two square off in the "Pali vin Galu", where they attempt to outargue the other.

"This is a focused endeavor", Cliwen said. "We can't have any distractions or disruptions. So, at this point, we will kindly ask you to leave the hospital and return tomorrow. Late morning at the earliest."

"Actually, make it early afternoon", Kara said. And Cliwen agreed.

Herrin and I stood up, shook their hands, thanked them before letting go, and then we left.

"You haven't been on campus lately. Would you like a tour of the changes?", Herrin asked on our way out.

"I can't think of a better distraction. But only if you have the time to spare."

He reminded me that it was Departure Day. On a Seros. "What else is there to do?"

We spent a few hours strolling around the university. Much of it was familiar. Other parts were unrecognizable.

Farhearth still pretends to be three institutions in one. They're still using the same triangle emblem. Education, Advancement, and Sport. Really though, instruction (education) and research (advancement) are connected. Faculty teach the subjects they study. I always encountered questions and limitations in the classroom that informed my research. And my research informed my instruction. I think it's more reasonable to see it as a two-institution school: there's the academy, which is responsible for all education and advancement, and then there's athletics, in which young adults play with balls. And the two institutions meet in no middle. No relationship at all but for proximity and finances.

While I taught here, I saw athletics gradually isolating itself from the academy. Every year, a starker and starker division was created between the two. And still today, they seem to be steadily separating. Mitosis of a kind. The student athletes can scarcely attend classes anymore owing to overlapping schedules, and the athletics personnel refuse to collaborate with the researchers.

This seems unsustainable for athletics, given that they bring in no money. Tuition pays for their budget in full. And the costs are not negligible. It's a strain long felt by the faculty. Like rearing a child who grew into an adult but never became independent. And those costs seem to get bigger every year. Everyone knows athletics would collapse the day it emancipated itself from its benefactor. So they don't. They *operate* independently, but they syphon oxygen from the blood of the host. That's how it worked when I was here, and from what Herrin showed me this morning, it still works that way today. The only new construction anywhere belonged to athletics. There were fields and buildings and monuments cropping up everywhere. But the only notable change in the academy itself was decay.

Also, the cats are still there. The feral cats. Every one of them as skittish as a finch. Impossible to touch. Back when I was a student, they went around spraying every piece of nature so if you tried to smell the aroma of a magnolia or lilac, you got a noseful of cat piss instead. But there was one cat that worse than all the rest. In grotesqueness, he had no peer.

You know when an animal is so utterly ugly people mistake it for being cute? This cat was even uglier than that. And it was fooling no one. That bulbous, swollen-shouldered, bandy-legged, scowling catball couldn't go five seconds without squirting stinky pheromone onto something formerly lovely.

Drop for drop, I doubt there's ever been a raincloud that could compete with its urethra. At some point, I named the creature "Hideous Gross Thing" and it caught on. At least among my friends and colleagues.

When I saw the feral cat den, I looked for Hideous Gross Thing, but I didn't see it. That probably means it is no longer among us. May it rest in peace. Decomposition surely made its form less grotesque, so I know the world it left behind has seen its peace enhanced.

As Herrin and I were walking by the cat corner, I saw someone I recognized. She was sitting on a stump, reading a book, surrounded by the skittish ferals. Which were rubbing against her legs and meowing.

Her face was immediately familiar, but I couldn't recall how I knew her. So, I didn't approach her. Herrin and I just kept walking. But then Herrin was stopped by a group of students. A whole classroom worth. All of whom had very important questions.

"Professor Herrin!", they chanted asynchronously.

As Herrin answered them, I stared off into space and tried to remember how I knew that young woman on the stump.

"What is her *name*?", I whispered to myself several times. And the answer remained hidden.

Then it occurred to me: it's because I don't know her name. I forgot to ask. That was the woman who escorted us to the "Fentin Infirmary" after I asked for directions to the Commons Hospital. The kind, gentle one who jumped when I spoke.

That must have been on Lyros. Earlier this week. It feels like a month ago.

Once I had solved the mystery of the familiar stump sitter, I returned my attention to Herrin. And I heard him radiating compassion to each student. In the way that he always does. You can practically capture the gushing of his warmth on a thermometer.

The students, though. Their smiles were like garlok ears. Any kindness was a ruse. Or at least that was true for a couple of them. The rest were polite. But you're more affected by the impolite ones. In this case, the impolite two. As those two turned from Herrin's sight, their expressions quickly curdled. Their faces were unclothed of all glee and only a naked bitterness remained.

But, again, all the others seemed perfectly lovely.

Every one of us is filled with benevolence and enmity, prejudice and empathy, truth and hypocrisy. And it requires constant effort to nurture the kinder natures in ourselves.

The equation can be balanced on either side. Older generations seemed to work harder on suppressing their less wholesome inclinations, as opposed to overemphasizing their wholesomest. You don't see them smiling theatrically at every passerby. But nor do they scowl behind their backs.

But the smile before the scowl is the worst. It's not as much a smile as it is a docile exhibition of their teeth. And an inch behind that expression festers prejudice and enmity. Then they turn their heads from visibility and their lips slither back over their incisors.

But what could have caused such indignance? Is it because they didn't quite understand what they thought they did? Or they had some extra work to do? Extra pages to read? Extra self-betterment to enact?

They have been victimized! They don't see themselves as crybabies; they see themselves as martyrs. Let their cause be known.

Again, all the others seemed perfectly lovely. They just escape your memory quicker. Because they don't deliberately haunt you.

Although I must admit, neither of this morning's students was anywhere near as egregious as that violet-draped queen bee I saw on the day we arrived.

The one with the gaping void where empathy should be.

That's how far my mind had rambled – beginning with the kind cat woman and ending with the cruel hornet – when I heard Herrin say, "I can be there in ten minutes. You go on ahead."

Then he turned to me. Which cast a sudden light on my mind's unsupervised wandering. And I realized I have some of my own compassion to work on if I want to live up to Herrin's standard.

"Something has come up", he said. And then he explained that he needs to take care of some things.

"Even on Departure Day?", I asked. "On a Seros, no less?", I finished.

He smiled. I smiled. Both genuine. Then we said our temporary farewells, having agreed to meet for breakfast tomorrow.

Now I'm back at the inn.

On the way here, I stopped to see Rorrik. He wasn't there, so I left a note.

Which he must have seen. Because he just arrived.

Seventy-Seven

Seros, Third Lufoa, Day Six. Night.

The newsletter about the Pendelhall tournament was published. It celebrated all the tournament winners, but mostly fencing. On the front page, there was a large drawing of the tournament winner. Beside it, there was a description of his physique and fighting style. Just like my front-page paragraph so many years ago, the writer made a comparison to an animal. Unlike my front-page experience, this year's winner wasn't disgraced by that comparison.

Dwarves were handled insensitively, though. And it went on about pianos and ships in an absurd way. The whole paragraph was whimsical fairytaling in the place of real reporting. I get the impression news is no longer read by the public unless it is sufficiently entertaining. At that point, if there's still room for truth, you can squeeze some in... but not too much.

Here's what was written beside the depiction of this year's fencing winner:

Styravesa's stride is long, and seldom minded, so his knees are scarred with the punctures of dwarf teeth. Styravesa's hands are broad; they span two piano octaves, but he knows no instrument and he settles every quarrel with fists. So, they're as scarred as his knees. Styravesa's back is as straight as the mast of a Ryndor ship and vast as a full-wind sail; standing at full height, he blots out the sun like an eclipse. And Styravesa's attack is as fierce as a mighty hymog; each swing connects with the power of a felling crack.

That was it. Word for word. I guess "dwarf teeth" is marginally better than children's teeth. I wonder how many alternative populations were considered before the author committed to that one.

The article itself was longer. That's just what was said on the first page. Which is the only page I read. Which concluded with the animal comparison. I'm not saying a hymog is the most graceful or regal creature out there, but it's better than a hairless nihox.

Now that I'm thinking about it, the nihox would have been a better depiction of Styravesa than me. Purely on matters of physical resemblance.

His stature may not have been blotting out any suns, but it was impressive. Although I still think I could have won in a hymogian clash of our swords.

Maybe I'm overestimating myself. I'm not saying I would have won. He's a good foot taller than me. Definitely has me on reach. But I would bet the horse from the carriage that I could *heave* with more might. And I might have stood a chance had we faced each other, given that heaving was his primary strategy. But I doubt I would have made it that far. The opponent pairings determine much of the rankings. There's no way I could have bested Rorrik that day, and bad luck would have probably paired us early.

In the end, beating Rorrik is a front-page feat no matter the circumstances. Styravesa earned it.

Also, had he lost, it would be Rorrik's likeness on the cover of the newsletter. And there would be people pointing and swarming and accosting. Having a sailboat giant with knee bites on the cover permitted Rorrik and me to stay relatively invisible. Which permitted us to spend the evening watching and listening to the chattering students.

Some were patient and contemplative, but others spoke with such urgency. Despite having nothing to say. It was like the conversational equivalent of young Harthy lutists. Those parading novices whose notes come so quickly – squeezing eight of them into every bar – but they say so little. Desperate to outplay the Laberi, they only betray their insecurity.

I become more averse to this every year. I see it in writing, too. I'm presented with enormous paragraphs of tiny thoughts, and I find them painful to read. But in speech, it's even worse. It feels like the inverse of an eating contest. How many empty calories can you *expel* in ten minutes?

We did run into a couple of familiar faces while we were out.

First: Ariem. The cat woman. I remembered to ask for her name this time. She was at the eatery where Rorrik and I went for dinner. Municipal Grocery. It was the one eatery that was open.

We approached, I reintroduced myself, and we sat near her. She was sitting in front of a gigantic tome, struggling to read its faded and damaged pages while taking sporadic swigs from a mug of lavender tea. It was her third cup. She volunteered that information after I solicited her advice on what to order. Her fourth cup arrived shortly after. And I watched her dissolve so many granulated seasonings into it that the water level rose.

"I saw you earlier today", I said. "On the other side of campus. With a bunch of cats."

"I saw you, too. You had some cats of your own."

I didn't remember interacting with any cats. My confused look said as much.

"You couldn't see them. Because cats are sneaky like that. And they're nosy. And sometimes they're curious. So they'll follow you. And sneak wherever you go. They must have found you interesting."

I didn't know how to respond, so I asked, "Are any of them your pets?"

"I don't think cats can be pets. From their perspective. But I do feed them. And at breakfast, most of them bring me gifts."

"What do they bring you?"

"Whatever they think I want. Usually, it's leaves. Probably because they see me looking at trees so much."

"Can you look at money and train them to fetch it for you?", I asked.

"There's no controlling cats. Where they *should* be doesn't determine where they go. And what they take isn't up to me. I just accept the gifts, whatever they are. And then I feed them."

"Do you have a favorite?"

"I don't have a favorite, but I've been spending the most time with Moibel."

"Which one is that?"

"The really scrangly one", she said. And I think I knew what she meant. She went on to explain that she's knitting him booties because his feet had been hurt in an accident. And she has no experience knitting, so it's been difficult, but she's committed to making booties that will fit him.

There's an old Western expression I learned from Rorrik that applies here: "Nursing the fly."

Literally, it describes someone who's nursing a fly back to health. Which will probably die of old age in a period of hours anyway. But as a figure of speech, it's about people pouring themselves into pointless things.

I always find it sad, but in a tender way.

Listening to Ariem talk about the scrangly cat booties felt like that. It was so heartrending, I couldn't listen anymore, so I changed the subject. "What are you reading?", I asked while pointing at her book.

She was studying botany. She described it for a minute. Her tone revealed that she empathizes with nature as if born of and bound to it.

Then the food came. Which ended the conversation. Rorrik and I were too busy eating to speak.

When we were done, we thanked Ariem for the company, excused ourselves, and started our walk back to the inn. And the stables. Rorrik is still sleeping in the wagon.

Along the way, we ran into the *other* familiar student: the bragger boy with the bracelets. Except he wasn't wearing bracelets this time. Plenty of other jewelry. Just no bracelets.

"A year's worth of food for the average Harthy", he said to his coterie in a tone that rivaled Lanko's conceit. We missed the context, but after he said it, he twisted a ring on his pinky. Rorrik and I exchanged a look. The same look we would have exchanged upon hearing a Lanko victory speech.

Then Sir Pinky Ring managed to outdo his own conceit: "And I bought *two*. In case I ever lose one."

Rorrik and I exchanged a second look. It was the same one we would have exchanged had Lanko's victory been in a rigged match against the creature from Thorn.

"Lanko has put the Nightmare Incarnate to sleep! He has set famine upon the seeds of the Sower of Cruelty! He cut the head from the Thief of Life slithering in the grass! The Giver of Death has been given death at last!"

That's the best I could do. Lanko would do much better. But it turns out Sir Pinky Ring can do *even better*.

He displayed his unparalleled pomposity with what he bragged about next: his sword. The same sword as last time, I think. The legendary one that's imbued with the spirit of its maker or some such nonsense.

After he swung it around with the bungling flamboyance of The Boy King, he said, "The ghost of a rogue couldn't pilfer with as much grace."

Then the boy – who owns not one but *two* groceries-for-a-year pinky rings – told a story – the most boastful tale I've ever heard – about how he stole it… from a family of modest means… who would have never parted with it.

After mocking their finances, he said, "But no lock, coffer, or hiding place is safe from the likes of me." Then he unloosed another uncoordinated flurry of attacks on the air.

Stealing from those with lesser means is just cruel. I guess that's how society has always functioned. But the rich don't usually boast about their thievery. They pretend everyone benefits. "It's good for *society* that I hold this position of power" or "my wealth feeds so many mouths" or "If it weren't for me, there would be twenty fewer employees in the East." All hillians pretend to have accrued their wealth honestly. And to be using it ethically. That's ugly, but it's not *as* ugly as a rich kid bragging about stealing from the poor. Which is nowhere near as ugly as *how* this kid was bragging. He's smarter, swifter, more cunning and courageous than Lanko has ever claimed to be.

In my experience, humility is the sign of real heroism, meekness a common trait of the mighty, while arrogance is how the oblivious reveal their oblivion. Just peruse the history of every continent. Examples abound.

The inventors of the iron berserker put considerable effort into downplaying its importance, while the smith who designed the dastard's dagger (I'm sorry, the "Sun's Sword") proclaimed it "a pivotal moment for civilization!"

The people who boast about their skills are never the ones who possess them. If they did, they'd understand how much of a burden talent is, and they'd try to conceal it. In the interest of energy conservation. The moment people discover you have a useful set of skills, the requests for your time multiply like an invasive species.

Expectations of this kind are the tribulations of the talented. It's a rare curse to be blessed with. And this bedazzled sword thief has no such curse. That's why he has the free time to boast. And he thinks it makes him look fancy. Elite. Respectable. But none of that can be bought. Despite all his wealth, dignity is a bauble he'll never wear.

Seventy-Eight

Aldos, Third Lufoa, Day Seven. Morning.

It's early. Darkly early. But the moon is once again nearing its full bloom. So one candle is sufficient for me to write.

I fell asleep without too much trouble. Satisfaction is a much better sedative than frustration. But anticipation is a mighty expergefactor. So here I am, writing in the candlelight. And the moonlight.

I think Cliwen and Kara are going to have the answer I've been looking for. They each have two terminal degrees. Cliwen is a physician and apothecarist. Apothecarist first, physician second. Similarly, Kara was an herbalist first and became a physician second. If my experience so far has taught me anything, it's that narrow education begets narrowminded physicians. And this is not a limitation that applies to Cliwen and Kara. I can't imagine a two-person team with a more comprehensive background. I'm familiar with their work in numerous disciplines. They're cobbling the frontier in all three divisions of medicine. And based on our conversation yesterday, they don't perceive any division or discipline as better or worse than others. Diagnoses are only accurate or inaccurate; prescriptions are only appropriate or inappropriate. There are some patients who are best treated by a physician over the other branches, just as there are patients who are best treated by an herbalist or apothecarist. Despite this, the latter two divisions are commonly regarded as sub-physician in their standing.

In part, herbalists have a reputation for ingesting and smoking their own inventory. And every apothecary has a record of "misplacing" medicines that are not authorized for public provision. But at least neither of these classes has ever bled a patient to death. Which physicians still do at least monthly.

Excepting extraordinary blood pressure or excesses of iron or red blood cells, I can't think of a condition that could be palliated by a bloodletting. Yet its practice has not fallen from favor. Acne? Convulsions? Fever? Gout? Indigestion? Pneumonia? Shepherds' fever? Nothing we can't treat with a little venesection. Fetch me my thumb lancet!

I understand where this belief came from. Cyn and I studied it extensively. Aloxa adle – "the first disease" – was reported in Roden's Compendia to be cured by "breathing the patient's vein until unflushed."

The reasoning was reasonable for the time. Roden observed that menstrual pains were always relieved following blood loss. This elimination of blood must therefore be a natural defense mechanism, purging the noxious agent. If not *all* of it, at least enough for the body to neutralize the rest on its own. "The fairer sex appears more susceptible to lunar toxicity; fittingly, she hath developed a conduit for expulsion", he wrote.

When Roden noticed the onset of aloxa adle and menstruation had a similar presentation of symptoms, he tested his theory. And it apparently worked. "After three days, the bled patient hath regained her color, and the pale pallor never encircled her throat."

Today, aloxa adle is assumed to be shepherds' fever. Roden's description of the symptoms and their time course both match. Cramping precedes the pale wreath by several days. And once the wreath appears, survival is unlikely. Especially if you're short on blood.

In the years since Roden, we've learned that blood functions as a medium. Just like paper, it enables the book to be written. To ensure the stories of our lives continue to be told, it's important to have enough pages in our veins. So why in all of Gaea's green goodness would any physician drain a patient's life into a dirty basin? For the same reason they enact every other treatment: out of confidence in themselves. That's why physicians have always killed more than they've cured. Whether by bloodletting or any of the unscientific drivel that Cyn's physicians so brazenly declared, self-assurance is the most dangerous trait any clinician can possess. The herbalists and apothecarists may miss opportunities to cure at times, but their misses are relatively benign.

Perhaps I'm biased. I grew up in a medical botanist's house. Back when it was still distinct from herbalism. Among the fundamental tenets of our family was a respect for Gaea. "The body has a natural wisdom", my mother would say any time we were sick or injured. "There's no better medic in Farhearth." She would then explain that every body knows how to heal... provided its environment is right. Just as every plant knows how to grow... as long as *its* environment is right. But placed in the wrong soil or the wrong climate, we wilt. "Half of healing is finding where you belong."

Even though I studied an entirely different subject at Farhearth, I still believe in my mother's principles. And I retain a fascination with the world's flora. Plants have to accumulate nutrition, attract pollinators, battle predators. And they don't have legs to flee or fists to fight. They're paralyzed in their stations. And yet they survive. Century after century, they thrive. By way of alchemy, synthesizing a unique chemical for every purpose... which we may *repurpose*.

Nature has had a long time to perfect its healing. Millions of years perhaps. There's no way of knowing how long, but it's certainly longer than the short thousands we've been intervening, as though we know better. So I think it's wise to consider patients from the perspective of herbalism. Which is why I'm thankful that Kara is on Cyn's case.

I'm too nervous and eager to say anything coherent. I've been trying to pass the morning with writing. But it's not working. If anything, it seems to be slowing the passage of time.

I'm going to go see if Rorrik is awake.

Seventy-Nine

Aldos, Third Lufoa, Day Seven. Noon.

We'll be leaving for the hospital soon. In an hour or so. I feel like I've already been awake and active for a whole day. But it's only noon.

I went down to the stables early. To the wagon. Where Rorrik was sleeping. The horizon was glowing, but just barely.

"Are you awake?", I whispered.

Silence.

That can almost always be interpreted as "no, I am not awake", but I wanted a verbal answer. So I whispered again. "Are you awake?"

Silence.

"Are you awake?", I whispered a third time. A little bit louder.

That woke him up. But it didn't startle him. He was coherent enough to realize anything he said would have the double meaning of "yes, I am awake." So, instead, he asked, "Is something wrong?"

"No, everything is okay." And then I explained that I could use his company. So he got up and sat on the edge of the wagon with me, chatting until it was time to meet Herrin for breakfast.

Now that Departure Day had passed, everything is open again. I didn't have much of an appetite, but I managed to eat some boiled pink mallard eggs. Then the three of us walked around campus until lunch, where I had a fried blue mallard egg. It was bland. Breakfast was, too. If we wanted a real meal, we could have gone to Arxey's. But we opted for convenience instead.

We just finished eating. And Herrin just left. He had an errand to run before we go to the hospital. He'll meet us there. And Rorrik is currently ordering a second lunch. So I'm writing.

I learned a lot about contemporary Harthy culture on this morning's walk. Here are some of my observations:

Many of the Harthies seem pathologically concerned with their reputations. They're either counterfeiting a greater-than-themselves image or pretending their mediocrity is already marvelous. Mostly, I just feel bad for them. Their insecurity must hurt an awful lot. But my sorrow is balanced with annoyance.

Among the marvelous mediocre, the word "brave" has really eroded in recent years. "That's so brave", I heard students tell each other after signing up for a class or speaking up for themselves or piercing some irregular bit of flesh.

Bravery is not simply the absence of cowardice. Yes, it would be cowardly to opt out of wearing those socks for fear of the public's disapproval. That doesn't mean it's *brave* to wear them. No more than is emaciation the absence of morbid obesity, or destitution the absence of Thevroan prosperity.

Can you imagine what Mizjak would think about that definition of bravery? Without hesitation, he confronted the horror from Thorn in single combat. Despite certain death, he remained undaunted in his duty. Compare that to today's Harthies. Wearing two different colored socks: so brave. *So* brave.

Among those fabricating a greater-than-themselves facade, I saw at least a dozen Harthies pretending to read the classics. Not useful academic works like Rouska or Carrin. Or Pirazok or Pizarok. Or Amaral or Lightner or Lan. Definitely not Gundric or Aetheldorf. Not even Maren. Instead, they were carrying around Bergeron or Cleworth or Waldock. In a very exhibitive way. Not *actually* reading them; just being *seen* with the books. To me, that reveals their illiteracy. Just as the fanciest instruments belong to the most dreadful musicians. And those with the fanciest swords tend to be the worst fencers (like the boy from yesterday). You can't buy skill. You can only buy baubles.

The same is true for those attempting to be perceived as deep and interesting. Nothing is more boring than the attempt to be interesting. And nothing is more shallow than the attempt to be deep. People who squander their lives curating a reputation do not have the priorities of someone who will actualize his or her potential.

We listened to some of the conversations. It corroborated our assumptions. It was how they described their triumphs. Farhearth has become a land of futurists. The type of people who declare their ambitions as a surrogate for actual accomplishment. Magnificent feats they will *soon* achieve. Just wait, you'll see! My success is as certain as the rising sun! Among these Harthies, "I'm going to" means "I wish I could." As in: "I'm going to write a novel." Or: "I'm going to win the Pendelhall tournament next year." Or: "I'm going to buy a Thevro mansion by the time I'm twenty-five." And so on.

When people say, "I *aspire* to", that's a softer claim. And soft speech harbors more honesty. It's the hardness of "I'm *going* to" that thwarts follow through. To declare an accomplishment is to forbid it. The declaration is satisfying enough; by the time the sentence ends, the reward has already been received. So why go through all the effort to actualize it?

If "I'm going to" turned out to be true one in ten times, Farhearth would be overrun with legislators, lawyers, physicians, professors, inventors, scientists, and Bonstans. And celebrated writers, singers, and artists. Public figures, all. Half of them would be triple crown winners. And *all* of them would live in castles and palaces. The consequent shortage of cobblers and cartwrights, shearers and broggers, butchers and grocers, tailors and mercers, furners and farmers, farriers and boonmasters, barbers, barm brewers, masons, maderers, well sinkers, pikemen, hoymen, and a hundred other essential lines of labor, would bring about the collapse of society. And there would certainly be no night soilmen. But despite the grand promises of Farhearth's young, there continues to be a robust workforce doing the most important work. *And* the most unimportant work, such as political campaigning. We were harangued by uncountable campaigners this morning.

We were *also* harangued by a larger-than-usual mob of "the end is at hand!" bellowers. They used to appear one at a time on busy street corners while a major event was underway. The Farhearth Faire, a rowanoki championship, the mayoral inauguration. But the movement seems to have gained members in my absence. This morning, while no event of any kind was taking place, there were droves of them shouting portents about the collapse of Farhearth. And a few stragglers shouting more extreme warnings: Gaea itself is on the brink of obliteration! The delusion of the apocalypse-mongers can be seen in their expressions. It's mostly in the eyes. Just like the addled patient whose face is dressed in the wrong emotion... which I wrote about a few days ago. It doesn't require much medical expertise to distinguish sanity and insanity in the clinic. And on the street corner, it doesn't take a degree in Druinian eschatology to disregard the doomsaying. Even if there *are* a bunch of cryptic catastrophes buried in Druin's passages, why would we believe them over the uncryptic claims of the natural sciences?

The *moderate* doomsayers, though – those who merely portend the collapse of Farhearth – sounded reasonable to me. The premise wasn't prophetic in a mystical sense. If today's youth are true to their word, society *is* doomed. That doesn't seem fetched from afar. But I suspect a much more likely fate is that the next generation of burlers and brayers, gardeners and gummers, plumbers, puggers, and peagers will simply be dispirited, having failed to actualize their grand, certain-as-the-sunrise ambitions.

Although, given my experience on this trip in Farhearth so far, I don't think I'd intervene in the collapse. Seems better to just let doom run its course. Then rebuild it from the rubble.

More common than the doomsayers were the fundraisers. Everyone was "raising money" for some cause. And I couldn't get past the euphemism. "You mean *taking* money?", I wanted to ask my solicitors. "Requesting that I *give you* money?" *Raising* means something else.

More common than the fund-raiders were the promoters of the "campus hall forum on ethical course content". I must have been invited by half a dozen students. It takes place tomorrow night. Hosted by the Student Congress Against Menace.

More common than the creepy assembly invitations were campaign posters. Some "Pro This"s, some "Anti-That"s. Although "I'm pro" always implies the opposing candidate is anti. Especially about issues in which no candidate has ever been opposed. Such as education, opportunity, health, and safety. "I'm pro-progress!" implies the opposition is an enemy of advancement. You see it in every election. And it's never been anything but silly.

Each campaign year, no matter how many candidates are running, there are only two distinct mayors:

The first option is an unabashed rich man who preserves the wealth of the wealthy by ignoring the poverty of the impoverished. The second option is a theatrically abashed rich man who pretends to care about the impoverished to keep them complacent. He realizes there are a lot more poor people than there are rich. And he maintains the wealth of the wealthy by placating the impoverished.

I voiced that opinion to Rorrik and Herrin after we saw a poster for one of the current mayor's rivals.

Herrin made a much better point: "Ceryd is going to be reelected no matter who runs against him. Reputation is the only thing that could end his reign, and his reputation has already survived four terms."

"How?"

"He's a storyteller. That's how you get the public to pay attention these days. And in every story he tells, he is a wise and patient hero and victim. What does that tell you?"

"He's a liar?"

"Precisely. No life story can be told both neatly *and* honestly. Every time an experience unfolds, we find ourselves creased. Just like the paper on which our stories are written. If you're not a fool or the bad guy in *any* of your tales, you're not telling the truth. You're hiding your crinkled and crumpled past. And over the last eight years, Ceryd has told a thousand stories… without a single pleated page."

Herrin went on to explain how Ceryd is terribly ineffective in office. "But it doesn't matter. Because securing power and wielding it are different tasks. He may be a bungler at the latter, but he's a master at the former. So there's no getting rid of him."

It had never occurred to me how flawed our political structure is in the East. By way of comparison, if you had to be a renowned cobbler to compete in sprinting, we'd have some uninspiring athletic records. The same can be said about any other sport or profession. If fencers had to smith their own swords, either the swords or the swordsmen would be lousy.

Then the conversation returned to the university itself. And I mentioned to Herrin that a lot of the students seem like they could serve society better in other ways. Off campus. "So why are they registering for classes?", I asked.

"For some of them, this is all they *can* do", Herrin said. Then he mentioned that a great many grass grads *are* fulfilling their indentured years off campus.

I know *on* campus they're working as lobbyists. But what role are they serving *off* campus? I was about to ask, but then I saw someone I recognized: Violet. Or whatever her real name is. The young woman I saw wearing a violet dress on the day I arrived. She was hanging a Student Congress Against Menace poster on a tree trunk.

"Is that the future of Farhearth politics?", I asked.

"Unfortunately, those politics are already here. They may not have the titles of proper offices, but they have just as much power. And they're not afraid to abuse it."

"What do you mean?"

Herrin suggested we take a closer look at the poster.

So we did… as soon as Violet moved on from her tree… and began to violate a different one with another poster.

It's a meeting that proposes the enforcement of new prohibitions on both course content and educational materials. Book bans, in other words.

Beneath that was a list of researchers and professors that the organization was demanding be terminated. The list was long. And I recognized some of the names. Kind-hearted, hard-working people with decades of academic and charitable contributions to the institution.

"Adon's aphids!", I said, genuinely stunned. Too stunned to come up with a less hackneyed response.

Herrin smiled and replied, "I'm just glad I'm not listed among the damned. So far, I've been lucky enough to be ignored. Well, luck and caution both."

"Cautious about what?"

"Speaking up. These days, the most honest and innocuous comments can place you on the reaper's list. Especially if what you say is true. Nothing will sentence your career to the scaffold quicker than the truth."

I didn't want to say "Adon's aphids" again. And nothing else came to mind. So I just looked back to the poster. And stared at the list of names. Silently.

After ten seconds or so, Herrin interrupted my silence: "Lunch?"

"That sounds good. Where?"

He suggested the place where I got the blue mallard egg. And where Rorrik just finished his second lunch.

And now it's time to leave. We'll meet Herrin at the hospital.

Eighty

Aldos, Third Lufoa, Day Seven. Night.

I retained my hope and wits during all the hours before breakfast, throughout every bite of breakfast, every step of the walk between breakfast and lunch, every bite of lunch, and every word of my postprandial journal. And for most of the walk to the hospital. I was about fifty feet from the front doors when I started to panic.

Rorrik managed to keep me *nearly* calm.

When we walked into the lobby, Herrin was there waiting. He gave me a hug. As though I hadn't seen him in a month.

"No word from Cliwen or Kara yet", he said. "But I already spoke with the receptionist at the scheduling counter. They know we're ready. And I don't have any other commitments until this evening. So I'll stick around as long as it takes."

It didn't take long. Ten minutes later, I saw Kara.

"We'll wait here", Herrin said. Maybe it was Rorrik. Or maybe neither of them said that. I was far too anxious to maintain any situational awareness. I don't even remember walking to Cyn's room. I would have no idea how to find it again. Couldn't tell you what floor it was on. No recollection of what the room looked like. The only thing I remember is the conversation with Cliwen and Kara. They were relaxed and reassuring. Clear and thorough in their communication. Unhurried in their manner. Everything a physician should be and seldom is.

And they did give me an answer. Finally. And it made sense. They thought of things I didn't. They tested things I wouldn't know to test. They retested things I wouldn't know to doubt. And I trust their diagnosis. Completely.

But it belongs to Cyn. This is her story. It's not mine to disclose.

As for the prognosis, with a lot of therapy, there's a tiny bit of hope. That gave me more confidence than they intended to convey. An *ordinary* person would have a sliver of hope, I reasoned. But Cyn is not an ordinary person. And neither does she deserve ordinary hope.

I left Cliwen and Kara's office with a swirling typhoon of emotions, but chief among them was a feeling of gratitude.

It's not the best answer, but I'm grateful that Cyn and I finally got what we came for, and we can put the mystery to rest. And leave this place behind. And I, for one, don't plan on returning.

I doubt Cyn will either. Ever since I met her, she's expressed a desire to return to Cinderheim. After she's learned everything she can about science and medicine. To bring that knowledge to her community. To bring healing to her home.

Although she can't voice it, I know that's where she would prefer to be now. Family and familiarity are far more therapeutic than any medication sold in the apothecary. (Especially the prescriptions I filled a couple of days ago.)

I consider Cyn a part of my family, but there's something unique about blood. The same is true for one's childhood home. There's something safe about it. And that sort of safety, surrounded by blood relatives, is what she needs now. As my mother used to say, half of healing is being where we belong.

I had no words for Herrin. Other than "thank you" while I was hugging him.

"Let me take care of this bill", he said before I let go of the hug.

Instead of responding, I just kept hugging. I produced no rebuttal. Not even a feeble one as a polite gesture.

Eventually (*very* eventually), the hug ended.

And then we left the hospital. All four of us. Herrin, Rorrik, Cyn and me.

"I really should get to work", Herrin said.

I figured that was the case. And he was just neglecting his duties for my sake. By extension, for Cyn's sake.

We hugged once more. Then he left. And Rorrik helped me get Cyn into my room at the inn. She's lying in the bed.

I'll sleep on the floor tonight.

And Rorrik is back in the wagon. Still sleeping at the stables.

Soon, Cyn and I will start our trip south. The long journey to Cinderheim. To take her home. Not tomorrow, though. Tomorrow, I need to stock up on supplies. I'd do my stocking at Estevro, but it's in the opposite direction. Too far to justify the trip. So we'll get everything we need here. Then leave the following morning.

I don't know how much longer Rorrik will be staying. No one ever knows with him. But I could use his help tomorrow. My attention will be divided between Cyn and preparation for the trip. It would be difficult on my own. The journey itself won't be any easier, but I'll confront those challenges as they arise.

As for tonight, I'm going to stop writing. My emotions are still swirling with the dizzying intensity of a typhoon. But the hour is late. So I'm going to close my eyes and hope those winds die down.

Eighty-One

Lyros, Third Lufoa, Day Eight. Morning.

Rorrik showed up early. With breakfast. "Delivery", he said when I opened the door.

While we ate, I asked for his help preparing.

"Of course", and so on.

He's never been to the South, though. Not even to Moonkruug. Lum's city. He's passed the Salt Road Bridge countless times on his journeys from the West to the East and back to the West. But he's never *crossed* that bridge. So, he doesn't know how to prepare for a trip south of it.

Although on this trip, Cyn and I have no need to take the Salt Road Bridge. We won't have to enter Thorn at all. Bonstan's new bridge will allow us to cross the strait directly from Charwarg to Baguzu. Which should save us a couple hundred miles.

The first leg of our trip will be along the Grass Road to Charwarg. It'll take longer than cutting across country, but I don't want to bounce Cyn around in the carriage. From Charwarg to Baguzu. From Baguzu to Moonkruug. From Moonkruug, we'll head south, along the Wren Ridge, toward an old, abandoned outpost. Perigee. According to my father's maps, we should be able to get water there. Then southwest from Perigee to Cinderheim.

Maybe four hundred and thirty miles in all. And just as many to get back. Plus a few more to Estevro.

But once we're out of the East, food isn't guaranteed. For Wylmot either. Unless he enjoys dead grass. Scant patches of it. It's not a nourishing land.

Normally, when I travel, I eat the staples of my destination. After a prolonged stay in Ryndor, I'll have consumed an entire school of fish. In Pendelhall, it's elk, sweet bean pastes, and dense, salty pastries. In Farhearth, it's a little bit of everything. Lonvaraka and Charwarg are mostly street vendor meals, except Lonvaraka is way better. In the West, it's just fruits and vegetables. And in the South, it's mostly inedible. Bad food and very little of it. So there's a lot of stock to stock up on before we go.

"What do you mean bad?", Rorrik asked. "Southern food is popular here, isn't it?"

I forgot how little he knows about the South. So, I explained:

"The Southern *style* of food is. But the Southern *style* is considered a *delicacy*. Which always means bad food consumed in expensive moderation. No one ever enacts gluttony upon a delicacy. Even if they can afford it, the experience is too punishing. And Farhearth's delicacies are superior imitations of their Southern equivalents: bad cactuses, bad root tubers, and a lot of snake meat. Which isn't *that* bad. But it *is* scary."

"What kind of snakes?"

"Not the same as you get here. Here, it's just harmless garters. I wouldn't even mind a splitjaw or thunder constrictor. Those aren't scary when they're cubed in a stew. But the most common meat on the Southern menu is the viceroy viper. It's one of two species of the Southern mountain viper."

Rorrik asked about it. And I got carried away describing every detail I know, all of which I learned from Cyn:

"The crowned viper is the most poisonous of all known snakes. Its skin wears regal, striped robes, and gleaming atop its head is a golden circlet. Those are the ornaments of warning. And every member of the animal kingdom takes notice of its grandeur. But one member has taken keener notice than the rest: the viceroy viper, imitator of the crowned viper. Except it isn't poisonous."

"What's a thunder constrictor?", Rorrik interrupted. "A big Southern snake", I said, and then immediately returned to the topic of the vipers:

"Once upon an earlier age, it was easy to distinguish them. The stripes were plain, and it wore no crown. It looked like a peasant of the same community. But today, not even the snake hunters can tell the difference. In the old days, they were called greater and lesser mountain vipers, and the lesser vipers were hunted aggressively. Those that resembled the crowned viper even a *little* bit were left alone. The lesser vipers were so abundant, one needn't take risks. But over time, they grew less abundant. So, hunters began capturing the lookalikes. At first, it was strictly the ones wearing cheap attire. Obvious imitators. Then those, too, grew scarce. The only lesser vipers left were near-perfect clones. And the hunters continued. Until only the perfect clones remained. Which, today, go by the name viceroy vipers. Maybe once a week, one of the mountain vipers they catch for dinner wears a true crown."

"How do they tell which is which?", Rorrik asked.

"Release them into an enclosed space with another animal – something other than a clergy camel – and wait twenty minutes. If the animal is dead, it was a crowned viper."

"What do they do with it then?"

"I don't know. Kill it, probably. Or recapture it and sell it to a Guzu peddler, who peddles it to a poisoner, maybe? I don't know."

"I meant the dead animal. What do they do with the carcass?"

"Dinner. Instead of the snake. Then a new animal will be penned in its place. And that animal will endure more snakebites until it, too, meets its unmaker."

"Why do they use a dinner animal to test the snake? Why don't they just eat that in the first place?"

"Other animals aren't abundant enough. If they were made into a daily meal, they would go extinct."

"So why don't they just use something abundant to test it? Like rats?"

"The vipers eat them whole. Without releasing any venom at all. The animal has to be sizable. Even then, the vipers decide how much poison to release. If they don't perceive a threat *and* they don't perceive food, they won't attack. Goats don't work because they don't goad the snakes. And chickens goad way too hard; afterward, they can't be salvaged for food. Clergy camels goad just the right amount, but they're immune. So baldwolf turns out to be the test animal of choice. Pen the two creatures together, wait a while, and then you'll know whether your next meal is a snake or a wolf."

"Is the wolf good meat?"

"I wouldn't know. I'm not a Southerner. Every wolf that's served as food is filled with poison. The Southerners have adapted to it. Those who couldn't survive the poison were suffocated out of their lineage. It only took a couple of generations. Today, with few exceptions, all of them can tolerate modest doses. Cyn can handle it. Lum could probably handle it, too. I think he has some south-of-the-meridian ancestry. But not me. My ancestral trees have not been pruned with such selective pressures, so I'd stop breathing within an hour of biting into the wrong steak."

"So meat's off the menu. What about plants?", Rorrik asked.

"That menu isn't much better. Unless you enjoy bitter cactus. Or you can endure the stony tubers. Those mostly grow in the higher latitudes, though, which is why they've become Eastern delicacies. Travel farther south and you get into the deep menu. Carrot berries, drought grapes, and furnace fruit. The berries are poisonous, the grapes are impossible to swallow without a lubricant, and the molten pulp is just ash."

There are a few more foods I could have mentioned but didn't. Other kinds of cactus. Some peppers that will blister your mouth. And *some* edible meat, but unless it's served in the shape of a lizard, you have no idea what kind of animal your food came from, or how old and maggoty it was before it was burned black.

I could have mentioned the apocra fig. Which has no business growing in the Southern climate, but it somehow manages to. It's rare though. Not just seasonal. It scarcely offers its fruit. So I can't count on it. For the bulk of the Southern continent, all I can count on are carrot berries, drought grapes, furnace fruit, and "long meat". Thus, preparing for a journey through the sunbaked clays and endless sands involves careful packing.

"Are horses okay in the South?", Rorrik asked.

"Because of heat, thirst, and insufficient food?"

"Because of the vipers."

"Oh, I think so", I said. "I can't be sure, but I'm confident. There shouldn't be any vipers on the road. The Salt and Stone Circle runs two hundred horses two hundred miles on those roads every year, and vipers are the least frequent cause of death. But if there *are* any loitering in our path, I should see them well before they pose a threat."

The conversation would have continued. Indefinitely. But I wanted to write before heading out.

And now it's time to do that.

It's time to start packing. Carefully.

Eighty-Two

Lyros, Third Lufoa, Day Eight. Afternoon.

Trip preparation has been difficult. For me, at least. I was out for over five hours and managed to purchase nearly nothing. Rorrik was more successful.

My plan was to buy all the food while he picked up the supplies. Then we could stock up on water tonight. Each take some canteens out and fill them. Then each take some more out and fill those. And so on.

We left shortly after 7:00 this morning. Separately. I took the wagon while Rorrik went on foot.

The supply markets are all over the place, plenty of them near the stables, and Rorrik has spent the last several days wandering around this part of the city, so he knows where everything is. Matches to start fires, knives to carve meat (if I manage to capture and kill any meals along the way), cooking utensils (assuming there will be food to cook), and an absurd number of canteens. "And medical supplies", I said before we parted. "Just the disposable stuff. Pick up whatever you can find."

I'll need more supplies than I mentioned, but those were all my suggestions. In small part, my mind was preoccupied with my own shopping list. In larger part, Rorrik knows how to pack for a long journey. With the exception of intercontinental transportation workers – my father, for example – Rorrik has traveled more miles than anyone I've ever met. He knows what supplies I'll need. Better than I know my own needs.

I was nurturing some frustration when I returned to the inn, having failed to find what I was looking for. But then I saw two large boxes of supplies sitting on the floor. One was filled with canteens and waterskins. The other was neatly packed. I assume it contained everything else I would need. On top of that box was a large pile of socks. "Twenty-five extra pairs", Rorrik said.

He was at the table, eating a sandwich.

He took a bite, then spoke through his food: "A hundred miles into the trip, you'll be glad to have them." He swallowed that bite, took another, and then spoke through that one, too: "Did you get all the food you need?"

"Almost nothing", I said. And then I explained:

I can't get what I need from the eateries. Powdered food, dried meat, and all the other invincible foods can only be picked up in the agricultural market. Which is at least two miles away. Four-mile round trip, maybe five. And if I'm buying a hundred pounds of food, I'm not going to carry it all the way back to the inn. So, I took the wagon. But when I pull it up to a shopfront, they see it and think I have money. And their prices reflect that. The same thing happens when people see my house. It's not fancy, but it's nice enough, so people think I have disposable wealth, and they try to dispose it from my purse. But the house and wagon are both red herrings.

The wagon was inherited. And it was built by my heirs. I could never afford to purchase it. And the only way I was able to afford the house was by forgoing any home at all for over two years. I was living in my office, and several times a week, I would pretend to be a recruit, so I could dine at the visitors' eatery for free. One saves money. Enough to purchase my house… provided I get it in a state of disrepair, and my father helps with the repairs.

Today, I eke by. Nearly every bite of food – for Abbie, Wylmot, and me – comes from my yard. Books and furniture aside, my only real possessions are rocks. Which I take from the ground. Whatever wealth I have resides in shallow pockets. And the physicians at "Fentin Infirmary" were not kind to the contents of those pockets.

So, this morning, when I pulled my fancy wagon up to a shop and attempted to buy a hundred pounds of food, the shopkeeper quoted the you-look-like-you-can-afford-it price. And that made it unaffordable. I need to keep *some* money for emergencies and ongoing travel expenses.

"Will you come with me tonight?", I asked Rorrik. "We'll park the wagon around the corner, out of sight, and then one of us can walk to the shops?"

"How about I head out now? You stay here."

"If someone doesn't stay with the wagon, everything will be stolen."

"Don't worry. I won't lose anything. Just tell me what you need."

I don't know how Rorrik plans to accomplish this. But he always finds a way. So I ripped a blank piece of paper from this journal and began writing items. Things that would travel well. Dried horrux, butter berries (skin on), various powders. And I wrote quantities next to each.

Then Rorrik asked, "How about *actual* butter? And carrots?"

Initially, I dismissed both. "Carrots are too light on calories and butter melts into hot, greasy milk."

But then I changed my mind, realizing the carrots will be good for Wylmot and the butter will be good for Cyn. She'll need plenty of "liquid" calories. So, I added both to the list.

Once it was done, I looked it over. To see if I could think of anything else. I prefer food that perishes. It feels healthier. Food that's as durable as rocks, enduring month after month without rotting, doesn't seem nourishing. But I can't take my garden with me. So the page was filled with immortal foods.

Deciding it was complete, I handed the list to Rorrik, gushed some gratitude, and reached for my purse.

"I'll cover it", he said with a tone of finality.

I protested his charity. But his finality held strong.

I succumbed. And thanked him. With a depth and earnestness that can only be expressed by the newly penurious when they receive meaningful help.

Rorrik folded the list, put it in his pocket, and left. Then I returned to Cyn. We ate. And afterward, I sat down to write this journal.

Rorrik isn't back yet. I thought he would be by now. If nothing went wrong, he should have been back an hour ago.

Even if he comes up short on a couple of items, there are places along the way I should be able to replenish the pantry. Maybe we'll run into Lonvaraka. Depends on where it is. We can eat there, but we can't stock up as everything is perishable. *Quickly* perishable. Nourishing, but only if eaten immediately. Same with Charwarg, butcher capital of the East. Although we can probably buy some fruits and vegetables there. Once we reach Baguzu, I'll be able to restock the immortal inventory. And there will be plenty of tavern calories in Moonkruug. Liquified bread. That'll meet most of our nutritional needs. But once we're south of Moonkruug, lizards are the best we could ask for. So I hope Rorrik didn't run into any problems.

Eighty-Three

Lyros, Third Lufoa, Day Eight. Night.

Rorrik made it back to the inn shortly after I finished writing. It took him a while to find a few of the items, but he managed to get everything on the list. And he managed to get all of it at a discounted rate. Without losing any of it.

"How?", I asked.

"I told the merchants I was starting a delivery business, and I was looking for a permanent supplier. And I *might* have implied I would be back every week to make larger and larger purchases, assuming the business grows. But only if I was happy with the price."

A small laugh started tumbling around inside my chest. Instead of letting it loose, my throat clenched around it, restraining it to a smile.

"And it worked?", I asked through that smile.

"The wagon is all stocked up."

"I really appreciate everything you're doing. This would be so much harder without your help."

I intended to express more gratitude, but as my throat relaxed its restraint of my laughter, it left behind a lump. An emotional globus. Like how an oyster converts a sand grain into a pearl.

Until that moment, I had been distracted by responsibility. Preparation for the trip. Tomorrow, a difficult journey begins. Rorrik and I will part before. Cyn and I will part after. And then I'll begin the long hike back home. Alone.

I wasn't thinking about any of that. Because I had a task to focus on. Once the task was complete, I found myself unable to think about anything else. So, I sat with Cyn and Rorrik. And I expressed how much their friendships have meant to me over the years… by telling Cyn the story of how I met Rorrik and telling Rorrik the story of meeting Cyn.

"I hate to interrupt this moment", Rorrik interrupted, "but we should fill the canteens before it gets too late."

"I'd forgotten about that", I said. "I would have been traveling dry if you didn't remind me. Can I ask for your help one last time?"

"Of course."

Rorrik knew the best place to fill them. He had found it on his campus walks. It wasn't far from the stables. With each of us taking four canteens per trip, it didn't take long. But plastered all around the pump were posters for the Student Congress Against Menace event. We discussed it the entire time.

How disturbing it would be. How angry, sad, creepy, and absurd it would be.

By the time we had finished filling our canteens, we had talked ourselves into attending. "Only for a few minutes", we reasoned. "Just to see what it's like", we reasoned some more.

So we returned to the inn, dropped off the last batch of full canteens, and told Cyn we would be heading out once more "to go to a political assembly run by hostile students... only for a few minutes... just to see what it's like."

Then we left for the amphitheater. Which turned out to be the poster capital of the world.

Nearly every vertical surface was defiled by an advertisement for *something*. Mostly for this event. But whenever any event is over, nobody seems to take the posters down. They just plaster new ones on top, making thicker and thicker walls of paper. So, I ripped the superficial layer from one such wall to see what was underneath. It was an advertisement for the Singing Sisters. From a couple of weeks ago. I ripped that one down too... and took it:

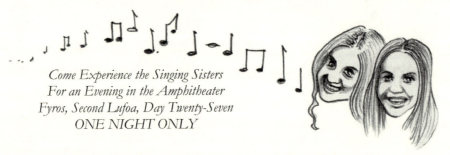

Come Experience the Singing Sisters
For an Evening in the Amphitheater
Fyros, Second Lufoa, Day Twenty-Seven
ONE NIGHT ONLY

Those are the same sisters whose countenances *also* grace the most common *Wanted* posters in town. Although they aren't wanted by law enforcement. Rather, it's Atrok-Ilrum who will pay dearly for their singing heads.

Half an hour before tonight's meeting started, the amphitheater was already packed. With anger. It wasn't that full of *people*, but everyone present seemed to pulse with the fury of a dozen justice-seeking vigilantes… who had been waiting there all day, warming up their tempers. Like angry afternoon clouds gathering up rain in anticipation of the night's storm.

Prior to any big rowanoki match, crowds of belligerent fans will show up to the venue – before it opens – to begin their ale-addled, pre-contest rallying. This was similar. Except here, the crowd was *more* obnoxious. And I realized I would have a difficult time connecting with any of these students. I would have to become a person I find boring to be perceived as funny, a person I find tedious to be companionable, and cruel to be respected. That's not me.

A few minutes later, the event started. And the host took the stage.

It was the creature in the violet dress. Somehow, I knew it would be her.

Except tonight, she was wearing a gown so angelically white, it wouldn't have looked out of place had she affixed clip-on wings. But underneath was a vile, gnarled vulture. Whose name, I learned, is Morga.

Morga repressed her vulturous personality and spent the evening portraying herself as a one-faced non-shrew. She smiled at everyone. Almost believably. She praised the institution. Almost believably. And she thanked those in attendance who held contrasting views, as they ensured a diverse perspective was represented. That last part wasn't as believable, but taken as a whole, her act was compelling.

Rorrik and I had planned to watch the event from a distance. And leave early. As soon as our curiosity was sated.

We stayed for the entire event. And we were right up front, listening intently. To Morga. Whose mouth sounded at least as parched as the Southern sands. If I closed my eyes, the voice was being emitted from a different creature. The image in my mind was a desiccated, old hag. Which wasn't unsettling. Actually *watching* Morga speak is what unsettled me. Everything about her looked girlish and inexperienced. Except one thing: her eyebrows were those of someone three times her age. It made her appear both young and old, innocent and guilty, harmless and dangerous. Impossible to interpret.

But her words were clear enough: anyone who has ever wronged her (or her parents or brother or companionable allies; "friends" feels like a euphemism) is a villain. And we must eradicate villains from campus.

People used to protest organizations. In formal public chamber meetings. That's what activism was in my time. What I saw tonight was *person* picketing. A vicious effort to ruin human beings. Not just ruin their day, but their lives. Weed them out of society forever. It reminds me of childhood in the garden, with my mother yelling "get it by the root!" so the weed can never grow back. And over what?

In most cases, it was a tiny fragment of a story that clearly contravenes the context from which it was quoted.

I guess this isn't new. I was a child when Aetheldorf was exiled. He fled the continent long before any student union had formed. Left for Whitebone. And what was he exiled for?

An honest reading of his work portrays him as a champion of immigration, especially welcoming to those who overcame adversity along their journey. A slightly less fair interpretation claims he was declaring Harthy superiority.

Less than a month ago, Cyn and I sat in my study discussing this very topic. The unjust interpretation of Aetheldorf's work. Or rather, Cyn talked while I nodded along. To paraphrase her paraphrasing of his premise in *Exodus*:

Our most curious and ambitious ancestors are those who refused to settle. Those who continued to explore. Hill after hill, shore after shore. Until they decorated our maps with all nineteen settlements that we've inherited today. The final ornament hung was Farhearth. So its inhabitants must have been the *most* curious, the *most* ambitious. And they must have passed those traits onto their offspring. But since the breadth of Gaea had already been mapped, the sons and daughters of the final settlers aimed their curiosity and ambition inward. Into the frontiers of human understanding. In doing so, Farhearth became the womb of the sciences. And its residents the… impregnators?

At the time of its publication, no student was bothered. Professorial words and published works were regarded as well-intentioned wisdom, meant only to foster discussion. And Aetheldorf had a lot of words and works under discussion at that time. Many of which seemed thornier than that one. So… who called for his exile upon the publication of *Exodus*?

Hillians. Who else? Wealthy elites who felt their eliteness was cast in doubt.

But their call for Aetheldorf's termination didn't go anywhere. Because they were only calling with their voices. In public chamber meetings.

Until Aetheldorf published *Aphorisms*. Which directly attacked his attackers. And Aetheldorf's wit was sharp; it made a precise incision into hillian pride. It opened with a chapter called Hubris from on High. Again, I'll provide a summary of Cyn's summary from a month ago:

The child bit by a snake learns to spot the hidden coils lurking in the brush. The explorer who eats an eldritch berry and soon spews torrents of vomit will never forget the look, smell, or taste of that fruit. And the student who fails a course with an incorrect answer will remember that material long after every correct answer has faded from recollection. Therein lies the difference between the rich and the poor. It is only through challenge and struggle that lessons burrow into memory. And where is the hardship in bought success? Prosperity armors us against pain and failure. Thus, true learning belongs to the downtrodden. It is the fate of the uptrodden to spend their elder years short on memory, bereft of wisdom. And it is hubris that fills those holes.

When that book went into print, hillians did more than speak out on the public chamber floor. They boycotted the institution. And they weren't just boycotting matriculation. Thevro was the sole supplier of Farhearth's paper. Or at least the timber to make it. And until the institution righted this wrong, it wouldn't receive a flip penny of tuition nor a thin splinter of birch.

What were they demanding? Aetheldorf's execution was too much to ask for, but termination wasn't enough. So, deportation became the resolution.

Off to Whitebone Aetheldorf went. He could have gone to any other city in the East. Thevro aside. Or back to the West. But he chose to explore a new frontier, add a twentieth settlement to our maps. "Aetheldorf chose exodus", as *The Poorman* put it one Seros morning. It was a poetic end to his career. According to that article, which was published when I was a wee, illiterate babe, numerous Harthies followed Aetheldorf on his voyage to Whitebone, and they were calling it "New Farhearth". According to the *Thevro Chronicle*, the tally of followers was "zero", and Aetheldorf was not expected to survive his solitary crossing of the Eldsyn Bay.

Whatever the truth, Aetheldorf was the first faculty member to lose his job over the publication of a theory. And in the long aftermath, every one of his works was banned. They still are.

The dismissal of a Ranked Professor over an academic idea, and the banning of those ideas from university bookshelves, was unsettling to the remaining faculty in all nine colleges.

But after that incident, other than a lingering reluctance to criticize Thevro, a few decades passed without further censorship.

Until now. Those decades are clearly over. Censorship is back on campus. And it's bolder than ever. But this time, it's not a city imposing it. It's kids. More specifically, it's the Student Congress Against Menace.

Rorrik and I watched the organization demand the immediate Aetheldorfing of numerous faculty members. "Disciplinary dissolution", as they called it. Nomenclatorial objections aside, if these students get their way, there will be an enormous surge in the population of Whitebone.

It makes me wonder: if Farhearth had stood its ground when Aetheldorf was under attack – forgone paper for a decade or so, weathered the tuition famine, tightening the belt around the belly of their endowment, and gone to war on Aetheldorf's behalf – would the university be a different place today?

I suspect so. Because it's never war that plunges us into an age of darkness. It's an unfortunate way to learn, but socially sanctioned killing has taught us half of what we know about physiology and psychology, and it's hastened the advancement of science and technology. War hurts while it's being waged, but the tragedy inspires innovation.

What cripples progress is the exile of our heroes. Our pioneering thinkers. When we silence them – out of fear that their ideas may be too persuasive to defend against – we expel a voice of reason from discussion. The real cruelty is not inflicted on *them*, but on society itself. Which is rife with tribulations. And what is the most effective solution to *any* social problem? Conversation. Perhaps war is the second best. "Disciplinary dissolution" is not third best. It does not reduce violence, it sustains it. We celebrate the Great Armistice – more than a hundred years without open conflict between nations – but that doesn't mean we've stopped conquering. We're just targeting individuals instead of armies. Individuals whose logic and reason we fear.

If Farhearth's administration yields to the Student Congress Against Menace, Aetheldorf's cave will soon be an academic metropolis… for those who can endure the eternal Arzox.

Rorrik and I approached Morga after the meeting. And congratulated her on her hard work. We were feigning as much sincerity as we could. But sincerity typically blows the cover of dishonesty. Morga smiled and portrayed civility. I think she could tell, though. It wasn't in her expression. It was in her fumes. Like a malicious aura. Odorless and invisible, but you can sense its presence.

When morbidly venomous people radiate their mood, everyone in the room can feel it. And Miss Violet was like a Mulgothan bog of cantankerousness before we even greeted her. Rorrik's compliments just functioned as fuel, increasing the emission of those noxious fumes.

"I really wish you had the authority to execute most of these professors", Rorrik said. And then he decided to keep going: "A beheading or a hanging, maybe a quartering. But even that feels too gentle. Better than they deserve. I really believe that. You're sure doing a good thing here."

Rorrik wanted to keep taunting her. Poking at her composure. Seeing if he could make it burst. But I felt like I was suffocating. So I politely excused us from her company. "I'm sorry to interrupt, but we have other commitments. And I'm sure you do too. Please forgive our intrusion." And then I bowed a little. Not a full-bodied bow, as my back is too stiff for that. Probably from sleeping on the floor. Most of the bow happened above the shoulders, but it was polite enough.

And then we left. Rorrik returned to the stables, and I went back to the inn. With Cyn. For our last night in Farhearth. Forever, I hope.

Rorrik and I didn't talk about tomorrow. There was never a moment where it felt right to broach the topic. But I think I know what morning will bring.

He's never been to the South. Not once. And I don't expect him to forfeit his lifelong abstinence now.

I'm sure he'll be on some other quest by the time Cyn and I begin ours.

I'll find the wagon as I left it. Tidy, ready for travel, with no evidence that Rorrik had been there. Except for the supplies. He always erases his tracks from one adventure before embarking on the next. All he leaves behind is his breath. As scentless as the wind. Lingering, reminding you of his absence. Like a lonely silence haunting the air.

That will be the extent of Rorrik's company as Cyn and I begin our own journey. Not just gazing at all the old stones that line my sill, but embarking on a new adventure beyond the glass.

Eighty-Four

Fyros, Third Lufoa, Day Nine. Morning.

I didn't sleep well. The moon seems to have returned to its full brightness. Last night, it hung low in the sky, like a lamp in the darkness, its silver beams chasing away the creeping gloom and staining the world with a sterile pallor.

I guess it's supposed to reach its full bloom this evening. I'm not particularly fluent in astronomy, so I never know when it's truly full or merely *nearly* full. But last night, it was so stuffed, it looked like it was ready to burst. And yet it held itself together.

It kept the room sufficiently lit while haunting the night dwellers outside. Illuminating them as if under the sun, revealing their movements to all the other skulkers of the Untolled Hours. Which resulted in excesses of chirping, some growling and howling, and occasional hissing. The window was open, so the cacophony was as clear as it was raucous.

Light and noise aside, it was my second night sleeping on the floor. Which is usually the worst. The stiffness of the previous night hasn't yet departed, and the adaptation of the third hasn't yet arrived.

Eventually, a few beams more radiant than the moon's began to pass through the window.

That's when I heard a knock on the door.

It was the unmistakable ring of iron bones against cheap cottonwood.

It tolled three times. Boldly.

With a beaming grin and a concealed tear, I opened the door.

And Rorrik walked past. Without a word. Because his knuckles had already knocked everything he intended to say.

I didn't think either of us would ever persuade the other into allegiance, but I guess this settles our conflict. It doesn't end with me in pursuit of vengeance. Instead, Rorrik has chosen a less thorny path.

But then a thought occurred to me: "We'll need more food", I said.

"I already took care of that. It's why last night took so long. I doubled the list you gave me."

"What about waterskins?"

"I took care of that, too. I already filled half of them before you and I filled our first."

I gave him a hug.

Before letting go, I said, "We should go to Arxey's for breakfast. I've been wanting an omelet."

"I was going to suggest that if you didn't."

And now it's time to leave.

Life is strange. All of the unexpected turmoil. And the unwelcome changes. I can't believe it wound up this way. But I'm grateful that Rorrik is with me. I'm grateful our bond has remained intact.

The longest and most trying voyage, as a thousand clichés have informed us, begins with a single step. And then another. And another. And eventually, one finds a lifetime imprinted on the soils and sands behind us.

The first cliché descended from Old Adonian. The thousand contemporary, cringe-inducing derivatives have yet to improve upon that first idiom:

"Only Time can traverse the World."

Or maybe it's time *travels* worlds. Or something. Old Adonian is impossible. Time takes a lot of steps. That what it means.

I just checked with Rorrik.

This: Oko Gael lok kavra Galea.

And today, our time takes its first steps. Together.

To be continued in:

The Crown and the Caged God
Book One, Part Two: Bridges and Bonds

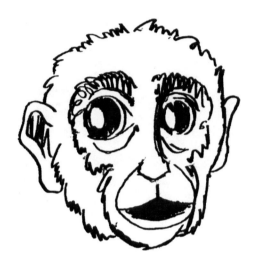

Made in United States
North Haven, CT
02 June 2024

53233145R10212